3D Printing: Applications in Medical Surgery

3D Printing: Applications in Medical Surgery

Volume 2

Edited by

Vasileios N. Papadopoulos

*Professor of Surgery
1st Surgical Department
Aristotle's University Thessaloniki
Thessaloniki, Greece*

Vassilios Tsioukas

*Electrical Engineer, Professor
School of Rural and Surveying
Aristotle University of Thessaloniki
Thessaloniki, Greece*

Jasjit S. Suri

*Global Biomedical Technologies, Inc.,
California, United States*

ELSEVIER

Elsevier
Radarweg 29, PO Box 211, 1000 AE Amsterdam, Netherlands
The Boulevard, Langford Lane, Kidlington, Oxford OX5 1GB, United Kingdom
50 Hampshire Street, 5th Floor, Cambridge, MA 02139, United States

Notices

Practitioners and researchers must always rely on their own experience and knowledge in evaluating and using any information, methods, compounds or experiments described herein. Because of rapid advances in the medical sciences, in particular, independent verification of diagnoses and drug dosages should be made. To the fullest extent of the law, no responsibility is assumed by Elsevier, authors, editors or contributors for any injury and/or damage to persons or property as a matter of products liability, negligence or otherwise, or from any use or operation of any methods, products, instructions, or ideas contained in the material herein.

ISBN: 978-0-323-66193-5

Publisher: Sarah Barth
Acquisitions Editor: Jessica L. McCool
Editorial Project Manager: Samantha Allard
Production Project Manager: Kiruthika Govindaraju
Cover Designer: Alan Studholme

Working together
to grow libraries in
developing countries

www.elsevier.com • www.bookaid.org

Contents

Contributors

Maria V. Alexiou, BSc, MSc
Molecular Biologist and Geneticist, Surgical Department, School of Medicine, Faculty of Health Sciences, Aristotle University of Thessaloniki, Thessaloniki, Greece

Panagiotis E. Antoniou
Senior Postdoctoral Researcher on Medical Physics, Biomedical Engineering and Digital Healthcare Innovations, Lab of Medical Physics and Digital Innovation, Department of Medicine, School of Health Sciences, Aristotle University of Thessaloniki, Thessaloniki, Greece

Keyoumars Ashkan, FRCS, MD
Department of Neurosurgery, King's College Hospital London, King's College London, London, United Kingdom

Alkinoos Athanasiou
Department of Neurosurgery, AHEPA University General Hospital, Aristotle University of Thessaloniki (AUTH), Thessaloniki, Greece; Lab of Medical Physics, School of Medicine, Aristotle University of Thessaloniki, Thessaloniki, Greece

Bakopoulou Athina
Department of Prosthodontics, School of Dentistry, Faculty of Health Sciences, Aristotle University of Thessaloniki (A.U.Th), GR, Thessaloniki, Greece

Panagiotis D. Bamidis
Professor of Medical Physics, Medical Informatics and Medical Education, Lab of Medical Physics and Digital Innovation, Department of Medicine, School of Health Sciences, Aristotle University of Thessaloniki, Thessaloniki, Greece

Petros Bangeas, MSc
Department of Surgery, Aristotle University of Thessaloniki, Thessaloniki, Greece; Doctor, Academic Researcher, 1st Surgery Department, Papageorgiou Hospital, Thessaloniki, Greece

Alexandros Brotis
Department of Neurosurgery, Larisa University General Hospital, University of Thessaly, Volos, Greece

Hadjichristou Christina
Department of Prosthodontics, School of Dentistry, Faculty of Health Sciences, Aristotle University of Thessaloniki (A.U.Th), GR, Thessaloniki, Greece

Angelos Daniilidis, MD, PhD, MSc, BSCCP, DFFP, MIGS
2nd Department of Obstetrics and Gynaecology, Hippokratio General Hospital, Aristotle University of Thessaloniki, Thessaloniki, Greece

Efterpi Demiri
Professor in Plastic Surgery of Aristotle University of Thessaloniki, Chief of the Department of Plastic Surgery, Papageorgiou Hospital, Thessaloniki, Greece

Dimitrios Dionyssiou, MD, PhD
Associate Professor in Plastic Surgery, Aristotle University of Thessaloniki, Thessaloniki, Greece

Konstantinos Fountas
Department of Neurosurgery, Larisa University General Hospital, University of Thessaly, Volos, Greece

Kleanthis E. Giannoulis, MD, FRCS, FEBS
Associate Professor of Surgery, Aristotle University of Thessaloniki, Thessaloniki, Greece

Grigoris F. Grimbizis, MD, PhD
1st Department of Obstetrics and Gynaecology, Aristotle University of Thessaloniki, Thessaloniki, Greece

Ion-Anastasios Karolos, PhD
Rural and Surveying Engineer, School of Rural and Surveying Engineering, Aristotle University of Thessaloniki, Thessaloniki, Greece

Ioannis Magras
Department of Neurosurgery, AHEPA University General Hospital, Aristotle University of Thessaloniki (AUTH), Thessaloniki, Greece

Bousnaki Maria
Department of Prosthodontics, School of Dentistry, Faculty of Health Sciences, Aristotle University of Thessaloniki (A.U.Th), GR, Thessaloniki, Greece

Laura Stone McGuire, MD
Department of Neurosurgery University of Illinois at Chicago, Chicago, IL, United States

Torstein R. Meling
Service de Neurochirurgie, Hôpitaux Universitaires de Genève (HUG), Geneva, Switzerland; Faculty of Medicine, University of Geneva, Geneva, Switzerland

Alessandro Moiraghi
Service de Neurochirurgie, Hôpitaux Universitaires de Genève (HUG), Geneva, Switzerland

Dimitrios Nikas, MD
Department of Neurosurgery University of Illinois at Chicago, Chicago, IL, United States

Koidis Petros
Department of Prosthodontics, School of Dentistry, Faculty of Health Sciences, Aristotle University of Thessaloniki (A.U.Th), GR, Thessaloniki, Greece

Christos Pikridas, PhD
Professor, Rural and Surveying Engineer, School of Rural and Surveying Engineering, Department of Geodesy and Surveying, Aristotle University of Thessaloniki, Thessaloniki, Greece

Stavros Polyzoidis, MD, PhD
Department of Neurosurgery, AHEPA Hospital, Aristotle University of Thessaloniki, Thessaloniki, Greece

Constantine P. Spanos, MD, FACS, FASCRS, MBA
Doctor, Surgery, Aristotelian University, Thessaloniki, Greece

Marianna P. Spanos, BA
Center for Human Genetics, Cambridge, Massachusetts, United States

Georgia-Alexandra Spyropoulou, MD, PhD
Associate Professor in Plastic Surgery, Aristotle University of Thessaloniki, Thessaloniki, Greece

Theodoros D. Theodoridis, MD, PhD
1st Department of Obstetrics and Gynaecology, Aristotle University of Thessaloniki, Thessaloniki, Greece

Andreas I. Tooulias, MD, MSc
General Surgeon, HPB Fellow, Surgical Department, School of Medicine, Faculty of Health Sciences, Aristotle University of Thessaloniki, Thessaloniki, Greece

Antonios Tsimponis
Plastic Surgeon, Department of Plastic Surgery of the Aristotle University of Thessaloniki, Thessaloniki, Greece

Vassilios Tsioukas, PhD
Electrical Engineer, Professor, School of Rural and Surveying Engineering, Aristotle University of Thessaloniki, Thessaloniki, Greece

Georgios Tsoulfas, MD, PhD
Associate Professor of Transplantation Surgery, Chief of the Department of Transplantation Surgery, School of Medicine, Faculty of Health Sciences, Aristotle University of Thessaloniki, Thessaloniki, Greece

Lazaros Tzounis, PhD, Diploma Engineer
Department of Materials Science & Engineering, University of Ioannina, Ioannina, Greece; Mechanical Engineering Department, Hellenic Mediterranean University, Heraklion, Greece

Introduction

Ion-Anastasios Karolos, PhD [1], **Vassilios Tsioukas, PhD** [2], **Christos Pikridas, PhD** [3]

[1]*Rural and Surveying Engineer, School of Rural and Surveying Engineering, Aristotle University of Thessaloniki, Thessaloniki, Greece;* [2]*Electrical Engineer, Professor, School of Rural and Surveying Engineering, Aristotle University of Thessaloniki, Thessaloniki, Greece;* [3]*Professor, Rural and Surveying Engineer, School of Rural and Surveying Engineering, Department of Geodesy and Surveying, Aristotle University of Thessaloniki, Thessaloniki, Greece*

Medical imaging industry is undergoing a dramatic transformation driven by three main technological trends: artificial intelligence (AI) using software-based solutions, augmented reality (AR), and additive manufacturing (AM) redefining the medical imaging workflow. These emerging technologies have the potential to take personalized medicine to the next level in the near future. However, to achieve this, physicians need to collaborate with a variety of engineers and data scientists.[1] Medical experts should be able to bring their expertise to the process of the AI, AR, and AM development and engineers should be able to translate their inputs into medical applications. This collaboration of the individual scientific discipline could create new specialties in medicine in the future, as the demands on the handling of these emerging technologies would increase. Along these lines, a radiologist of the future should understand the basic structure of a medical imaging deep learning annotation algorithm, in order to improve it, by using retraining processes, and thus eliminating the errors on medical reports. At the same time, radiologists should be able to implement the segmentation process of the greyscale CT or MRI images, transforming them to multicolor 3D models suitable for AR headsets and 3D printers. On the other hand, a surgeon should be capable of using these AR or 3D printed models for preoperational planning and clinically assisted navigation surgery for better definition of the patients' organ's (such as vessels or tumors) internal anatomy in real time, without reference to previously obtained 2D radiological data. The optimization of the interaction between these three distinct technologies will be the key for a smooth transition of medical technology to the Fourth Industrial Revolution (Industry 4.0). Of course, the main task of every scientist through this transition is to fully ensure and guarantee the effectiveness of the above technologies, especially when they are intended to make decisions concerning human lives.

At this point, it would be very crucial to analyze the current state and challenges of AI, AR, and AM technologies having to do with medical applications separately

3D Printing: Applications in Medical Surgery. https://doi.org/10.1016/B978-0-323-66193-5.00001-0

and to further investigate the interaction between them, with a view towards optimizing the future of the healthcare system. This chapter is intended as a brief introduction to these technologies with a more detailed approach to follow in the next chapters of this book.

Artificial intelligence in medical imaging

Today, radiological imaging data are growing continuously at a disproportionate rate when compared to the number of available well-trained readers in a hospital. This factor has contributed to a dramatic increase in radiologist workloads. Studies report that an average radiologist must interact with one image every 4 s in an 8 h workday. As radiology involves visual perception as well as decision-making, errors in medical reports are inevitable, especially with this workload conditions.[2]

As a solution, deep learning research in medical imaging is rapidly increasing and has given rise to new, nondeterministic algorithms that do not require manual explicit feature definition. The underlying methods of deep learning have existed for decades. However, only in recent years, there are sufficient data and appropriate computational power available. In past years, most of this research was performed in isolation and with very limited primary medical imaging datasets. This often led to implementation of overly simplified AI models that met accuracy requirements only in narrow use cases. Nowadays, this scenario has changed as with the advent of big data and with Moore's law broken and computational capability ever increasing, AI models that can save humans and make medical experts more efficient and effective are increasingly becoming the norm.[3] Over the next 5 years, we will see the rise of the "smart AI hospital," growing by workflows incorporating thousands of AI models. A smart workflow like this can be described based on the following ten distinct steps, always using specific restrictions in how data are transmitted (high-quality data encryption and decryption), as respecting patient data privacy is paramount:

- The patient visits the radiology department of the hospital for a medical test,
- The radiologist applies an imaging modality protocol like CT, MRI, X-ray, or ultrasound to the patient,
- The DICOM image series are automatically uploaded to the central picture archiving and communication system (PACS) server of the hospital,
- The central PACS server communicates with the AI annotation server, which includes AI pretrained models and special hardware accelerated graphics processing units (GPUs) modalities,
- The AI annotation server consists of tools to draw closed boundaries around the patient's internal organs like the liver, pancreas, or spleen, isolating them from the rest of the dataset on every single 2D slice of the DICOM series,

- Subsequently, the same software tools annotate the boundaries of the internal anatomic structures of the patient's organs like vessels or abnormalities such as tumors,
- A deep learning segmentation algorithm inside the AI server receives the extreme points of the organs, vessels, and possible abnormalities and transforms them to 3D .stl models,
- The anatomic 2D extreme boundaries, the 3D models, and a detailed medical report of the patient with the size and exact location of the possible abnormalities return to the PACS server,
- The radiologist evaluates the final exported boundaries of the organs and abnormalities, with manual annotation tools on the PACS viewer, in case of errors or partial annotation (for example, correction of extreme points of the liver parenchyma and tumor), since deep learning models, by their nature, are sensitive to the data used to train them and annotation accuracy might be lower than originally achieved with the training data,
- The radiologist's manual corrections transfer back to deep learning algorithm for retraining process and better diagnosis results in the future.

To better understand how such a form of workflow becomes applicable sooner than we thought, it is worth mentioning the recent example of the COVID-19 pandemic. GPU hardware companies, such as NVIDIA, have released pretrained models for volumetric 3D annotation of lung region from CT DICOM series in order to detect inflections from SARS-COV-2 virus in a faster and more reliable manner.

Augmented reality in surgical guidance

AR describes an environment in which virtual and real elements appear to coexist. To interact with these virtual elements in the physical world, the user must wear an appropriate mixed reality, head-mounted display. Mixed reality headsets, like the well-known Microsoft HoloLens, are becoming increasingly popular in healthcare, particularly in surgical navigation guidance. Mixed reality headsets could replace the classic medical monitors on every surgical specialty in the near future, solving many malfunctions faced by many surgeons today. Examples of such malfunctions are found in minimally invasive surgery. In laparoscopy, surgeons often operate on patients with a misalignment between their vision line and hand placement due to monitor positions. Recent studies show that a disrupted visual motor axis during a lengthy surgery can lead to a variety of problems including low-quality ergonomics and overall surgical performance, spatial disorientation, and finally increased risk of serious iatrogenic injuries. AR headsets could solve the above problems in the future and can be converted to virtual surgical aids with immersive fluoroscopic, CT, and endoscopic views, giving surgeons a great deal of spatial awareness.[4] AR headsets could also help in the area of general surgery, which even today follows more conventional operative modes. One example is surgical intervention for hepatic tumors. Traditionally, surgeons use Doppler ultrasound to confirm the locations of blood vessels and tumors inside the liver parenchyma, which cannot otherwise be detected with the naked eye or by palpation during the excision. However, this technique is not 100% reliable. In some operations, surgeons found the results from the Doppler too inaccurate and would prefer to skip it in favor of investigating its location by measuring distances on 2D slices of the patient's CT scan. In a more advanced approach in the future, surgeons could have an anatomic, multicolor 3D reconstruction liver model, with delineation of the hepatic and portal veins, based on the patient's CT scan, using a similar AI procedure as described above.[5] As a next step, this liver model could be uploaded to the surgeon's AR headset and during the operation deploy a virtual representation of the internal structure of the liver with great spatial accuracy. In this manner, the surgeon in combination with a suitable haptic system that would accompany his tools could project the tumor's location and vessel's topology in real time and complete the resection or ablation of the tumor with great precision, reducing the risk of extensive hemorrhage and minimizing the loss of healthy liver parenchyma.

Additive manufacturing on presurgical planning

AM, also known as 3D printing, has tremendous potential in the area of medical imaging and preoperational planning these days. With the advent of a wide range of low-cost (up to 6000 euros) fused deposition modeling (FDM) technology printers, which are based on the extraction of thermoplastic material in the form of filament, the 3D printing of internal human organs on an original scale has become easier and more affordable than ever. Furthermore, the release of water-soluble thermoplastic material of the polyvinyl alcohol (PVA) type, which is used on the construction of supporting structures of complex anatomical models, was decisive. But the number one feature that is currently missing from 3D printing in medicine is the reliability of FDM technology regarding the production of multicolor models. Many models of 3D printers from different manufacturers such as Prusa MK3S with MMU2S and XYZ da Vinci Color tried to bring multiple colors to the AM process. The da Vinci color, for example, includes a white polylactic acid thermoplastic extrusion head and an ink cartridge that works with classic inject technology, which has the ability to color any outside layer of the 3D printed model. On the other hand, Prusa's MMU2S kit has an intelligent system that can alternate up to five different color shade filaments of thermoplastic material. Both of the above 3D printer multicolor model kits have various advantages and disadvantages. The XYZ has the ability to create millions of different colors, but with the lack of PVA supporting structures, the Prusa can only produce up to four different colors with PVA compatibility (Fig. 1.1).

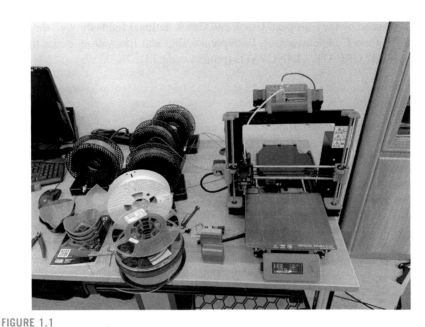

FIGURE 1.1

Prusa MK3S with MMU2S kit for multicolor 3D printing.

However, they both share a disadvantage and that is the lack of reliability in alternation and mixing process of colors. The result of this situation can lead to failure to print or printing durations up to 7 days with several large intervals of manual user interaction. Of course, the solution to the above problems has been given by PolyJet 3D printing technology, which can combine in the same printing process multiple polymers with different mechanical characteristics and color shades or even with full transparency. However, the cost of a PolyJet 3D Printer can reach 400.000 euros.

With the further "democratization" of 3D printing in the future, any surgeon will be able to print stunning anatomical models with low cost and effort, suitable for timely, preoperative planning. After all, this is what today's technological trends show, with recent examples like multimaterial multinozzle 3D printing (MM3D) technology being very encouraging. MM3D is a new technique created by researchers at the Wyss Institute and Harvard's John A. Paulson School of Engineering and Applied Sciences, allowing the switching between up to eight different inks 50 times per second, helping the creation of complex, high-quality 3D objects in a fraction of the time currently required by other FDM methods.[6] The inks can have different colors or even can be total transparent.

Overall, as bright and promising as the future looks, the key remains the collaboration between engineers and physicians, so that the marriage of medicine and technology can reach its full potential. The chapters that follow in this book would give us examples of these collaborations and the amazing things that they can accomplish.

Co-financed by the European Union and Greek national funds through the Operational Program Competitiveness, Entrepreneurship and Innovation, under the call RESEARCH? CREATE - INNOVATE (project code:T1EDK-03599).

References

[1] URL1: https://developer.nvidia.com/clara-medical-imaging.

[2] Hosny A, Parmar C, Quackenbush J, Schwartz LH, Aerts HJWL. Artificial intelligence in radiology. *Nat Rev Cancer*. 2018;18(8):500−510. https://doi.org/10.1038/s41568-018-0016-5.

[3] URL2: https://devblogs.nvidia.com/deploying-healthcare-ai-workflows-with-the-nvidia-clara-deploy-application-framework/.

[4] Al Janabi HF, Aydin A, Palaneer S, et al. Effectiveness of the HoloLens mixed-reality headset in minimally invasive surgery: a simulation-based feasibility study. *Surg Endosc*. 2020;34:1143−1149. https://doi.org/10.1007/s00464-019-06862-3.

[5] URL3: https://radiopaedia.org/articles/couinaud-classification-of-hepatic-segments.

[6] URL4: https://wyss.harvard.edu/news/multimaterial-3d-printing-manufactures-complex-objects-fast/.

3D printing and nanotechnology

Lazaros Tzounis, PhD, Diploma Engineer [1,2], **Petros Bangeas, MSc** [3]

[1]*Department of Materials Science & Engineering, University of Ioannina, Ioannina, Greece;*
[2]*Mechanical Engineering Department, Hellenic Mediterranean University, Heraklion, Greece;*
[3]*Department of Surgery, Aristotle University of Thessaloniki, Thessaloniki, Greece*

Introduction to additive manufacturing technologies and rapid prototyping

The rapid prototyping has dramatically expanded over the last 20 yrs, with the two-dimensional (2D) and three-dimensional (3D) printing processes to be in the forefront and the most promising technologies among others.[1,2] 2D and 3D printing are additive manufacturing (AM) processes based on sequential addition of (nano-) material layers offering the opportunity to print either 2D parts (thin or thick films/layers as self-standing films or coatings) or bulk 3D parts and components made of different (nano-)materials with variable mechanical and physical properties.[3,4] Namely, the global sales in 3D printing (products and services) rose by 21% from the market in 2017 (https://www.forbes.com) reaching 7 B$, while the total AM market only for the automotive sector is expected to grow from 1.5 B€ in 2018 to 5.3 B€ in 2023 and 12.6 B€ in 2028 (https://www.smartechpublishing.com/news/smartec-report-automotive-additive-manufacturing-market/).

Roll-to-roll and sheet-to-sheet 2D AM

The 2D AM processing could be a continuous process otherwise defined as roll-to-roll (R2R) or sheet-to-sheet (S2S), both of which allow a continuous deposition of materials as inks/pastes, melts, etc., onto rigid or flexible substrates (glass, plastic, metallic foils, textiles, etc.). In a R2R process, the materials are deposited in motion between two moving rolls named as unwinder and winder. R2R is an important class of substrate-based manufacturing processes in which additive and subtractive processes (e.g., laser scribing) can be used to build components in a continuous manner. R2R is a process that combines many technologies to produce rolls of finished material in an efficient and cost-effective manner with the benefits of high production rates of mass quantities. High throughput and low cost are the factors that differentiate R2R manufacturing from conventional manufacturing, which is slower and more expensive due to the multiple steps involved. Today, roll to roll (R2R) processing is applied in numerous manufacturing fields such as (i) coating of textiles (e.g., using a bath coating technology otherwise known as dyeing process),[5] (ii) prepregs for advanced carbon fiber—reinforced polymer structural composites (bath or slot-die deposition of epoxy onto fabrics),[6] and (iii) packaging, i.e., smart packaging (e.g., slot-die, gravure, bath coating, screen printing, flexography of inks, varnishes),[7] flexible and large area printed electronics (e.g., slot-die, gravure, bath coating, screen printing, flexography, inkjet printing of electronic inks and pastes),[8–10] thin-film batteries[11] and (bio-)electrodes (e.g., slot-die, screen printing),[12] textiles for wearables (e.g., inkjet printing, screen printing, and flexography),[13] membranes (e.g., slot-die),[14] etc. The global R2R technology market is expected to reach 35.69 B$ in 2023, expanding at a compound annual growth rate of 13.5% from 2015 to 2023 (http://www.mobilecomputingtoday.co.uk/4572/global-roll-roll-r2r-technology).

Fig. 2.1 demonstrates (A) a schematic of a R2R AM process, as well as (B) a representative R2R printing/coating line produced by FOM company (FOM Technologies, Denmark); while in (C), a schematic of a S2S printing coating AM process is depicted, and in (D), a S2S printing slot-die and blade coating machine produced by Coatema printing technologies company (Coatema Coating Machinery GmbH, Germany) is depicted.

3D AM

3D printing is an AM process based on sequential addition of material layers offering the opportunity to print 3D parts and components made of different materials with variable mechanical and physical properties.[15] The first 3D print was

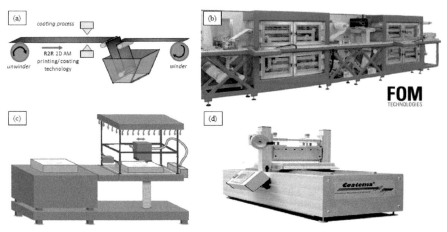

FIGURE 2.1

(A) Schematic of a roll-to-roll (R2R) additive manufacturing (AM) process, as well as (B) a representative R2R printing/coating AM line; (C) a schematic of a sheet-to-sheet (S2S) printing coating AM process, and (D) a S2S printing slot-die and blade coating machine.

reported by Hideo Kodama in 1982.[16] Since then, 3D printers have become much more accessible and are now able to print with a multitude of materials including metals, wood products, and thermoplastics such as polylactic acid (PLA) and others. In addition, there are various techniques for printing solid materials in 3D, including as shown in Fig. 2.2A: inkjet 3D printing, Fig. 2.2B: fused deposition modeling (FDM), Fig. 2.2C: stereolithography, and Fig. 2.2D: selective laser sintering, electron-beam freeform fabrication, and direct metal laser sintering, among others.[16]

Fig. 2.3 demonstrates (A) the flowchart of a 3D printing AM process including the generation of the computer-aided design (CAD) model (in a CAD-specific software, e.g., SOLIDWORKS, AutoCAD, 3D Builder) toward exporting it to an stl. file capable of being communicated with most of the 3D printer software for further the printing process (printing process has to be simulated, process parameters to be chosen, etc., from the printer software) (http://reprap.org/wiki/CAM_Toolchains). In

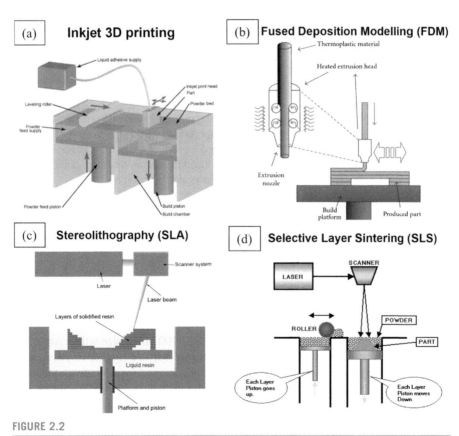

FIGURE 2.2

(A) Inkjet 3D printing, (B) fused deposition modeling (FDM), (C) stereolithography (SL), and (D) selective laser sintering (SLS).

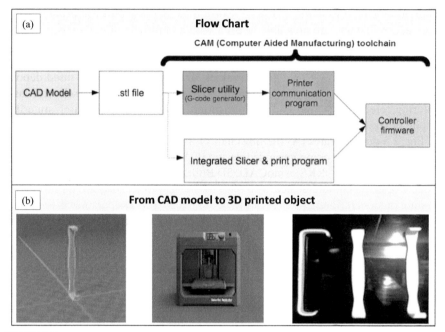

FIGURE 2.3

(A) Flowchart of a 3D printing additive manufacturing process including the generation of the computer-aided design (CAD) model toward exporting it in an stl. file capable of being communicated with most of the 3D printer software for further the printing process; (B) CAD model of a surgery retractor as well as a 3D fused deposition modeling printer deployed to print the objects shown on the right-hand side of the image.

Fig. (B), a CAD model of a surgery retractor is depicted, as well as a 3D FDM printer for thermoplastic materials (MakerBot Inc., USA) used to print the objects is shown on the right-hand side of the image.

Introduction to nanotechnology and applications
Nanoparticles

Nanoparticles (NPs) are particles in the range of $1-100$ nm in size with a surrounding capping agent or otherwise known as stabilizer, surface ligand, or passivating agent.[17] The capping agent is an integral part of nanoscale matter, fundamentally affecting all of NPs' properties, while it could be of various chemical compounds, i.e., ions, inorganic molecules, and organic molecules, endowing to the NP the appropriate surface chemistry endowing colloidal stability as well as proper surface functionalities for interaction with other substances. In nanotechnology, a particle is defined as a small object that behaves as a whole unit with respect to its transport and properties, while the type of NP element as a function of the size and morphological characteristics could give a great variety of different properties (catalytic, sensing, electrical and thermal conductivity, bactericidal, etc.).

Fig. 2.4 shows, representatively, scanning and transmission electron microscopy images (SEM, TEM images) of different NP types with different shapes, namely 1D, 2D, and 3D NP geometries with different sizes and aspect ratio (length/diameter). Fig. 2.4 summarizes NPs, i.e., multi-walled carbon nanotubes (MWCNTs)[18,19] and graphene monolayers (from the authors' library of TEM images and materials' microscopy investigations), silica (SiO_2),[20] Fe_3O_4 superparamagnetic NPs and Fe_3O_4@SiO_2@Ag core–shell–satellite NPs,[21] Au@Ag core–shell NPs,[22] and polymeric spherical NPs loaded with pharmaceutical substances (carriers for drug delivery applications) deposited onto electrospun nonwoven fabric biodegradable polymeric fibers (used as scaffolds for controlled drug release).[23]

Nanotechnology

Nanotechnology refers to the technology that is implemented at the nanoscale and has various applications in the real world.[24]. Unique physical and chemical properties of nanomaterials can be exploited for applications that the whole scientific society could benefit, i.e., electronics and biomedical devices. Nanotechnology represents thus a "megatrend" and has become nowadays a "general purpose" technology.

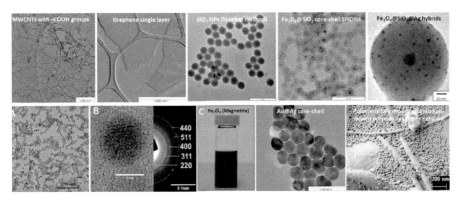

FIGURE 2.4

Representative scanning and transmission electron microscopy images of nanoparticle (NP) structures: multi-walled carbon nanotubes (MWCNTs), graphene monolayers, silica (SiO_2), Fe_3O_4 superparamagnetic NPs. (A) Low magnification image; (B) High magnification image together with the selected area diffraction pattern; (C) Nanoparticles in water dispersion, Fe_3O_4@SiO_2@Ag core–shell–satellite NPs, Au@Ag core–shell NPs, and polymeric NPs loaded with pharmaceutical substances (drug delivery) deposited onto electrospun nonwoven fabric biodegradable polymeric fibers (as scaffolds).

Nanotechnology is manipulating the matter on an atomic, molecular, and supramolecular scale, while it targets precisely manipulating atoms and molecules for fabrication of macroscale products (nano-enabled), also now referred to as molecular nanotechnology.[25] A more generalized description of nanotechnology was subsequently established by the National Nanotechnology Initiative, which defines nanotechnology as the manipulation of matter with at least one dimension sized from 1 to 100 nm. This definition reflects the fact that quantum mechanical effects are important at this quantum-realm scale, and so the definition shifted from a particular technological goal to a research category inclusive of all types of research and technologies that deal with the special properties of matter that occur below the given size threshold. Nanotechnology may be able to create many new materials and devices with a vast range of applications, such as in nanomedicine,[26] nanoelectronics,[27] energy production,[28–30] and consumer products.[31] However, nanotechnology raises many of the same issues as any innovative technology, including concerns about the toxicity and environmental impact of nanomaterials, and their potential effects on global economics, as well as speculation about various doomsday scenarios. These concerns have led to a debate among advocacy groups and governments on whether special regulation of nanotechnology is warranted. Basic research and development as well as research on potential safety issues of nanotechnology, workforce development, and education and curriculum should be continued.

Nanotechnology is more specifically defined as the design, characterization, production, and application of structures, devices, and systems by controlling shape and size at the nanometer scale.[32] It is now generally accepted that for a component or material to be considered as nano at least one critical dimension or manufacturing tolerances has to be below 100 nm, down to the size of atoms (~ 0.2 nm).[33]

Fig. 2.5 illustrates everyday examples of things that fall in the macro- to nano-size range.

Fig. 2.6 illustrates some nano-enabled structures that form well-ordered domains. Namely, an SEM image is depicted of SiO_2 spherical NPs that can self-assemble into hexagonally packed structures (left-hand side),[20] and TEM images of a block copolymer (BCP) with spherical morphology in which spheres are arranged into a hexagonally packed structure (middle image),[34] and finally a BCP with lamellar morphology that the lamellae have been oriented/aligned using a shear force field with potential nanoelectronics, thin-film nanotemplates with anisotropic magnetic, electrical properties, etc., applications.[35,36]

Namely, the revenues from nano-enabled products continue growing, with over 200 B$ in 2012 in the United States alone and over 700 B$ worldwide. This represents an impressive return on investment.[37] At the same time, due to a variety of potential applications (including industrial, defense), governments have invested billions of dollars in nanotechnology research, while just in 2012, the United States invested 3.7 B$, Europe 2.1 B$, and Japan 750 M$.

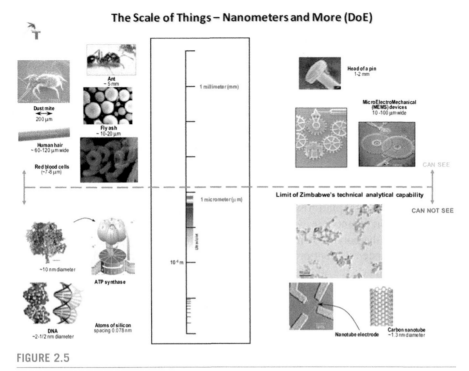

FIGURE 2.5

Scale of things from macro to nano size.

The figure is courtesy of the DoE, 2006 (Malanowski and Zweck, 2007).

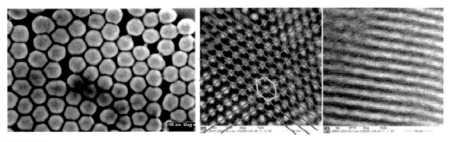

FIGURE 2.6

SiO_2 spherical nanoparticles that can self-assemble into hexagonally packed structures (left-hand side scanning electron microscopy image); a block copolymer (BCP) with spherical morphology, in which spheres are arranged into a hexagonally packed structure (middle transmission electron microscopy (TEM) image); and a BCP with lamellar morphology that lamellae have been oriented/aligned using a shear force field (right-hand side TEM image).

3D printing and nanotechnology

AM has become very popular in the past decade and has received a lot of attention from researchers in many fields because of the ability to create functional parts in a wide variety of materials.[38] 3D printing is a significant technological attainment that could be deployed for a variety of applications in the medical field, overcoming existing limitations and providing significant improvements to the state-of-the art technologies.[39] Multifunctionality through embedding of nanomaterials can further extend capabilities of nanocomposites to properties such as gradients in thermal and electrical conductivity, photonic emissions tunable for wavelength, and increased strength and reduced weight.

Among AM techniques, FDM uses feedstock thermoplastics, which then are extruded onto a build platform.[40] To improve the properties of the polymeric matrix, particle reinforcements are widely used due to their low cost and the ease to be dispersed into the polymeric matrix.[41−43] According to their type, they have the potential to enhance different properties of the final composite and add new functionalities. For instance, the addition of iron or copper particles to acrylonitrile butadiene styrene (ABS) can contribute to thermal conductivity and the improvement of the storage modulus, while it reduces the coefficient of thermal expansion. An Al or Al_2O_3/Nylon 6 composite exhibits reduced frictional coefficient. $BaTiO_3$ in ABS or $CaTiO_3$ in polypropylene dispersion can offer enhanced dielectric permittivity and controllable resonance frequency. MWCNTs and their surface functionalization affect the thermoelectric properties of melt-mixed polycarbonate nanocomposites.[44] Apart from the traditional particles, numerus nanomaterials can offer exceptional mechanical, electrical, and thermal properties to the polymeric matrix.[45] The addition of several nanomaterials for the production of composite parts utilizing 3D printing is also capable to increase the tensile strength.[46] For example, composite parts with 5 wt% titanium dioxide (TiO_2), 10 wt% carbon nanofibres, or 10 wt% MWCNTs exhibited an improvement of the tensile strength by 13.2%, 39%, and 7.5% in comparison with neat polymer parts, respectively.[47]

Apart from the mechanical enhancement, the addition of the NPs in the polymeric matrix can contribute to the improvement of electrical and thermal properties. Gnanasekaran et al. applied 3D printing of carbon nanotube (CNT)- and graphene-based conductive polymer nanocomposites by FDM.[48] They used dispersions of CNTs and graphene (G) in polybutylene terephthalate (PBT). The results showed that electrical conductivity increased from 1×10^{-13} S/m for neat PBT to 11×10^1 S/m for 3D-printed polymer nanocomposites with CNTs and 1 S/m with dispersed graphene. Additionally, they assessed thermal stability by conducting thermogravimetric analysis. They presented that the addition of conductive fillers enhanced the thermal stability, as both the onset and the maximum degradation temperature shift to a higher value. More specifically, a weight loss of 5% occurred at 303 °C, 339 °C, and 332 °C for the PBT, PBT/CNT, and PBT/G, respectively. Inlet guide van was fabricated from Glenn Research Center by using FDM process with Ultem 100 and chopped carbon fiber (CF) with operating temperature reaching 400°F. CF-reinforced polyether ether ketone composites with 50% less weight than aluminum was fabricated by Impossible Objects company, with heat resistance at about 482°F, while maintaining two-thirds of the aluminum's strength.[47] This composite material has been printed as demonstrator airfoil, rotor support arm, and air intake (Fig. 2.7).

The specific and closely linked dependencies of production processes, materials, and component design represent a challenge. The method of layer-wise construction enables the direct production of complex 3D geometries in a single production step and without time-consuming process and tool planning. The higher the geometric complexity of the component, the greater the advantages of additives over conventional manufacturing. The abovementioned properties open up new possibilities for structural optimization, especially in lightweight construction (Fig. 2.8). Nearly any structure that has an adaptation of the design depending on the load situation and the stress distribution can be produced. In this context, with the increasing possibilities of AM, research has focused in particular on cellular lightweight grid structures in combination with sandwich construction. This concept is based on the principle of inserting material only at places where it is required for force transmission or from an electromagnetic point of view.[49] Thereby, parts of the object with high material concentration are replaced by complex cellular structures.[50] The production of such structures is difficult or impossible with conventional methods, so that only the additive procedures make an economic conversion of such concepts possible. J.F. Christ et al. fabricated FDM 3D-printed nanocomposites of thermoplastic polyurethane (TPU)/MWCNT with various MWCNT content up to 5 wt%.[51] The results showed that the material strength, initial elastic modulus, and electrical conductivity enhanced with the increased addition of MWCNT filler. Also, different MWCNT

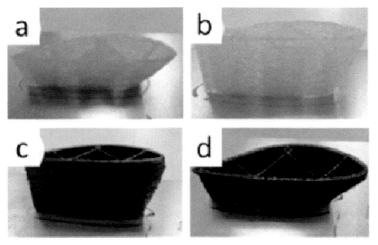

FIGURE 2.7

3D printed airfoil demonstrators based on the glass fiber (A and B) and carbon fiber (C and D) formulations.

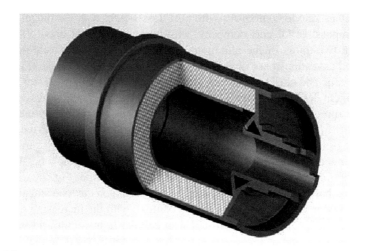

FIGURE 2.8

Optimized H13 rotor shaft with lattice structures for lightweight design optimization.

contents can provide different ranges of flexibility and sensitivity, offering tunable properties for particular applications. TPU/MWCNT 3D-printed nanocomposites can also be used as excellent piezoresistive feedstock for strain sensors. Other potential applications are in the fields of wearable electronics, soft robotics, and prosthetics (Fig. 2.9).Chizari et al. developed highly conductive nanocomposite materials (up to 5000 S/m) for three-dimensional (3D) printing of 2D and 3D structures with applications in liquid sensing and electromagnetic interference shielding.[52]

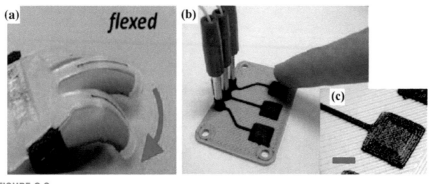

FIGURE 2.9

3D-printed carbon black/polycaprolactone composite for (A) piezoresistive sensors, (B) capacitive sensors, and (C) macro image of the printed sensor pads (scale bar 5 mm).

3D printing and nanotechnology toward biomedical applications: recent trends and challenges

3D printing FDM method could allow direct printing of nanomaterial-modified filaments, to bring a new paradigm for nanocomposite functionality in bulk 3D objects.[53]

A novel development accomplished with 3D printing process was a formatting glove with embedded programmable heater, temperature sensors, and the ability of thermotherapeutic treatment via associated control electronics.[54]

Palmiga (a Sweden company; https://palmiga.com/) developed and characterized soft and flexible conductive 3D-printed surface electromyography (sEMG) sensors/electrodes. In comparison to the gold standard Ag/AgCl gel electrodes, there was no significant difference in the EMG signal amplitude under the same conduct area. The sensors were capable of distinguishing several levels of muscle activity of the biceps brachii. This gives 3D-printed sEMG electrodes a high potential for creating personalized sensing structures, for example, in prosthetic and orthotic contexts[55] (Fig. 2.10). Palmiga also constructed flexible force sensor by 3D-printed conductive TPU. The capacitance of the sensor changed due to an applied sinusoidal force. The experiments were established using an oscillatory readout circuit consisting of only an operational amplifier and a frequency counter based on an Arduino Nano. This indicates the possibility to implement low-cost capacitive sensors into 3D-printed objects, which is especially interesting for customized robotic and prosthetic applications.[56]

Recently, AM has been intensely investigated for surgical implants, tissue scaffolds, and organs.[57] Till now, the most important application of 3D printing in the medical field is the design and development of medical devices and instrumentation.[58,59] For instance, surgeons are using patient computed tomography—derived 3D prints for better preoperative planning to plan surgical approaches,[60] plan complex operations,[61–63] and/or for surgical educational proposes.[64] 3D models of

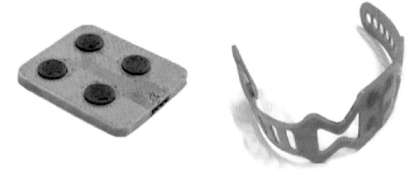

FIGURE 2.10

Photograph of 3D-printed electromyography electrodes using flexible conductive filaments (thermoplastic polyurethane/carbon black based).

patient-specific anatomy such as dental crowns and biological scaffolds are already being used for human implants.[65–67] There is, however, scant literature to date for the production of surgical instruments and equipment by 3D printing.

Within the surgical realm, PLA and polyglycolic acid have been intensely investigated for biodegradable implants and suture material, such as Vicryl (Ethicon, New Brunswick, NJ).[66] PLA has been proven to be safe for surgical implantation as it is a biocompatible and biodegradable polymeric material; it cost effective and safe and therefore could be suitable for printing surgical instruments. Surgery equipment should also have the ability to be sterilized as it is of paramount to its application. PLA is extruded at temperatures well above 120°C, rendering possible its exposure and application for steam sterilization or even for dry heat sterilization at 170°C.[67] However, research has found that autoclaving compromises the structural integrity of PLA.[66,68,69] Minimal degradation of PLA polymers has even been shown in vitro, when physiological conditions are simulated for days to weeks.[70] Although lower temperature methods of sterilization such as ethylene oxide "gas" sterilization did not impact PLA strength, harmful levels of ethylene oxide residue are a serious concern. Alternatively, glutaraldehyde, an effective sterilant at room temperature, has been shown to retain the greatest PLA strength when compared with other chemical sterilants.[71] Considering a surgery instrument, it should be sterile and exhibit potentially resistance to biofilm formation. This is because a surgery that involves a cut (incision) in the skin can lead to a wound infection after surgery. Surgical wound infections may have pus draining from them and can be red, painful, or hot to touch.

An important issue in 3D-printed biomedical objects is to endow antimicrobial properties to the final object. For this purpose, polymeric materials have been modified by incorporating antimicrobial agents in their bulk structure, for example, by solvent of melt mixing, or by depositing thin AM films onto their surface yielding the desired properties. Various antimicrobial agents have been extensively studied, and results indicate the capability of preventing the growth of pathogenic microorganisms, such as bacteria, fungi, and algae.[72–74] Namely, silver, copper, metal salts, quaternary ammonium compounds, polyhexamethylene biguanides, triclosan biopolymer chitosan, N-halamine, etc., are some of the AM agents that could be introduced in a polymer matrix or be deposited as thin films on polymeric material surfaces.[75] Among the abovementioned antibacterial agents, silver has been widely used due to its broad spectrum of antibacterial activity and its low toxicity toward mammalian cells.[76] The release of silver ions is believed to be the main reason for its antibacterial properties. Ionized silver is highly active, as it binds to tissue proteins and brings structural changes to the bacterial cell wall and nuclear membrane, leading to cell distortion and death.[77] Due to their small size, silver nanoparticles (Ag NPs) have emerged as a new generation of antibacterial agents with unique properties for diverse medical applications.[78] In the past, different strategies have already been proposed and investigated for the incorporation of Ag NPs in plastics or the deposition of thin films consisting of silver. The incorporation of silver in a polymer matrix by solvent mixing could be found elsewhere,[79] while deposition of silver on the surface of various substrate materials has been reported using magnetron sputtering,[80] ion beam−assisted deposition process,[81] dip coating using colloidal silver,[82] and sonochemistry deposition methods.[83,84] From the latter wet chemical deposition processes, the sonochemical process is very promising due to the versatility as well as the possibility to stabilize the NPs onto the polymer substrate surface due to the fact that the polymeric chains are partially swollen during sonication and the silver ions are penetrating into the polymer chains and getting entrapped and further reduced during sonochemistry.

Future perspectives: advancements beyond the state of the art

Surgical equipment like for instance an antimicrobial retractor could be fabricated by 3D printing the 3D object and subsequent deposition of a nanolayer of a specific antimicrobial agent. A lot of attention has been paid already to achieve planar surfaces, bulk materials, textiles, etc., with antimicrobial properties, especially in the health and hygienic field. More specific, the 3D objects could be produced at a specific use case and by design as well as patient specific. As PLA has been proven to be safe for surgical implantation, it can be selected for various future applications as it is a cost effective, safe, and environmentally suitable material for printing a surgical instrument. Ag NPs could be deposited in a wet deposition method via a versatile sonochemical protocol, yielding extremely reactive antimicrobial surfaces. The antimicrobial retractor must be strong enough to retract human tissue, must be hypoallergenic, and must tolerate repeat sterilization. Finally, it must be at least equivalent in cost, strength, and accessibility when compared with a standard stainless steel Army Navy retractor to be considered as a substitute.

Fig. 2.11A shows the process for printing a PLA surgical retractor, as well as the method for sonochemically immobilizing Ag NPs, while the chemicals and the protocol followed to achieve high-quality monodispersed Ag NPs immobilized onto the retractor surface are illustrated in Fig. 2.11B.

The optimization of 3D FDM AM processes via online monitoring and modeling approaches has the potential to provide high-quality components with built-in functionalities for multiple applications in various fields such as health, automotive, aeronautics and aerospace, consumer goods and electronics, industrial equipment and tooling, construction, and energy. Additionally, Three dimensional (3D) fused deposition modelling (FDM) additive manufacturing (AM) further developments at process and process optimization and process monitoring control level, as well as at materials level will improve the reliability, the quality and the accuracy as well as the multi-material capabilities through printed processes of nanocomposite filaments as fast as standard materials by avoiding process related issues.

Impact of the combined 3D printing and nanotechnology in biomedical and other applications

3D AM of multifunctional nanocomposite thermoplastic filaments and 3D-functionalized printed components will have enhanced mechanical, electrical, surface,

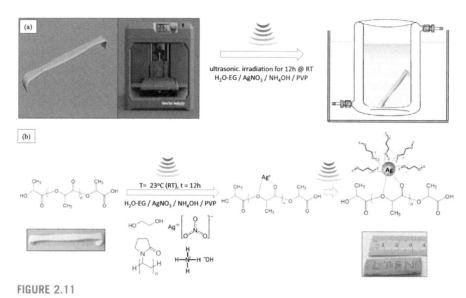

FIGURE 2.11

(A) Process for printing a polylactic acid surgical retractor, as well as the method for sonochemically immobilizing silver nanoparticles; (B) chemicals and the protocol followed to achieve high-quality monodispersed Ag NPs immobilized onto the retractor surface.

and durability properties, providing improved efficiency, quality, and reliability of the final product, while using fully reprocessable and recyclable materials reducing the environmental impact could result in minimizing the manufacturing cost by 40%−50%. Especially in the biomedical sector, the combination of 3D AM and nanotechnology could positively influence societal and economic challenges. The vision for 2030 foresees that Europe will improve its leading role in AM, greatly impacting on the competitiveness of European industrial sectors. AM will improve the quality of life of European citizens in terms of retention of high-quality jobs in Europe; availability of customized, cleaner, safer, and affordable products; increased access to cleaner energy; mobility; and effective and personalized medicine.

Improvement of the efficiency, quality, and reliability of the products

The sustainable development of material depends not only on the superior quality of the products but also on the reduction of environmental impacts throughout the life cycle. The emerging technology of AM has prosperously focused on an advantage of personalizing the products according to the demand that are socially, economically, and environmentally feasible. 3D-manufactured products can be hugely adaptable to the improved mechanical properties regardless of their complexity. This certainly allows the prospect to design well-detailed products with enhanced quality and reliability. This also helps companies to reassess their design and products and be environmentally and economically efficient throughout every life cycle stage. According to Verhoef et.al, 40% saving in construction materials can be achieved, as demonstrated by a Chinese manufacturer of 3D-printed houses.[85] This established concept can be readily further visualized to improve the efficiency, quality, and reliability of the product by at least 40% in other applications. This could be met by focusing on competence of circular economy, i.e., increase in recycling rate extremely, which provokes using less material in the feedstock and generates less waste. This also includes the need of more efficient manufacturing systems, introduction of new composite materials, and adopting efficient business models. Previously, life cycle assessment (LCA) has shown that the estimated savings in the production and use phases of a product due to AM are in the ranges of $113−370 billion and $56−219 billion, respectively, by 2025 (https://www.ifm.eng.cam.ac.uk/uploads/Research/CTM/working_paper/2015-03-Despeisse-Ford.pdf).

Better use of raw materials and resources with reduced environmental impact and to lower cost

AM may play a lead role in the circular economy, for example, by producing high value-added products from recycled or bio-based powders and enabling full reuse of AM by-products in new products. The exploitation of the full potential of AM will also lead to resource and energy saving in the whole value chain and in particular in manufacturing and transportation, thus contributing to the environment (Fig. 2.12). Additionally, AM technologies can contribute to the availability at low cost of highly efficient green energy solutions (e.g., renewable energy components), thus contributing to the EC 2050 low-carbon economy roadmap (https://ec.europa.eu/clima/policies/strategies/2050_en).

The concept of circular economy also makes better use of materials. Previously, approximately 35% of the energy needed for processing was saved with AM

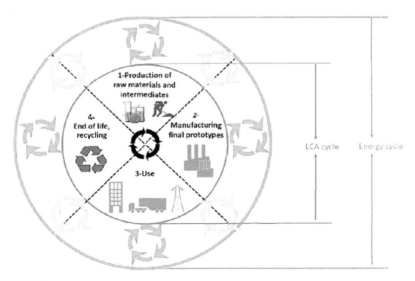

FIGURE 2.12

Circular energy economy.

process. The LCA methodology will help fully compare the existing technologies and intensify their concept for the efficient use of energy and raw material. Through LCA, material efficiency can be monitored or foreseen, opening door to the future analyses of new components and materials. The price of 3D printers is predicted to be decreased by 78% by 2022 in comparison to 2012. This is enough motivation to execute materials inspection for new composites and nanocomposites, applicable for AM. Additionally, the reduction in primary energy supply could be one of the key focuses of this work (*Baumers, M., (2011) Energy Inputs to Additive Manufacturing, Wolfson, Loughborough, UK*).

Summary and conclusions

In this chapter, an introduction to 2D and 3D AM processes as well as to nanotechnology has been given, with a specific focus on combining the 3D printing with nanotechnology toward "smart" and multifunctional nanotechnology-enabled, 3D-printed objects. Throughout the whole chapter, many examples of nano-enabled 3D objects are described; however, special attention is given on biomedical objects and potential products, i.e., EMG sensors, surgery equipment, 3D-printed gloves with embedded programmable heaters, and temperature sensors for thermotherapeutic treatment. It is of utmost importance that more researchers need to become engaged to realize the mutual benefits of nanotechnology and AM. Despite early successes, challenges in the application of nanomaterials to AM are nevertheless numerous: several nanomaterials are yet to be applied in an AM context; there is little information on the interaction of nanocomposites with 3D printing material; and standardized process parameters and synthesis methods for different nanomaterials and processes do not yet exist. Both the nanotechnology and AM communities could benefit from increased scholarly interactions and collaborations. Only through such greater engagement between the nanotechnology and AM communities can the promises of 3D printing of multifunctional nanocomposites be realized.

Acknowledgment

L. T. gratefully acknowledges the Bodossaki Foundation for financial support.

References

1. Vaezi M, Seitz H, Yang S. A review on 3D micro-additive manufacturing technologies. *Int J Adv Manuf Technol.* 2013;67(5):1721−1754.
2. Takagishi K, Umezu S. Development of the Improving Process for the 3D Printed Structure. *Sci Rep.* 2017;7:39852.
3. Lewicki JP, et al. 3D-Printing of meso-structurally ordered carbon fiber/polymer composites with unprecedented orthotropic physical properties. *Sci Rep.* 2017;7:43401.

4. Pitsalidis C, et al. Transistor in a tube: a route to three-dimensional bioelectronics. *Sci Adv*. 2018;4(10):eaat4253.

5. Tzounis L, et al. Fiber yarns/CNT hierarchical structures as thermoelectric generators. *Mater Today: Proc*. 2017;4(7, Part 1):7070−7075.

6. Felisberto M, et al. Carbon nanotubes grown on carbon fiber yarns by a low temperature CVD method: a significant enhancement of the interfacial adhesion between carbon fiber/epoxy matrix hierarchical composites. *Compos Commun*. 2017;3:33−37.

7. Kang H, et al. Fully roll-to-roll gravure printable wireless (13.56 MHz) sensor-signage tags for smart packaging. *Sci Rep*. 2014;4:5387.

8. Kapnopoulos C, et al. Fully gravure printed organic photovoltaic modules: a straightforward process with a high potential for large scale production. *Sol Energy Mater Sol Cell*. 2016;144:724−731.

9. Kapnopoulos C, et al. Gravure printed organic photovoltaic modules onto flexible substrates consisting of a P3HT:PCBM photoactive blend1. *Mater Today: Proc*. 2016; 3(3):746−757.

10. Tzounis L, et al. Perovskite solar cells from small scale spin coating process towards roll-to-roll printing: optical and morphological studies. *Mater Today: Proc*. 2017;4(4, Part B):5082−5089.

11. Schmitt M, et al. Slot-die processing of lithium-ion battery electrodes—coating window characterization. *Chem Eng Process: Process Intensification*. 2013;68:32−37.

12. Bariya M, et al. Roll-to-roll gravure printed electrochemical sensors for wearable and medical devices. *ACS Nano*. 2018;12(7):6978−6987.

13. Karim N, et al. All inkjet-printed graphene-based conductive patterns for wearable e-textile applications. *J Mater Chem C*. 2017;5(44):11640−11648.

14. Kellenberger CR, et al. Roll-to-roll preparation of mesoporous membranes by nanoparticle template removal. *Ind Eng Chem Res*. 2014;53(22):9214−9220.

15. Bangeas P, et al. Three-dimensional printing as an educational tool in colorectal surgery. *Front Biosci*. 2019;11:29−37. https://doi.org/10.2741/e844.

16. Rankin TM, et al. Three-dimensional printing surgical instruments: are we there yet? *J Surg Res*. 2014;189(2):193−197.

17. Tzounis L. Chapter 9 - Synthesis and processing of thermoelectric nanomaterials, nanocomposites, and devices. In: Beeran Pottathara Y, et al., eds. *Nanomaterials Synthesis*. Elsevier; 2019:295−336.

18. Tzounis L, et al. Highly conductive ultra-sensitive SWCNT-coated glass fiber reinforcements for laminate composites structural health monitoring. *Compos B Eng*. 2019;169: 37−44.

19. Tzounis L, et al. P- and n-type thermoelectric cement composites with CVD grown p- and n-doped carbon nanotubes: Demonstration of a structural thermoelectric generator. *Energy Build*. 2019;191:151−163.

20. Tzounis L, et al. Controlled growth of Ag nanoparticles decorated onto the surface of SiO_2 spheres: a nanohybrid system with combined SERS and catalytic properties. *RSC Adv*. 2014;4(34):17846−17855.

21. Tzounis L, Logothetidis S. $Fe_3O_4@SiO_2$ core shell particles as platforms for the decoration of Ag nanoparticles. *Mater Today: Proc*. 2017;4(7, Part 1):7076−7082.

22. Contreras-Caceres R, et al. Polymers as templates for Au and Au@Ag bimetallic nanorods: UV−vis and surface enhanced raman spectroscopy. *Chem Mater*. 2013;25(2):158−169.

23. Pappa AM, et al. Oxygen-plasma-modified biomimetic nanofibrous scaffolds for enhanced compatibility of cardiovascular implants. *Beilstein J Nanotechnol*. 2015;6: 254−262.

24. Tzounis L, et al. The interphase microstructure and electrical properties of glass fibers covalently and non-covalently bonded with multiwall carbon nanotubes. *Carbon*. 2014;73:310–324.

25. Karalis G, et al. A carbon fiber thermoelectric generator integrated as a lamina within an 8-ply laminate epoxy composite: Efficient thermal energy harvesting by advanced structural materials. *Appl Energy*. 2019;253:113512.

26. Perli MD, et al. Synthesis and characterization of Ag nanoparticles for orthopaedic applications. *Mater Today: Proc*. 2017;4(7, Part 1):6889–6900.

27. Borges BG, et al. Surface, interface and electronic properties of F8:F8BT polymeric thin films used for organic light-emitting diode applications. *Polym Int*. 2018;67(6):691–699.

28. Papageridis KN, et al. Comparative study of Ni, Co, Cu supported on γ-alumina catalysts for hydrogen production via the glycerol steam reforming reaction. *Fuel Process Technol*. 2016;152:156–175.

29. Charisiou ND, et al. An in depth investigation of deactivation through carbon formation during the biogas dry reforming reaction for Ni supported on modified with CeO_2 and La_2O_3 zirconia catalysts. *Int J Hydrogen Energy*. 2018;43(41):18955–18976.

30. Charisiou ND, et al. Ni supported on $CaO-MgO-Al_2O_3$ as a highly selective and stable catalyst for H_2 production via the glycerol steam reforming reaction. *Int J Hydrogen Energy*. 2019;44(1):256–273.

31. Wise K, Brasuel M. The current state of engineered nanomaterials in consumer goods and waste streams: the need to develop nanoproperty-quantifiable sensors for monitoring engineered nanomaterials. *Nanotechnol Sci Appl*. 2011;4:73–86.

32. Royal Society, Royal Academy of Engineering. *Nanoscience and Nanotechnologies: Opportunities and Uncertainties*. Royal Society; 2004.

33. Malanowski N, Zweck A. Bridging the gap between foresight and market research: integrating methods to assess the economic potential of nanotechnology. *Technol Forecast Soc Change*. 2007;74(9):1805–1822.

34. Carrasco PM, et al. Thermoset magnetic materials based on poly(ionic liquid)s block copolymers. *Macromolecules*. 2013;46(5):1860–1867.

35. Wode F, et al. Selective localization of multi-wall carbon nanotubes in homopolymer blends and a diblock copolymer. Rheological orientation studies of the final nanocomposites. *Polymer*. 2012;53(20):4438–4447.

36. Tzounis L, et al. Shear alignment of a poly(styrene-butadiene-styrene) triblock copolymer/MWCNT nanocomposite. *Polymer*. 2017;131:1–9.

37. Bhushan B. Introduction to Nanotechnology. In: Bhushan B, ed. *Springer Handbook of Nanotechnology*. Berlin, Heidelberg: Springer Berlin Heidelberg; 2017:1–19.

38. Bangeas P, et al. Evaluation of three-dimensional printed models in surgical education: a paradigm of a new educational method for the simulation of surgery environment. *HPB*. 2018;20:S779.

39. Malik HH, et al. Three-dimensional printing in surgery: a review of current surgical applications. *J Surg Res*. 2015;199(2):512–522.

40. Rodríguez José F. Mechanical behavior of acrylonitrile butadiene styrene fused deposition materials modeling. *Rapid Prototyp J*. 2003;9(4):219–230.

41. Tzounis L, et al. Influence of a cyclic butylene terephthalate oligomer on the processability and thermoelectric properties of polycarbonate/MWCNT nanocomposites. *Polymer*. 2014;55(21):5381–5388.

42. Papageorgiou DG, et al. β-nucleated propylene–ethylene random copolymer filled with multi-walled carbon nanotubes: Mechanical, thermal and rheological properties. *Polymer*. 2014;55(16):3758–3769.

43. Tzounis L, et al. All-aromatic SWCNT-polyetherimide nanocomposites for thermal energy harvesting applications. *Compos Sci Technol.* 2018;156:158−165.

44. Liebscher M, et al. Influence of the MWCNT surface functionalization on the thermo-electric properties of melt-mixed polycarbonate composites. *Compos Sci Technol.* 2014;101:133−138.

45. Terzopoulou Z, et al. Effect of MWCNTs and their modification on crystallization and thermal degradation of poly(butylene naphthalate). *Thermochim Acta.* 2017;656: 59−69.

46. Liebscher M, et al. Influence of the viscosity ratio in PC/SAN blends filled with MWCNTs on the morphological, electrical, and melt rheological properties. *Polymer.* 2013;54(25):6801−6808.

47. Wang X, et al. 3D printing of polymer matrix composites: a review and prospective. *Compos B Eng.* 2017;110:442−458.

48. Gnanasekaran K, et al. 3D printing of CNT- and graphene-based conductive polymer nanocomposites by fused deposition modeling. *Appl Mater Today.* 2017;9:21−28.

49. Krenkel W. *Verbundwerkstoffe: 17. Symposium Verbundwerkstoffe und Werkstoffverbunde.* Wiley; 2009.

50. Lock C, Reinhart G. A meta-model for analyzing the influence of production-related business processes. *Procedia CIRP.* 2016;57:79−84.

51. Christ JF, et al. 3D printed highly elastic strain sensors of multiwalled carbon nanotube/thermoplastic polyurethane nanocomposites. *Mater Des.* 2017;131:394−401.

52. Chizari K, et al. Three-dimensional printing of highly conductive polymer nanocomposites for EMI shielding applications. *Mater Today Commun.* 2017;11:112−118.

53. Campbell TA, Ivanova OS. 3D printing of multifunctional nanocomposites. *Nano Today.* 2013;8(2):119−120.

54. Ota H, et al. Application of 3D printing for smart objects with embedded electronic sensors and systems. *Adv Mater Technol.* 2016;1(1):1600013.

55. Wolterink G, et al. 3D-printing soft sEMG sensing structures. In: *2017 IEEE SENSORS.* 2017.

56. Schouten M, Sanders R, Krijnen G. 3D printed flexible capacitive force sensor with a simple micro-controller based readout. In: *2017 IEEE Sensors.* 2017.

57. Nguyen D, et al. Cartilage tissue engineering by the 3D bioprinting of iPS cells in a nano-cellulose/alginate bioink. *Sci Rep.* 2017;7(1):658.

58. Sodian R, et al. 3-dimensional printing of models to create custom-made devices for coil embolization of an anastomotic leak after aortic arch replacement. *Ann Thorac Surg.* 2009;88(3):974−978.

59. Kurenov SN, et al. Three-dimensional printing to facilitate anatomic study, device development, simulation, and planning in thoracic surgery. *J Thorac Cardiovasc Surg.* 2015; 149(4):973−979.e1.

60. Bangeas P, Voulalas G, Ktenidis K. *Rapid Prototyping in Aortic Surgery. Interactive Cardio Vascular and Thoracic Surgery.* 2016.

61. Sodian R, et al. Three-dimensional printing creates models for surgical planning of aortic valve replacement after previous coronary bypass grafting. *Ann Thorac Surg.* 2008; 85(6):2105−2108.

62. Kolyva C, et al. A mock circulatory system with physiological distribution of terminal resistance and compliance: application for testing the intra-aortic balloon pump. *Artif Organs.* 2012;36.

63. Biglino G, et al. Virtual and real bench testing of a new percutaneous valve device: a case study. *EuroIntervention.* 2012;8.

64. Lioufas PA, et al. 3D printed models of cleft palate pathology for surgical education. *Plast Reconstr Surg Glob Open*. 2016;4(9):e1029.
65. Michael S, et al. Tissue engineered skin substitutes created by laser-assisted bioprinting form skin-like structures in the dorsal skin fold chamber in mice. *PloS One*. 2013;8(3): e57741.
66. Meseguer-Olmo L, et al. In-vivo behavior of Si-hydroxyapatite/polycaprolactone/DMB scaffolds fabricated by 3D printing. *J Biomed Mater Res*. 2013;101A(7):2038–2048.
67. Fedorovich NE, et al. Organ printing: the future of bone regeneration? *Trends Biotechnol*. 2011;29(12):601–606.
68. Rozema FR, et al. The effects of different steam-sterilization programs on material properties of poly(L-lactide). *J Appl Biomater*. 1991;2(1):23–28.
69. Kondor S, et al. On demand additive manufacturing of a basic surgical kit. *J Med Dev Trans ASME*. 2013;7(3), 030916-030916-2.
70. Weir NA, et al. Degradation of poly-L-lactide. Part 2: increased temperature accelerated degradation. *Proc IME H J Eng Med*. 2004;218(5):321–330.
71. Athanasiou KA, Niederauer GG, Agrawal CM. Sterilization, toxicity, biocompatibility and clinical applications of polylactic acid/polyglycolic acid copolymers. *Biomaterials*. 1996;17(2):93–102.
72. Gorenšek M, et al. Functionalization of polyester fabric by Ar/N2 plasma and silver. *Textil Res J*. 2010;80(16):1633–1642.
73. Cheng X, et al. Antimicrobial coating of modified chitosan onto cotton fabrics. *Appl Surf Sci*. 2014;309:138–143.
74. Shahid ul I, Shahid M, Mohammad F. Green chemistry approaches to develop antimicrobial textiles based on sustainable biopolymers—a review. *Ind Eng Chem Res*. 2013; 52(15):5245–5260.
75. Deng X, et al. Antimicrobial nano-silver non-woven polyethylene terephthalate fabric via an atmospheric pressure plasma deposition process. *Sci Rep*. 2015;5:10138.
76. Shrivastava S, et al. Characterization of antiplatelet properties of silver nanoparticles. *ACS Nano*. 2009;3(6):1357–1364.
77. Feng QL, et al. A mechanistic study of the antibacterial effect of silver ions on *Escherichia coli* and *Staphylococcus aureus*. *J Biomed Mater Res*. 2000;52(4):662–668.
78. Chaloupka K, Malam Y, Seifalian AM. Nanosilver as a new generation of nanoproduct in biomedical applications. *Trends Biotechnol*. 2010;28(11):580–588.
79. Sawant SN, et al. Antibiofilm properties of silver and gold incorporated PU, PCLm, PC and PMMA nanocomposites under two shear conditions. *PloS One*. 2013;8(5):e63311.
80. Chen Y-H, Hsu C-C, He J-L. Antibacterial silver coating on poly(ethylene terephthalate) fabric by using high power impulse magnetron sputtering. *Surf Coating Technol*. 2013; 232:868–875.
81. Jiang SX, et al. Surface functionalization of nanostructured silver-coated polyester fabric by magnetron sputtering. *Surf Coating Technol*. 2010;204(21–22):3662–3667.
82. Jeong SH, Hwang YH, Yi SC. Antibacterial properties of padded PP/PE nonwovens incorporating nano-sized silver colloids. *J Mater Sci*. 2005;40(20):5413–5418.
83. Ilana P, et al. Sonochemical coating of silver nanoparticles on textile fabrics (nylon, polyester and cotton) and their antibacterial activity. *Nanotechnology*. 2008;19(24):245705.
84. Nina P, et al. Depositing silver nanoparticles on/in a glass slide by the sonochemical method. *Nanotechnology*. 2008;19(43):435604.
85. Verhoef LA, et al. The effect of additive manufacturing on global energy demand: An assessment using a bottom-up approach. *Energy Pol*. 2018;112:349–360.

Three-dimensional bioprinting in medical surgery

Maria V. Alexiou, BSc, MSc [1], **Andreas I. Tooulias, MD, MSc** [2]

[1]*Molecular Biologist and Geneticist, Surgical Department, School of Medicine, Faculty of Health Sciences, Aristotle University of Thessaloniki, Thessaloniki, Greece;* [2]*General Surgeon, HPB Fellow, Surgical Department, School of Medicine, Faculty of Health Sciences, Aristotle University of Thessaloniki, Thessaloniki, Greece*

Introduction: 3D bioprinting technology in a few words and its evolution through the years

The need to overcome the restrictions of transplantation process such as the limited number of biocompatible donated organs, the increasing demand for organs, the transplants rejection, and/or the overall difficulties after transplantation has led the research to a new field knowing as tissue engineering[1] and regenerative medicine. Currently, the new applications adjusted in this field include three-dimensional (3D) bioprinting technology. Bioprinted tissues and organs will be greatly expected to eliminate this increasing organ shortage crisis that predominates.

The bioprinting technology was initially introduced as a method for fabricating tissue scaffolds and it has been applied for engineering a variety of tissue constructs such as the bone, skin, and cartilage.[2-4] In conventional tissue fabrication, cells are seeded onto the scaffold, which provides a microenvironment mimicking the properties of the real extracellular matrix (ECM), after the printing process. The emerging difficulty with this method is the inability to position different cell types in appropriate locations within the scaffold and control the cell migration. These parameters are crucial for the generation of complex tissues and/or organs in order to satisfy the transplantation requirements.

The limitations of scaffold-based tissue engineering were overcome with the evolution of 3D bioprinting, where living cells are directly disposed mixed with biomaterials in order to develop complex structures tending to mimic native tissues and/or organs. 3D bioprinting is defined as the precisely deposition of biocompatible materials and growth factors along with living cells layer-by-layer using the traditional 3D printing technology, which is mentioned as cell-laden printing.[5-8] It is well established that each human tissue is consisted of multiple and different cell types organized in an accurate and complex architecture. The 3D bioprinting methods allow for the organization of multiple cell types in predesigned positions with the contribution of computer-aided design (CAD) in a totally controlled way in order to generate 3D structures that maximally imitate the native tissue/organ characteristics.[5,9]

The trigger which gave birth to 3D printing technology was when Charles Hull invented a 3D printing method based on stereolithography (SLA) apparatus.[10] This major breakthrough along with the introduction of tissue engineering[1] laid the foundations of bioprinting, setting the goal to combine cells, and biomaterials for the fabrication of tissue analogues of custom-tailored shapes and sizes. A great number of studies and observations have been conducted through the years making 3D bioprinting a very promising and challenging tool for the development of organ-on-a-chip drug screening systems and fully functional tissues and organs.[11,12]

3D bioprinting methodology has already been applied for scaffold fabrication meeting the needs of tissue engineering. Regarding the use of living cells in the fabrication of complex tissue constructs, by the late 1990s, scientists mentioned the development of 2D bioprinting systems combined with living cells by the use of micropositioning methods.[13] In 2004, a scientific team with Roth at the head achieved to print cells employing an inkjet printer filled with collagen.[14] Taking this great progress into account, Boland and his colleagues focused their research on the printability of mammalian ovary cells and as a result the first patent for inkjet bioprinting of viable cells is a reality.[15,16]

Mironov and his scientific team developed tube-shaped tissues (e.g., blood vessels) through printing layers of cell aggregates and gel alternatively.[17] One year later, Mironov, Forgacs, and their colleagues brought to the forefront and applied for a bioprinting-related patent that includes self-assembling cell aggregates and modeling methods in order to produce an engineered tissue with the desired 3D structure.[18] Inspired by this work, one of the pioneers of bioprinting, the research company Organovo, was founded in 2005, and in 2009, the first world's commercial 3D bioprinter, NovoGen MMX (Organovo, United States), was available.[19] Several studies have been conducted resulting in the use of multicellular spheroids, the scaffold-free printing of blood vessels, and the commercialization of printed liver cells.[20,21] Common goal until nowadays is the evolution of 3D bioprinting process from a research tool to an efficient process for the fabrication of viable and functional tissues and organs. However, despite the significant progress of the researchers worldwide, there are few reports concerning the clinical applications of bioprinted constructs.

In general, 3D bioprinting process consists of three stages: prebioprinting, bioprinting, and postbioprinting.[17,22,23] Major components that are crucial for the execution of the bioprinting process are the suitable bioinks, the appropriate bioprinting process (modality), and a functional 3D bioprinter.

In this chapter, the latest advances in the use of the 3D bioprinitng will be discussed, including the processing, the used bioprinting modalities, the criteria of the most convenient bioink's selection, and the recent clinical applications.

Classification of 3D bioprinting methods

The bioprinting could be divided into inkjet-based bioprinting, extrusion-based bioprinting, laser direct-write bioprinting, photocuring-based bioprinting, and cell ball assembling bioprinting. Among them, the inkjet-based bioprinting, the extrusion-based bioprinting, and the laser direct-writing bioprinting are the most widely used. Each method influences positively or negatively the cell viability and integrity during the process. In the sections below, the characteristics of the existing bioprinting methods are cited.

Inkjet-based bioprinting

In order to form the desired 3D structure, the inkjet-based bioprinting method utilizes bioinks, instead of ink, deposited repeatedly in the form of droplets at predesigned locations in a moving stage.[24,25] The desired 3D structure is printed using the conventional layer-by-layer approach as a series of consistent and fusing together droplets using the thermal heater method[15] or the piezoelectric actuator method.[26-28]

Inkjet-based bioprinting technology was introduced in 2003 and constitutes the first bioprinting attempt,[29] which is mainly used for printing small scaffolds. Since then, Ciu, Boland, and their colleagues printed hamster ovary cells in 2005,[30] and a few years later, in 2009, it was Boland and Cui[31] who constructed a structure that resembles the blood vessels using human microvascular endothelial cells. The wide use of this bioprinting modality emerged from the fact that it is an inexpensive, non-time-consuming method and the printing properties (e.g., printing speed, resolution, size, position of droplets) can be easily electronically controlled.[32]

The inkjet bioprinter can be used for printing different types of cells that allows the cell-cell interfaces printing, as well as for heterocellular tissue engineering[33,34] and for the creation of complex structures.[35,36]

On the other hand, there are some limitations that restrict its use. The inkjet bioprinters use bioinks of low viscocity due to the small squeezing force of the nozzle, resulting in a limited capability of processing high-density cells.[37] The preference of low viscous bioinks creates structures of weak strength and limited ability for perfusion and/or implantation. In addition, denaturalization of the biomaterials, cell lysis, and damage in cell viability is possible to occur probably due to thermal or mechanical properties of the inkjet bioprinter (for example, the applied voltage in piezoelectric bioprinter is about 12−25 Hz).[34] Finally, it is very crucial for the ink droplets to be consistent and fused immediately with each other in order to avoid deformation and mechanical instability of the constructs.[2]

Extrusion-based bioprinting

The extrusion-based bioprinting method is considered to be the most widely used method of bioprinting. In this technique, the bioink is extruded out of a nozzle driven by pneumatic pressure[22,38,39] or mechanical force[40-44] via screws and pistons, in a totally controlled manner. The extrusion process produces filaments, instead of the droplets in the inkjet-based bioprinting method, resulting in the formation of a 2D model that under the appropriate processing produces the desired 3D structure. The first attempt for extrusion printing was performed in 2003[17] and since then plenty of reports mentioned the method in a variety of tissue applications.[45-49] The bioinks used for extrusion bioprinting have high density, which permits the printing of cell-laden patterns with enhanced ability for perfusion and/or implantation. Moreover, the bioinks should have fluid-like capacities in order to be extruded through the nozzle tip. In comparison with inkjetting, the choice of biomaterials is versatile. More specifically, viscous polymers, high cell density cell-encapsulated hydrogels, and thermoplastic biomaterials can be printed.[50-52] However, it is of notice that the resolution of this technique is low compared with the inkjet- and the laser-based bioprinting,[53] the nozzle becomes often clogged and the cell viability could be damaged in case of increased extrusion pressure.[54] It would be a very interesting challenge to find a balance between printing cells at high viscocity while protecting the cellular function and viability during extrusion.[55,56] It is worthy to report that it is simple and easily accessible method. An extrusion-based system can be developed in an easy way and with low cost by the suitable processing of a commercialized plotter or a desktop 3D printer.[57]

Laser direct-write bioprinting

The laser direct-write bioprinting was first introduced in 1999,[58] when Odde and his colleagues have used laser for cell patterning, and 1 year later, the same team[59] reported direct writing of living cells with the use of laser as well. Since then, plenty of reports have been followed regarding the development of the laser-assisted cell printing method.[60-66] This method is based on the principles of laser-induced forward transfer to transport droplets[67] and resembles the conventional typewriters. The main components of such methods include the use of a donor slide (or ribbon), a laser pulse, and a receiver slide. The top layer of the ribbon is a transparent glass coated with a thin layer of metal so as to absorb the energy of the laser protecting the cells from direct contact. The underlayer contains the bioink. Initially, a laser pulse is applied onto the top layer resulting in the formation of microbubbles, from the glass substrate in the underlayer containing the printable biomaterial. Subsequently, the absorbed laser energy forces the mixture of cells and cell encapsulation (a kind of hydrogel) to be vaporized forming droplets of the materials containing the cells. Then, the droplets are transported to the receiver slide and the 3D object can finally be printed.[67-69]

The laser-assisted bioprinting can be regarded as a nozzle-free inkjet-based bioprinting method. As a result, the problem of nozzle clogging no longer exists and the ability to position precise patterns for a variety of cells types and biomaterials is enhanced.[31] The laser bioprinting permits the printing of bioinks with high density and in high resolution.[33] The printing resolution is depended on the laser's energy and pulse frequency, the speed of the laser, the thickness of the layers, the distance between the donor and the receiver slide, and the bioink's viscosity as well.[70,71] Moreover, it permits a single-cell manipulation and the accurate control of the cell droplets positioning.[70]

However, there are some parameters that restrict its use including the low cell viability in the printed tissue constructs as a consequence of the laser's energy, the fact that it is an expensive method,[23,72] the fact that it is time consuming to spread the mixture of cells in each printing layer, and that there are no available commercialized laser-based bioprinters. It is very challenging for the applications of this method to be combined with a well-designed bioreactor or other biofabrication systems.[73,74]

Photocuring-based bioprinting

Photocuring-based bioprinting is a method that mimics the conventional printing of tissue engineering scaffolds where the cells are seeded onto the scaffold after the printing.[6-8] In photocuring boiprinting system, the use of UV light turns light-sensitive materials to be solidified layer by layer. One layer is solidified at a time regardless of the complexity of the layer's structure. The presence of the UV light restricts the use of this technique in printing cell-laden structures due to the damage that provokes in the cells. A lot of studies have been conducted in order to achieve simultaneous printing of cells and scaffolds by using less harmful light. Examining the viability of these cells, the results were very encouraging.[75,76] There are two different technologies of photocuring-based bioprinting resulted from the way of scanning: the SLA technology, where the bioink is cured point by point, and the digital light projection technology, where the bioink is cured plane by plane.[77] Many types of cells have been reported to be seeded onto the printed scaffolds and the HUVECs and HepG2 are indicative. Apart from the fact that generally this type of printing is time saving, convenient, and of high resolution, the choice of the materials and the selection of the light source should be very careful in order to avoid the cell damage.

Cell ball assembling bioprinting

A new approach has emerged in the field of tissue engineering called modular tissue engineering. Modular tissue engineering aims to recreate biomimetic macroscale structures by designing microscale structural features in order to fabricate modular tissues to use them as building blocks in order to fabricate larger tissues.[77,78] Between these building blocks, cell balls are used in bioprinting by a self-fusion process.[22,77,79,80] The cell ball assembling bioprinting is based on the creation of 3D structures by self-assembly and self-fusion process. More specifically, 3D constructs are manufactured by fusion of smaller discrete units. The basic blocking units involve microparticles, microfilaments, and planes. Each unit is glued together in order to fabricate a realistic 3D structure which can be achieved with different methods in inkjet-based, laser direct-writing, extrusion-based, photocuring-based bioprinting techniques. The cell ball assembling bioprinting is a scaffold-free method, which means that the fabrication of a 3D structure is based on the in vitro fusion of two adjacent cell aggregates.

Bioinks in 3D bioprinting

One of the crucial components of 3D bioprinting technology is the bioink that is used for the printing process. This bioprintable material is consisted of various biological factors such as cells, media, genes, growth factors, proteins, polymers, hydrogels, etc.

The bioinks used in 3D bioprinting for the development of cell-laden structures are divided into two categories depending on the use or not of a scaffold: the cell scaffold-based approach and the scaffold-free cell-based approach.[81] In the cell scaffold-based approach, the bioink consists of biomaterials and living cells. The cells are encapsulated in the biomaterial scaffold which will be biodegraded forcing the cells to proliferation, growth, and conquest of the space in order to form the desired 3D structure. On the other hand, in the scaffold-free cell-based approach, the cells (cell aggregates—spheroids), in the absence of scaffold, are directly printed resembling the real embryonic development. Specific cell types are printed at a time to form the primary tissues and finally these tissues form larger and more complex tissue structures.[82]

There are many preconditions that the bioink should fulfill in order to be selected. The bioink's selection is very crucial because the success of the bioprinting process is depended on these preconditions. The properties an ideal bioink should have are determined by the characteristics of the available bioprinters as well as by their biological status. The bionk's characteristics should be also adjustable to the requirements of the desired tissue and organ and modifiable in order to achieve efficiently the regeneration of the corresponding tissues and organs. Among others, some of the most important bioinks' properties include biocompatibility, biodegradability, and printability. In the section below, we will mention the overall requirements for the selection of the appropriate bioink.

If the preferable method is the cell scaffold, there are criteria for the selection of the bioink formulation concerning the nature of the biomaterial's properties (such as printability, biodegradability, mechanical properties) and its biological status (biocompatibility, cytocompatibility) as well.

The printability of the biomaterial refers to its ability to be disposed in a totally controlled way and subsequently form a designed structure via a fusion process. It is depended on the rheological properties of the bioink such as viscosity, gelation and shear thinning properties, yield stress, and shear recovery. These properties should be optimized in order to ensure the effectiveness of printability and the mechanical strength. Before printing, the biomaterial should be in liquid state while it is placed on the basic blocking units (microparticles, microfilaments, planes).[77] A very crucial feature of an appropriate biomaterial is its viscosity and the capacity to be tunable so as to be used by the different commercially available bioprinters and to be adjusted in the different printing conditions (e.g., temperature, shear thinning). It is considered that bioinks with higher viscosity form more stable 3D constructs when compared with lower viscous bioinks. However, the balance between the high viscosity and the printing speed requires attention so as to yield highly stable structures because the pressure applied may affect the cell viability. After printing, the printed units must glue each other through a sol-gel process, which imposes the material to be solidified/ gelatinized immediately after printing in order to maintain the shape and ensure the fusion. After that, the materials are stacked together through a layer-by-layer process deposition, and it is important for them to be stacked continuously in the vertical direction to keep the predesigned architecture. Apart from the printability, there are also other properties for the selection of the most suitable bioink. Mechanical properties of the material, such as high mechanical strength, shear thinning, stiffness, and elasticity, play very important role in the integrity, the cell survival, and the maintenance of the 3D shape of the printed structure (so as the internal design of the structure does not collapse during the layer-by-layer deposition).[83-85]

The mechanical strength of the printed object should mimic the properties of the native tissue in order to ensure the cell growth, proliferation, and tissue maturation.[86,87] Furthermore, the structure should be stabilized as soon as possible after printing within a postprinting maturation process. For example, the high viscous bioinks used in extrusion bioprinting need to have shear thinning in order to compensate the high shear stress applied during printing procedure. The major challenge for the candidate biomaterial is the ability to provide the environment which permits the cells to achieve their cellular function, retain their potency, and ensure their bioactivity after printing.[88] The properties of this artificial environment should be indicative of cell survival just like the native cellular environment does. The candidate biomaterial should be also biodegradable, biocompatible, cytocompatible, and immunocompatible as well.[84] The biomaterial scaffold ideally provides the environment for the cellular function. Once the cells grow and proliferate, the scaffold will be degraded, with the cells conquesting the space and producing their own ECM. It is of notice that the biomaterial and subsequently the biodegradation products should not be toxic or generally harmful for the cells disposed within the biomaterial and for the other neighboring tissues/cells.[84] In addition, it is prohibitive to create any immunological response to the host in case of in vivo implantation.[85] In order to be biocompatible and cytocompatible, the bioink material should also be favorable for cell adhesion and modification of the functional groups on their surface to include and deliver different biochemical signals or biomolecules.[89] Another desirable aspect for a bioink is the capacity to create the conditions for the permeability of oxygen, nutrients, growth factors, and metabolic waste, in order to enhance cell growth and metabolic activity.[82,90]

The bioinks used so far and their properties

As mentioned in the section above, the suitable bioink should satisfy specific preconditions that are also depended on the requirements of the desired tissues and organs as well. The widely used bioinks include tissue spheroids, cell pellets, tissue strands, and biomaterial scaffolds with encapsulated cells. The scaffolds include hydrogels, microcarriers (MCs) and decellularized ECM.[82]

The different human tissues have diverse properties and they are composed of different types of cells that achieve specific cellular function. In 3D bioprinting, different types of cells can be used according to the demands of the corresponding tissue. These cell's types include already differentiated adult and progenitor cells and stem cells as well.[91] Induced pluripotent stem cells (iPSCs), embryonic stem cells (ESCs), and extraembryonic cells have the ability to be bioprinted for developing a functional tissue and/or organ.[91]

There is a wide variety of biomaterials that can be used. There are two categories of biomaterials used in 3D bioprinting. The first category involves the natural and the second one the synthetic polymers. Natural biomaterials are subdivided according to their origin in these coming from proteins (silk, collagen, fibrin, gelatin) and those based on polysaccharides (hyaluronan, alginate, agarose, chitosan). Among them, the hydrogels are the most prominent mainly due to their unique properties, which satisfy the bioink's requirements (high water content, biodegradable, ideal for cell survival, adjustable mechanical and modifiable chemical properties, able to yield high resolution during printing).[90] In addition, the fact that they mimic the properties of living tissues make them suitable in the field of tissue engineering and regenerative medicine.

Even though an ideal bioink should not need any physical, chemical, or photocrosslinking modifications to become cell-friendly, natural and synthetic hydrophilic materials can be physically or chemically crosslinked to form hydrogels.[92] Even though, natural biomaterials are more preferable due to their cytocompatibility, their weak structure and the fact that they are degraded in a fast pace make the cross-linking necessary to enhance their mechanical strength. Physical, chemical, or covalent and enzymatic cross-linking are the main mechanisms of hydrogel gelation. Physical cross-linking (e.g., ionic) is performed during bioprinting and results in ignorable viscosity fluctuations but contributes in the fabrication of relatively weaker structures and cross-linking treatment can be reversible.[93] Chemical cross-linking needs considerable time of gelation that restricts the formation of multilayered structures.[93] Furthermore, it creates toxic crosslinkers that must be removed completely before the implantation.[82,94,95] Alternatively, photocross-linking (e.g., under light irradiation) is a way for instantaneous cross-linking, although the effect of the light and the time of exposure on cells need further consideration.[96] Even though enzymatic cross-linking is more preferable biologically, it is expensive and has a negative effect on the practicality of the process. However, the cross-linking mechanism is possible to affect negatively the cellular compatibility and the homogeneity of the biomaterial.[97,98]

The bioinks also should be affordable and abundant. Unfortunately, cell-laden bioinks as well as some natural hydrogels such as collagen and hyaluronan acid are relatively expensive. In general, printable biomaterials are limited with the synthetic polymers to be more available in comparison with natural polymers.

Synthetic polymers

The high mechanical strength, the ability of the mechanical properties to be totally controlled, the tunable chemical properties (response to PH and temperature, adjust their molecular weight and functional groups) and their printability are indicative advantages that support their use over the natural materials.[99,100] However, the disadvantage that limits their use is the inability to ensure the cellular proliferation/differentiation and promote the interactions between cells.[101] Among synthetic polymers, Pluronic and poly(ethylene glycol) (PEG) are the most preferable.

Pluronics, or poloxamers, are a class of synthetic block copolymers that consist of hydrophilic poly(ethylene oxide) and hydrophobic poly(propylene oxide), arranged in an A-B-A triblock structure.[102] The amphiphilic property enables this group to interact with hydrophobic surfaces and biological membranes.[102] The characteristic that allows its use in 3D bioprinting is the capacity to form self-assembling gels at room temperature and flow at 10°C.[103] There are two reports that mention the use of Pluronic for the fabrication of 3D structures. Wu and his colleagues printed microchannel with Pluronic in photopolymerizable hydrogel matrix in order to develop biomimetic microvascular structures.[104] Müller and his team, trying to develop more stable constructs, used acrylated Pluronic for the development of UV crosslinked constructions.[105]

PEG, which is a water-soluble polymer, constitutes one of the most widely used synthetic materials in 3D bioprinting technology. It is suitable for cell encapsulation and it can become more compatible by been functionalized with cell adhesion motifs.[88,106] It can be modified with acrylate groups in order to achieve satisfying printability.[107,108] For example, in extrusion-based bioprinting, the PEG-diacrylate and PEG-methacrylate polymers are usually used.[107,109,110]

PEG can be combined with a variety of other materials to achieve increased mechanical properties in 3D printing constructs.[111] The application of PEG is limited by not being biodegradable. However, there are synthetic biomaterials suitable for bioprinting applications such as poly(lactic acid), poly(lactic-co-glycolic acid), and poly(ε-caprolactone) (PCL).[112] Among them, PCL is more applicable due to its low melting temperature (60°C),[39] whereas the use of polylactone-based polymers is restricted because of the release of acidic products during degradation, which are inflammatory for the tissues. Recently, it was developed a photopolymerizable, thermosensitive, biodegradable biomaterial consisted of poly(N-(2-hydroxy-propyl) methacrylamide lactate) and PEG.[113]

Natural biomaterials

The major advantage of natural biomaterials when compared with the synthetics is their ability to mimic the ECM composition and the structure of native tissues. They also ensure the cellular integrity, they have the appropriate biocompatibility and biodegradability, and they have self-assembly abilities. However, their tunable properties are very low[114] and the structure's stability is endangered. In order to overcome this, the natural biomaterials are combined with other natural biomaterials or even with synthetic polymers. Natural polymers are mixed with synthetic materials or other natural biomaterials to produce new bioinks with modifiable properties.[115-117] Recently, a group of scientists reported a mixture of Pluronic and alginate in an effort to examine the effects of this combination on myoblast cell viability and alignment. The reported gene expression confirmed the cell viability.[118]

There is a wide variety of natural biomaterials used for 3D bioprinting applications. In the section below, we will describe the most commonly used.

Agarose-based bioinks

Agarose is the par excellence polymer with many applications in the field of medicine and biology mainly due to its gel formation properties.[119] It is a polysaccharide mainly sourced from red seaweed.[120] Agarose is a linear polymer consisting of the repeating unit of agarobiose, which is a disaccharide made up of D-galactose and 3,6-anydro-L-galactopyranose.[121-123]

Despite the biocompatibility, the excellent gelation, and the indicative mechanical properties, it is weak to support and enhance cell growth.[124] However, the fact that it can change its properties through chemical modifications and the observation that the combination of agarose with other biomaterials (alginate, collagen, fibrinogen) leads to stable 3D structures with observed cell viability triggered many scientific teams to investigate its use in 3D bioprinting applications.[125-127] The research of Gu and his team who developed functional neurons using a blend of agarose, alginate, and carboxymethyl-chitosan with human neural and iPSCs is very interesting. They achieved to form stable 3D constructs with encapsulated cells.[128,129] In another research, it was used with chemically modified agarose, carboxylated agarose, along with human mesenchymal stem cells (hMSCs) and the cell viability was even 95% more in comparison with agarose without any modifications.[130] A variety of reports investigated the use of agarose-based hydrogels as bioinks mixed with human cells or multicellular aggregates in 3D bioprinting, the printability, and the cell viability and the results are satisfying. In conclusion, it is important to use the agarose in combination with other hydrogels and/or modify its chemical structure in order to reinforce its properties and promote the cell proliferation/differentiation.[131-133]

Alginate-based bioinks

Alginate, also known as alginic acid or algin, is the most preferable biomaterial in 3D bioprinting. Being a polysaccharide refined from brown algae, it belongs to the natural polymers.[134] It is a hydrophilic linear copolymer whose blocking units, the monomeres $(1,4)$-β-D-mannuronate (M) acid and α-L-guluronate (G) acid, have distinct roles. The polymer is consisted either of homopolymeric blocks of consecutive G-residues (G-blocks), which enhance the gel formation, or consecutive M-residues (M-blocks) or altering M- and D-residues (MG-blocks), which contribute to the material's flexibility.[24,135] The alginate is immunoneutral after in vivo implantation and the solution's viscosity can be modified by altering the average molecular weight and the chain segment ratio.[136] Alginate with low viscosity can be used in inkjet-based bioprinting, whereas alginate with high viscosity can be used in extrusion-based bioprinting and laser direct-write bioprinting. It is worthy to mention that even though the degradation rate is slow, it can be ameliorated through oxidation.[134] Furtheromore, the chemical structure of alginate can be modified by adding cell adhesion signals making it more biocompatible and more suitable to promote cell adhesion. However, the chemical treatment may affect negatively the viability of the cells.[137] All these characteristics emerge alginate as the most suitable hydrogel for bioprinting of large tissues.[138,139] There are plenty of studies that mentioned the use of alginate, alginate-based biomaterials, and/or combination of alginate with different biomaterials.

Alginate-based bioinks were used with cartilage cells for printing of hollow constructs by forming vessels-like printable microfluid channels. These channels were able to support the cellular growth and permit oxygen, nutrients, and biomolecules transporting through the construct.[140] A bioink consisting of cartilage cells and alginate was also used in order to print tubular constructs with a triaxial nozzle assembly. The combination of the coaxial system along with the specific bioink was able to ensure the viability of the cells either during the printing process and the postprinting procedures.[141] Furthermore, high strength constructs having microchannels for the appropriate nutrient transportation were developed using alginate-based hydrogel as a biomaterial.[142]

There is a wide range of polymers that mixed with alginate to produce a variety of 3D printed constructs for tissue engineering applications, including gelatin,[143] polycaprolactone (PCL),[39,131,144] poloxamer,[145] and so on.

In 2016, alginate-based biomaterials were used so as to print 3D structures with live cells. In this study, the way in which the flow behaviors effect on different cell lines like Schwann cells, fibroblast cells, and skeletal muscle cells during printing was investigated.[146]

It is very important to mention that alginate was selected to be the biomaterial when human iPSCs and human ESCs were bioprinted for the first time and they differentiated into hepatocytes for the formation of 3D minilivers.[48]

In a detailed review of the literature, Gopinathan and Noh present comprehensively the variety of studies performed regarding the use of alginate in 3D bioprinting.[90] It is concluded that the advantages of alginate over the other hydrogels provoke the scientists to select it more often for research in the field of 3D bioprinting.

Collagen-based bioinks

It is well known that the collagen is the mayor structural protein of extracellular matrix.[147] It consists of amino acids bound together in a configuration to form a triple helix of collagen. Collagen, as an endogenous protein, is a biocompatible and biodegradable polymer and creates the conditions for the cells to adhere to and allow them to proliferate. These characteristics makes collagen a very promising candidate in the skin, bone, cartilage, and islets regeneration[53,148-150] and in 3D bioprinting applications in general either alone or combined with other biomaterials.[53,151,152]

One disadvantage is that its mechanical strength is low, and as a result, it cannot be used for supporting long-term tissue and organ cultures.[149] It has been mentioned although that collagen cross-linking by altering the temperature, PH, or by adding riboflavin[153-155] makes it more durable in tension and provides it with viscoelastic properties.[156,157] Likewise, the mechanical properties can be improved by adding polymers of different proportions.[157]

Yang and his colleagues used a combination of collagen, sodium alginate, and chondrocytes in order to form 3D cartilage structures.[127] They concluded that the specific combination is able to suppress the dedifferentiation of the chondrocytes, to increase cellular functions, and to ameliorate the structure's mechanical characteristics. All the above, it can converge on the characterization of collagen/alginate as the most preferable biomaterial for cartilage tissue bioprinting applications.

Another group of scientists used an alternative combination in a 3D bioprinting effort, collagen, and gelatin—crosslinked independently—and cultured simultaneously a mix of human endothelial and hMSCs. They mentioned the creation of stable 3D constructs with high biological activity and rheological properties. The incorporation of collagen increased the cell spreading and shear thinning of the bioink.[158]

In another study, scientists used collagen as the core biomaterial and alginate as sheath biomaterial with human stem cells. They observed increased mechanical properties and functional biological status that contributed to the presence of collagen and the expected differentiation of stem cells used in hepatocytes was achieved.[159] One year later, the same team used a bioink consisted of collagen and alginate crosslinked by polyphenol along with human adipose stem cells and mentioned higher viability and proliferative cells in comparison with the control alginate cell-laden structures.[160]

Gelatin bioinks

Gelatin is a water-soluble, nontoxic, immunoneutral, and biodegradable collagen derivative.[161] Despite these properties, gelatin gels are not stable at body temperature. In 3D bioprinting, gelatin cannot be directly used as cell scaffold and should be combined with other biomaterials. However, the gel formation can be achieved by adding methacrylate moieties to the amine side residues of the gelatin, and as a result, it becomes photocrosslinkable. A photoinitiator can meet this requirement.[162-166] The rheological properties of methacrylated gelatin (GelMA) could be modified through chemical treatment.[162,163] There are reports that mention the printing of high cell viability GelMA hydrogels for the development of cartilage and cardiovascular structures.[165,166] Recently, Pimentel and his colleagues reported the fabrication of vascularized constructs using modified gelatin (transglutaminase-crosslinked gelatin) which is promising for the fabrication of complex tumor models.[167]

Hyaluronic-based bioinks

Hualuronic acid or hyaluronan is another important component of the ECM and promotes the cell proliferation and migration.[168] It is a linear glycosaminoglycan with the disaccharides β-1,4-linked D-glucuronic acid (β-1,3) and N-acetyl-D-glucosamine to constitute the building blocks.[168] Being a natural biopolymer, it has excellent properties of biocompatibility and biodegradability,[169] but it is mechanically weak and its gelation properties are low.[170] This can be fixed through combinations with other biomaterials and various modifications.[171]

According to Ouyang and his research team, the use of hualuronic-based dual crosslinked biomaterial and simultaneously cell-adhesive oligopeptides results in the formation of 3D constructs with satisfying mechanical and cell adhesion properties.[172] 3D structures with enhanced mechanical properties and remarkable osteogenic ability were reported in another study where the chemical composition of hyaluronan-based hydrogels was altered by the presence of methacrylate followed by photocross-linking of the hydrogels. However, they mentioned an insignificant reduction in cell viability in a testing process with the use of hMSCs.[173] Stichler and his colleagues used a mix of hyaluronic acid and synthetic bioink materials modified through chemical and photocross-linking mechanisms. They demonstrated 3D constructs with enhanced chondrogenesis and stability.[174]

It is worthy to mention that multiple cell types are bioprinted by using blends of hyaluronic acid and various other polymers.[82] The viability and differentiation of human adipose stem cells were examined by Sakai and his team by using hyaluronan-gelatin based biomaterial with the contribution of visible light cross-linking and ruthenium-based complexes.[175]

Cellulose-based bioinks

Cellulose is a linear polysaccharide consisting of a great number of $\beta(1 \rightarrow 4)$ linked D-glucose units.[176] Its derivative, carboxymethyl cellulose (CMC) or cellulose gum, has been applied in 3D bioprinting. In order to be converted in a suitable hydrogel, some modifications should be applied (e.g., change the concentration, molecular weight, degree of methyl grafting, temperature of gel formation)[177] and appropriate combinations should be done. It has been noticed that the combination of nanocellulose with alginate demonstrated higher cellular function of iPSCs after printing than the nanocellulose-hyaluronic acid combination.[178] Law and his scientific team reported the use of hyaluronic acid/CMC bioink and examined the cell viability as well as the stability of the 3D printed structure under different hydrogel combination.[179] It was used for bone regeneration combined with bioactive glass for the fabrication of mechanically strong scaffolds.[180] Marksdtedt et al.[181] used nanocellulose/alginate-based bioinks for cartilage tissue engineering and Ávila et al.[182] printed human chondrocyte-laden nanocellulose hydrogels for 3D patient-specific auricular cartilage. Both works reported high mechanical abilities and cell viability after the printing process. In the latter work,[182] it is interesting that the redifferentiation of human nasal chondrocytes leads to the formation of neocartilage-specific ECM components.

Fibrin-based bioinks

Fibrin, also called Factor Ia, is a fibrous protein that participates in the clotting of blood. Its hydrogels result from fibrinogen through enzymatic treatment of thrombin, and they are biocompatible and biodegradable but they are mechanically weak.[31] There is a study where scientists used fibrin hydrogels mixed with PCL/

PLCL and formed 3D structures of urethra onto which they seeded multiple types of cells. The whole work was held in vitro and the properties of this hydrogel were investigated.[183] Fibrin/collagen gels have been printed in an effort to enhance vascularization relying on the ability of fibrin to bind to vascular endothelial growth factor (VEGF).[184,185] Furthermore, fibrin hydrogels have been already used for the printing of thick vascular networks and tubular tissue structures.[186,187]

It is very promising a study where the scientists used fibrin/hyaluronic acid hydrogels in order to encapsulate Schwann cells and examined the prospectives of this bioink in nerve regeneration.[188]

Silk-based bioinks

Another protein-based polymer is silk fibroin, and the silk-based scaffolds are usually used in 3D bioprinting applications.[189] It is usually used in combination with other polymers, and there are plenty of studies that examine the effectiveness of such hydrogels. Das and colleagues used mesenchymal progenitor cells and silk-gelatin hydrogels as bioink for the bioprinting of cell-laden structures through sonication and enzymatic cross-linking.[190] Rodriguez and his team supported that the use of silk and gelatin as biomaterials enhances the biocompatibility, the cell permeability, and the tissue integration in soft tissue reconstruction. The cross-linking was achieved physically with glycerol.[97] Another biomaterial with which silk fibroin can be combined is alginate, and their mix was used as bioink in a work based in inkjet printing.[191] Silk-gelatin bioinks have been used in skin regeneration methods where it was mentioned the addition of fibroblast growth factor-2 in the bioink before printing.[192] A combination of silk and the synthetic polymer PEG was also mentioned to exhibit significant printability with high resolution and to contribute to the maintenance of cell viability for a long period.[193] Recently, a new silk-based polymer, the spider silk proteins, gains ground but further investigation is needed.[194]

Extracellular matrix-based bioinks

ECM is a noncellular 3D macromolecular network consisted of collagen, proteoglycans/glycosaminoglycans, elastin, fibronectin, elastin, laminin, and a variety of other glycoproteins. ECM components form a network where cells reside in all tissues and provide the structural and biochemical support of the cells.[195]

In 3D bioprinting applications, decellularized extracellular matrix materials (dECM) have been used as bioinks. These materials are obtained from the desired tissues where the cells are removed through physical or chemical methods or by using biologic agents in a procedure that protects ECMs intactness.[196,197] High cell viability, intact cellular function, and printability of the structures after the printing process were remarkably observed by scientists who used decellularized extracellular matrix bioink for bioprinting of cell-laden constructs.[198] Likewise, viability of the printed cells is also protected when Ahn and colleagues developed a 3D method with heating modules, which totally controlled the stacking of the used cells.[199] Another team mentioned 3D printing of dECM containing dual stem cells for cardiac repair. They reported the ability of the structures to present fast vascularization with longer lasting cell viability.[200]

Although the use of dECM as biomaterial is very challenging as it provides the environment mimicking the native tissues, the isolation and quantification of DNA and ECM components are of high cost. In order to enhance the cytocompatibility, scientists formed a bioink derived from biological samples. For instance, they prepared decelularized liver matrix (dLM)-based bioink, which contains the intrinsic proteins of dLM and they demonstrated that it improves the compatibility of encapsulated cells.[201]

Cell aggregates as bioinks

A very promising option for used as bioink in 3D bioprinting technologies is the spherical cell aggregates (spheroids) consisting of thousands of cells. Spheroids are a type of 3D cell modeling that mimic the live cell's environmental conditions including the cellular function and the interactions between cells as well as the interactions between cells and the ECM.[202] Spheroids are seeded one by one onto biocompatible scaffolds and they are fused through a self-assembly process. Recently, a scientific group presented a novel tissue spheroids bioink for 3D bioprinting structures without the contribution of any scaffolds. These constructs are emerged as promising bioinks for articular cartilage tissue engineering in a process that includes generation of bioprintable tissue strands with rapid cell fusion by a self-assembly mechanism without chemical cross-linking, bioprinting in solid state without any liquid medium, and with the absence of a supportive molding structure during bioprinting for cell aggregation and fusion.[203] Finally, another group used poly(N-isopropyl acrylamide), a thermosensitive polymer gel, as a temporary substrate for the growth of the cell aggregates or cell sheets. The cell sheets were detached carefully from the substrate using mild heat in order to preserve the integrity of cell-matrix network.[204]

Cells in 3D bioprinting: stem cells, expansion, and differentiation process

The major advantage of 3D bioprinting compared with conventional tissue engineering approaches is the incorporation of cells and their directly disposition with biomaterials. One of the major bottlenecks of 3D bioprinting is the maintenance of cell viability and their long-term functionality during expansion and sequential differentiation. Scientists all over the world are trying to find optimum sources of cells and investigate the development of appropriate protocols for the isolation and expansion of these cells. It will be ideal to achieve the establishment of these protocols through rapid and inexpensive methods.

The in vitro expansion of cells is a critical process in 3D bioprinting, once it provides the conditions for obtaining the sufficient number of cells. These conditions should be optimized not only for achieving great rate of cell proliferation but also for providing the appropriate environment so as the cells to recapitulate their native function. The number of cells needed for 3D bioprinting is depended on the type of the 3D printer, and it can range between 1×10^6 and 1×10^8 mL^{-1}.[15,69,80,205] This amount of cells is necessary for the synthesis of the ECM, which is essential for ensuring the functionality of the 3D constructs. It is important that the cell expansion and the subsequent differentiation of cells into a specific cell type need to be performed under totally controlled conditions in order to minimize the potential complications. For example, the prolonged expansion of primary cells has been associated with chromosomal abnormalities, tumor development, and dedifferentiation.[206] Thus, it is essential to evaluate the cellular integrity and functionality of the 3D bioprinted constructs, especially these intended to be implanted in humans, by testing the viability, the genomic and phenotypic stability, and the cellular metabolism as well.[77]

In 3D bioprinting, progenitor cells as well as stem cells can be used. Stem cells are preferable due to their self-renewal and multilineage potency. The types of stem cells that are commonly used in bioprinting are mesenchymal stem cells (MSCs), ESCs and iPSCs.[207,208]

ESCs are pluripotent stem cells that constitute the cells of the inner cells mass of embryos at the blastocyst stage of development,[209] and they can differentiate into somatic cells of all three germ layers.[210] Despite the ability of ESCs to differentiate into any cell type making them the ideal source of stem cells, their application is restricted due to ethical controversy. Another important disadvantage of ESCs is the risk to exhibit immunogenicity because of their inability to readily control the differentiation process.

The iPS cells or iPSCs are pluripotent stem cells derived directly from adult cells through dedifferentiation into progenitor cells. The technology of iPSCs was introduced by Yamanaka and his colleagues in 2006, when he converted adult fibroblasts into iPSCs through the introduction of four transgenes (Oct 3/4, Sox2, Klf4, c-Myc) by retroviral transfection.[210] In 2012, Yamanaka along with Sir John Gurdon was awarded with the Nobel Prize "for the discovery that mature cells can be reprogrammed to become pluripotent."[211] Since then, more complex processes and a variety of factors including proteins, peptides, and chemicals were used in order to achieve efficient control of reprogramming.[208]

However, the high possibility of teratoma development in vivo restricts the clinical application of iPSCs and of ESCs as well.[212] Concerning iPSCs, the development of teratoma has been associated with the presence of undifferentiated cells. It is believed that the removal of these cells before the implantation would help to overcome this drawback.[213,214]

Another disadvantage of iPSCs application is that their use has been also associated with carcinoma formation as a consequence of the retroviral transfection. In order to make their application in regenerative medicine safer, new versions and virus free iPSCs have been developed.[215]

MSCs, also known as mesenchymal stromal cells or multipotent stromal cells, tend to differentiate into other mesenchymal or nonmesenchymal cell types in vitro such as osteoblasts, adipocytes, chondroblasts, myocytes, tendocytes, ligaments cells, smooth muscle cells (SMCs), endothelial cells, cardiomyocytes, hepatocytes, and neural cells.[216-220] MSCs can be sourced originally not only from bone marrow but also from tissues like the liver, lung, teeth, muscle, adipose, and perinatal/extraembryonic-associated tissues (amniotic fluid/Wharton's jelly, umbilical cord, placenta).[216,218-220] Each cell source determines the subsequent "fate" of the cells. For instance, it has been observed that the concentration of MSCs isolated from adipose tissue is significantly greater in comparison with the concentration of cells harvested from other tissues.[221] Furthermore, perinatal stem cells show great capability of expansion with the stem cells obtained from amniotic fluid being able to be cultured for over 300 cell cycles with a doubling time of 36 h.[208,222-224] Regarding the multipotency of perinatal stem cells is wider to that of "adult" stem cells. In addition to that, perinatal stem cells do not exhibit tumorogenic properties in vitro unlike ESCs and iPSCs.[208,222-224] The selection of cell source is very crucial as it has been mentioned that many cells in tissue constructs exhibited increased immune response after the implantation.[225] Regarding "adult" MSCs, there are studies that have shown that they present low immunogenicity and immunomodulatory properties when implanted in animal models.[226-228] For instance, it has been shown that the use of adipose-derived stem cells tends to exhibit immunosuppressive capabilities.[229,230] It is considered, however, that the autologous transplantation may eliminate the need of immunosuppression. It is well established that the state of stem cell's differentiation is related with the potency to become immunogenic. It has been mentioned that the undifferentiated MSCs tend to be more immune-tolerated when compared with differentiated stem cells. This behavior permits the undifferentiated stem cells to be successfully implanted and the possibility of grafts rejection is reduced.[208,231-233]

In previous section, the existing bioprinting modalities were described. Scientists have been made some observations concerning the possible effects of a specific bioprinting method on printed cell stemness. It has been observed that both mechanical and shear stress tend to trigger the stem cell differentiation. Mechanical stress could promote chondrogenic and osteogenic differentiation,[234] whereas shear stress stimulates the differentiation to endothelial cells and osteoblasts.[235] This can lead to the conclusion that possibly laser-assisted and inkjet bioprinting could prevail over extrusion bioprinting because the "gentler" low shear properties involved in the printing process is less likely to stimulate differentiation.[208] Furthermore, it has been demonstrated that laser-assisted bioprinting technique delivers undifferentiated MSCs to an alginate/blood plasma hydrogel and the scientists did not observe any change regarding cell viability, proliferation, apoptosis, and cell phenotype in comparison with unprinted cells.[236] Researcher teams all over the world should optimize the parameters of the bioprinting methods used and their properties in order to secure the viability and the differentiation of the cells.

The carefully selection of the bioink is critical for the successful differentiation of stem cells[72,237] as the cell growth and differentiation require "environmental conditions" that mimic the native ones. There are appropriate physical and chemical molecules that provide the corresponding microenvironment.[238] Specific signaling molecules, including bone morphogenic protein-2 (BMP-2),[239] epidermal growth factor[240] and Wnt proteins,[241,242] have been used to regulate and control the differentiation of stem cells in bioprinting.

In cases where the biomaterials and the bioprinting methods do not affect the cells lineage fate, the bioprinted cells can be differentiated through incubation in culture medium, which contains soluble factors such as growth factors and chemicals.[208] These soluble factors are optimized in order to promote lineage commitment and maturation into the desired types of cells. They can also be used in conjunction with bioprinting. The growth factors include transforming growth factor-β (TGF-β) superfamily, fibroblast growth factor (FGF), bone morphogenic proteins (BMP), Wnt signaling proteins, hedgehog proteins, and notch-1 ligands. It has been observed that TGF-β1 and BMP-6 are crucial for chondrogenic differentiation of MSCs.[243-245] Apart from signaling molecules that regulate stem cell differentiation, there are also growth factors that regulates cell's behavior and migration. In a study, Lee and colleagues bioprinted C17.2 neural stem cells along with collagen and VEGF releasing fibrin hydrogels.[185] They observed that the cells exhibited a tendency to migrate toward fibrin hydrogel containing VEGF and they presented a more differentiated like phenotype when compared with cells in VEGF-free scaffolds. Regarding chemicals as factors for controlling stem cell lineage, a mix of dexamethasone, ascorbic acid, and β-glycerophosphate,[246] a combination of isobutylmethylxanthine, indomethacin, and dexamethasone,[247] another combination of β-glycerophosphate, insulin, and dexamethasone[247] have been reported. Furthermore, the peroxisome proliferator activated receptor γ agonists rosiglitazone directs adipocyte differentiation of MSCs,[248,249] and the DNA demethylating agent 5-azacytidine stimulates adult human bone marrow MSCs to adopt a cardiomyocyte-like phenotype.[250] Bioprinting of iPSCs and ESCs along with RGD-coupled alginate hydrogels has been reported to differentiate into hepatocyte-like cells by incubation in the appropriate culture medium for over 17 days.[48] In this study, the differentiation process was initiated prior to bioprinting and then allowed to continue for 11 days after the printing process. Comparing the bioprinted and the nonprinted cells, both of them exhibited hepatocyte-like phenotype, indicating that the bioprinting did not influence at all the cellular differentiation.

Hydrogels can control the differentiation process by trying to mimic the ECM network where cells are located in contact with signaling molecules, tropic support, and topographical information. However, the fate of stem cells can be affected by the presence of different crosslinkers regarding the same bioink. It is reported that enzymatic cross-linking with tyrosine of bioprinted silk fibroin-gelatin hydrogels oriented the MSCs to differentiate toward chondrocytes, whereas physical cross-linking (e.g., sonication) promoted the differentiation into osteocyte.[190]

An important problem emerged from the prolonged expansion of some types of cells is the dedifferentiation of them. Several studies have proposed the use of polymer microspheres, which are called MCs in order to promote cell expansion. MCs provide a surface for cell growth and adhesion[251-254] and it is able to be modified in order to enhance cell attachment either by coating with molecules of the ECM or by manipulating the surface charge.[77] The addition of positively charged groups on the MCs surface resulted in increased stem cell adherence in comparison with the incorporation of ECM macromolecules.[255] However, when culturing human articular chondrocytes with MCs composed of collagen, the proliferative ability of the cells increased by 20-fold within 2 weeks.[256] When bone and cartilage cells were cultured on MCs in a bioreactor system, it has been observed the synthesis of new matrix, which is the main characteristic of the native tissues.[257,258] Apart from that, the use of MCs can be exploited as a delivery system for slow release of growth factors, which mimics the native cellular environment and as a result preserves the cellular phenotype and inhibits the dedifferentiation.[259] It is reported that these microspheres are able to support the proliferation and adhesion of MSCs without affecting their multipotency.[251] Furthermore, they could be useful for the modulation of stem cell differentiation within a hydrogel.[253] For example, there is the possibility of optimizing the size of MCs so as to regulate the stiffness of the polymer, the way of the cell's organization, and the surface growth area.[251,253] There are commercially available MCs consisted of either synthetic or natural polymers such as plastic, glass, dextran, cellulose, collagen, and gelatin[257,260] and their sizes range between 60 and 400 μm.[251,252,254] Apart from the use of MCs, the required environment for cell expansion could be achieved by the use of bioreactors, which are described in the section of postbioprinting below, or by a combination of them as it was proposed earlier.[257,258]

The maintenance of cell viability and the long-term cell functionality are the major concerns in 3D bioprinting. The processes performed during the stages of 3D bioprinting should be optimized in order to ensure these properties. Researchers have been investigating a variety of combinations of biomaterials and different cell types in order to explore their interactions. However, the results were controversial for different cell types with the parameters need to be adjusted depending on specific type of cells. For example, it was observed that the dispensing pressure applied in extrusion-based bioprinting affected the cell viability,[261] whereas the nozzle insulation enhanced the viability of HEK 293FT cells when they are bioprinted with a gelatin-based bioink.[262] There are plenty of reports that study the relation between different factors including viscoelasticity of the bioink,[263] shear stress,[264] bioink status,[265] photocross-linking mechanism,[266] gelation time and hydrogel viscocity,[267] and the way they affect the viability and integrity of the cells.

The three-dimensional bioprinting process

After the great and evolutionary advances of 3D printing technology, the introduction of 3D bioprinting technique about 15 years ago was considered to be a major breakthrough in order to overcome the bottlenecks of conventional tissue fabrication cell seeding.[268]

3D bioprinting is defined as the layer-by-layer deposition of cells and cell-laden biomaterials simultaneously in a precise position and cell arrangement.[269,270] The main goal is the construction of fully functional living organs and tissues in a totally controlled manner providing a system able to mimic native human tissues in vivo.[33,271] It is a high throughput, scalable, and highly reproducible technique. These characteristics are pivotal for industrialized mass production.[33] It is commonly accepted that the genetic evolution through the years resulted in human beings consisted of organs and tissues with a variety of different cell types defining the perfect function of the corresponding tissues and organs. In this regard, bioprinting could be the par excellence method for the organization of multiple types of cells in predesigned structural architecture resulting in functional tissue constructs.[9] Likewise, it is a promising tool for the creation of complex vascularized structures with heterogeneity in cell placements and ability to recapitulate the functionality of the complex human network. The effectiveness of the bioprinting demands the proper collaboration of a variety of associated sciences such as medicine, molecular and cellular biology, bioinformatics, mechanical/robotic/computing engineering, chemistry, and so on.

The whole 3D bioprinting process includes three interconnected and interdependent stages: the prebioprinting, the bioprinting, and the postbioprinting.[272,273]

The prebioprinting stage

The bioprinting stage is a very important preparation process that determines the properties of the ongoing bioprinted structure and aims to obtain high-resolution imaging models. The right selection of the procedures involved in this stage is critical for the bioprinting of 3D constructs that maximally imitate the native tissues and organs.

First of all, the acquisition of cells with adequate quantity and robustness through minimally invasive biopsy approaches is very important. The researchers are orientated in the development of appropriate protocols for the isolation and culture expansion of cells used in bioprinting. The methods investigated should ensure the cell viability and their long-term functionality during the process of differentiation, and they also should be cost-effective and time-saving.

The next step is the design of the bioprinted model through the generation of CAD. The data for the CAD are provided from high-resolution medical imaging techniques including X-ray, computer tomography, and magnetic resonance imaging.[274,275] These techniques are the most commonly used so far for the design of 3D structures, and they are informative of the tissue/organ anatomical architecture. The appropriateness of each method depends on which tissue is going to be bioprinted. Taking into account that in bioprinting, cells are directly disposed mixed with printable biomaterials, the imaging techniques should be enabled to provide data regarding the geometrical features of vascular network in order to ensure the efficient nutrient transport and by extension the cell viability. It is worthy to mention that the research is focused interestingly on the development of the molecular imaging which could be combined with the existing imaging techniques in order to provide more precise and functional information for the desired tissue.[276] Once the images of the desired structure is acquired, they are subjected to a necessary processing including image segmentation, feature extraction, data mining, and pattern recognition.[277,278] These steps lead to the generation of a CAD model, which later is converted to an STL format or a 3D graphics or a virtual reality modeling language.[279-281] Further analysis with suitable software is needed so as to have the computational blueprint of the bioprinted structure.

In the prebioprinting process, the processing of the model for biomimicry in order to give functional accuracy in the printed tissues and organs should be included. This is very crucial for the optimal fabrication of heterogenous tissues with complex vasculatory, circulatory, and neural networks. In order to meet the main goal of bioprinting, which is the fabrication of fully functional and viable tissues and organs that mimic the human's native structure, there are several parameters to be considered such as cell arrangement, ECM composition and physiology, and nutrient requirements.[270] The biomimicry approach would enable the comprehension of these parameters and those that would be critical for replicating activities such as cell proliferation, differentiation, migration, cell attachment, cell-cell interactions, and cell-ECM interactions. Another dimension of biomimicry would be the use of surface ligands for optimizing the attachment and proliferation abilities of the cells.[282] Likewise, according to the principles of biomimicry, the use of scaffold-free bioink should be investigated thoroughly as it provides an option more close to the native characteristics.[270]

There are variable studies in the worldwide literature describing processing modeling strategies for biomimicry among which fuzzy modeling approach is mentioned to be a very useful mathematic tool for biomimicry.[283]

The bioprinting stage

In this critical stage, the physical bioprinting process occurs and involves the selection of the suitable bioink, the design of the appropriate bioprinting modality, and the use of a bioprinter. The parameters that define the effectiveness of this stage include physicochemical (rheology, gelation), biological (cell integrity and viability, cell density, biocompatibility, and cytocompatibility), and process (duration of bioprinting, cost, use of radiation) factors.[93]

The properties required for the bioink's selection and the bioprinting methods are described in previous sections. In this section, we will describe the interactions between the components and mention some parameters that should be optimized in order to ensure the fidelity of the bioprinting process.

It is very challenging to embed cells in a bioink. First of all, when hydrogel-based bioinks are used, the concentrations of each ingredient should be precisely optimized in order to achieve effective bioprintability.[134] As mentioned above, an ideal bioink should not need any physical, chemical, or photocross-linking treatment to become cell-friendly, it should have the ability to be mixed homogenously with the other components and its formulation should contribute to the minimization of the encapsulation time.[284] A major bottleneck emerged from the use of cell-laden bioink is the fact that the cells should be suspended in an aqueous precursor solution, along with other water-only soluble ingredients.[284] The volume of suspension possibly could affect the stability and the strength of the hydrogel-based bioinks by altering the final concentrations of the cells and the hydrogels,[117] and it can increase the time needed for the cross-linking for the bioink affecting mechanical properties, swelling, and gelation time.[285]

In case of scaffold-free cell bioprinting, scientists have produced bioink solutions using ingredients within the culture media in order to avoid the starvation and hypoxia of cells resulting from the lack of adequate liquid precursor. An alternative method involves the use of microspheres filled with oxygen. These microspheres can be combined with bioink and allow the permeation of oxygen in order to avoid hypoxia and thus ensuring the cell viability during the bioprinting process.[286]

The homogenous mix of cells in the bioink is another challenge in the bioprinting process as the homogenously extrusion of the bioink is desired. It is possible for the bioink solution to have substantial chain entanglements. The presence of these entanglements restricts the uniform mixing of cells within the bioink. It is very difficult to break down such a structure and it is possible that even after the breaking down, cells accumulate in certain regions because of compartmentalization of polymers. To overcome this difficulty, mechanical mixing systems have been developed and are able to suspend the cells in a homogenous manner in fibrous hydrogels (e.g., collagen, methylcellulose, fibrin).[287,288] Undoubtedly, it is very important to be careful during the cell encapsulation in order to avoid any bubble formation within the bioink solution which could harm the bioprintability.

Another critical factor playing important role for the success of 3D bioprinting is the selection of optimum cell density. The cell density is dependent on the type of the bioink used, e.g., scaffold-free or scaffold-based cell bioprinting. It is expected that using scaffold-free cell bioprinting cells can be bioprinted at much higher densities and high cell density leads to faster tissue biofabrication.[207] However, using this approach, it is possible that the mechanical strength of the 3D construct may be at stake.[207] The selection of the appropriate cell density depends also on the tissue selected to be bioprinted and the amount of cells involved. There are several reports in the literature with detailed information about the number of cells in different tissues.[289,290] During the bioprinting process, there are conditions such as shear stress that damage the cellular viability.[291,292] Because of this, it is preferable to select bioinks of low viscocity and with low cell density ($<10^6$ cells/mL).[15,293] In laser-based bioprinting, a suitable bioink disposes a viscosity between 1 and 300 mPa s and medium cell density of $\sim 10^8$ cells/mL.[65,69] In extrusion-based bioprinting, high viscous bioinks ($3\text{-}6 \times 10^7$ mPa s) with high cell density are bioprinted.[294] Inkjet bioprinting is able to print bioinks with lower viscocity (<10 mPa s) and lower cell density ($<16 \times 10^6$ cells/mL) as well.[139] The cell density is also related with the mechanical properties of the hydrogels. In a study performed by Mauck and coworkers, constructs containing chondrocytes with low concentration (10×10^6 cells/mL) present greater stiffness in comparison to that with higher cell density (60×10^6 cells/mL).[295] Increasing the culture time of chondrocytes on agarose hydrogels, the constructs with higher cell density showed similar Young's modulus when compared with constructs with lower cell concentration.[295] Furthermore, the high cell density leads to an increase of bioink's viscocity, and it may affect its printability.[291]

There are also some parameters that should be optimized in order to ensure the bioprinting fidelity. Among them, the deformation because of the gravity, the hydrogel's fusion and the density of the cross-linking factor are involved. It is proposed that high crosslinker concentration increases the bioprintability, in contrast with low crosslinker concentration which results in reduced printability.[296] It is important to mention that the physiochemical properties of a bioink including its rheological behavior, the surface tension, the gelation kinetics, and the swelling ability define not only the effective bioprintability but also the maintenance of the postprinting integrity of the 3D structure.[291] The ability of these characteristics to be tunable plays very important role for the reproducibility of the bioprinting process. The use of physical and/or chemical elements can contribute to increased printability of polymers because of the incorporation of metal ions and glutaraldehyde in extrusion-based bioprinting.[45] Another example is the incorporation of Na^+ ions in gelatin hydrogels instead of Ca^{2+} and Fe^{2+}, resulting in altered profile of molecular interactions and improvement of the cross-linking density and mechanical strength of the gelatin gels.[297]

The cell viability and the long-term functionality of cells must be ensured in this stage as well. Despite the fact that the bioink properties is desired to be tunable so as to increase the bioprintability and achieve high printing resolution, these alterations may induce stress on the cells reducing their viability.[267]

Regarding the available bioprinters, the advance performed through the last decade in their technology is great. Persistent efforts are made in order to obtain bioprinters with the desirable compactness, suitable resolution, high printing speed, completely automated workflow, user friendliness, and undoubtedly to be affordable and versatile. Unfortunately, the interest for commercialization of 3D bioprinters is not kept as similar pace as the interest in exploring 3D bioprinting applications. However, the extrusion-based bioprinters are investigated more intensely in comparison with laser-based and inkjet-based bioprinters.

The postbioprinting stage

After being bioprinted, the 3D constructs need to be submitted through a postbioprinting process in order to obtain mature functional tissues. The conditions prevailing during postbioprinting process should mimic these of native environment. A major bottleneck in 3D bioprinting is the vascularization of the constructs since the presence of the vascular network provides with oxygen, nutrient, and metabolites all the regions of the designed structures. Such problems tend to overcome by performing postbioprinting in systems which control among other parameters the perfusion of the bioprinted constructs by recapitulating the mass transfer occurring in vivo and bioreactors in such system.

A bioreactor is defined to be a vessel where a biochemical process occurs by providing the environment to maintain and monitor vital parameters under precisely controlled conditions and allowing various stimuli to be exerted in order to regulate tissue maturation.[298]

A wide variety of different types of bioreactors as well as combinations of them have been used for the bone, skin, cardiovascular, and cartilage engineering applications including rotating wall, flow perfusion, spinner flask, compression, strain, and hydrostatic pressure.[299] The flow perfusion bioreactor seems to be an ideal system that allows the media to flow through the ECM of tissue constructs in order to enhance the fluid transport. Even though it is difficult to ensure the homogenous perfusion of media supply through a tissue construct, rotating wall and spinner flask bioreactors are demonstrated to ensure the media homogeneity.

The bioreactors used so far are designed to provide real-time monitoring and feedback control of conditions like temperature, PH, oxygen level, oxygen partial pressure (pO_2), levels of CO_2, concentrations of nutrients, and growth factors. These conditions should be maintained in bioreactors in order to optimize the cell growth. Furthermore, mechanical and biochemical regulatory signals should be exerted on tissue constructs in bioreactors for cells to encourage them to undergo differentiation and subsequently to mature into relevant tissues.[299,300] There are several bioreactors designed to exert mechanical stimuli such as compression, shear, and tension.[299]

There are several methods developed to exert mechanical, biochemical, or even electrical signals in order to accelerate the tissue maturation. In cartilage tissue engineering, enhanced mechanical strength is achieved when mechanical stimuli is applied to force the cartilage to produce a greater amount of ECM. In addition, mechanical stimulations promote the proper integration of cartilage constructs with host tissue. According to Correia and his colleagues, stimulation with 0.4 MPa pulsatile hydrostatic pressure or 1 Hz compression results in enhanced chondrocytes differentiation, glycosaminoglycans production, and ECM synthesis.[301] Wernike and his scientific team demonstrated that dynamic compression and low oxygen tension effect on a greater stability of chondrocytes phenotype.[302] Likewise, regarding cardiac engineering, the appliance of electrical or mechanical stimulation leads to improved tissue formation.[303]

It is worthy to mention that the conditions that dominate in bioreactors, the parameters should be modulated, and the exertion of stimuli depended on the properties of the desired tissue. Relevant with the recent advances in 3D bioprinting, many microfluidic perfusion bioreactors have been developed and promote the accelerated differentiation of bioprinted constructs into the desired tissues including heart[304,305] and bone[306] and the use of bioreactors for applications in clinical heart valve tissue engineering[307] has been reported.

However, despite these great advances, the majority of bioreactors have low volume output, and they are time-consuming and add significant cost regarding the filters used and the sensors integrated.[308] The development of bioreactors which will allow the creation of human-scale tissues and be capable for organ maturation would be challenging.

3D bioprinting applications

The major breakthrough of 3D bioprinting allows the placement of multiple types of high-density cells in predesigned precise locations in a manner that mimic the heterogeneous microarchitecture of the native tissues. Thus, it is a very promising tool for tissue and organ biofabrication. So far, numerous organs and tissues including the skin, cartilage, bone, cardiac tissue, liver, and vascular tissues have drew the attention, but the applications concern mainly drug screening and drug sensitivity testing.[68,309,310] The bottleneck of bioprinting is the efficient vascularization of the bioprinted constructs that restrict their clinical application. It is widely speculates that in the near future, bioprinting will result in clinically relevant volume of tissues with efficient vascularization ready for transplantation.

Even though bioprinting was initially applied for construction of tissue scaffolds, mainly bone scaffolds, in the sections below we will focus on bioprinted tissues and organs.

Tissue and organ bioprinting

Examples of bioprinting of hydrogels with one or multiple different types of cells were already mentioned. Successfully bioprinted alginate-hyaluronan hydrogels containing Schwann cells for peripheral nerve regeneration with enhanced structural integrity and satisfactory cell viability have been mentioned.[311] Complex heterogeneous tissue constructs containing three different types of cells has already bioprinted, and it was demonstrated that the cellular functions including cell survival, migration, and proliferation are preserved. Subsequently, the bioprinted mimics produced a vascularized bone tissue in vivo.[312] These examples and even more that are described in the section of bioinks used and their properties demonstrate that 3D bioprinting technology enables the fabrication of heterogeneous and complex tissue structures that resembles the native tissue architecture.

Cartilage: The technology of 3D bioprinting has been mostly applied to cartilage engineering since it is a tissue without apparent need for the presence of vessels. The currently used cartilage tissue engineering approaches do not succeed to perform tissue constructs that are identical to the original ones.[313] However, bioprinting is a very promising tool for the cartilage regeneration based on the major advantage of this technology, which is the accurate deposition of cells, biomaterials, and growth factors to the desired predesigned position. The maintenance of mechanical stability and integrity and the preservation of a long-term stability and integrity as well are crucial considerations for achieving cartilage engineering and regeneration through 3D bioprinting approach. Plenty of studies performed and include the printing of chondrocytes into hydrogel scaffolds. The resulted bioprinted constructs tested for cell viability with encouraging results.

Cartilage tissues have been biofabricated by bioprinting human articular chondrocytes with poly(ethylene glycol)dimethacrylate hydrogel.[107] The bioprinted constructs exhibited high mechanical stability, close to that of the native tissue, and excellent integration with the host tissue. Furthermore, after treating the constructs with growth and chondrogenic factors, satisfying cartilage formation was observed and the production of proteoglycan and glycosaminoglycan suggests a successive step toward cartilage regeneration. The formation of cartilage tissue was also accomplished by bioprinting chondrocytes encapsulated in alginate hydrogel and PCL and TGF-β was used as well.[314] The use of PCL contributed to greater mechanical strength, whereas the addition of TGF-β resulted in enhanced ECM deposition. In another study, the printed cartilage constructs consist of chondrocytes encapsulated in semiinterpenetrating hyaluronan and hydroxyethyl-methacrylate-derivatized dextran (dex-HEMA) hydrogel and presented mechanical stability and high cell viability.[169] Recently, an evolutionary approach that involves the use of MCs and the formation of MC-cell complexes resulted in increased mechanical strength of the printed hydrogels and higher cell viability within the hydrogels. Indeed, in 2014, Levato and his colleagues managed to print bilayered osteochondral models with the use of hydrogels incorporated with cell-laden MCs.[251]

Skin: The human skin disposes a multilayered architecture where keratinocytes and fibroblasts are the predominant cell types. There are several situations including burns or a variety of injuries that harm the skin, and the treatment approaches involve the transplantation of a donor's or animal skin. In order to overcome the limitations of the transplantation process such as immune rejection, the studies in the last years are focused either on the fabrication of artificial skin or on the skin regeneration via 3D bioprinting methods.[315-317] In the context of skin engineering, Lee and his scientific team printed a multilayered structure with high cell viability. The printed keratinocytes formed the epidermis, whereas the printed fibroblasts constitute the dermis resulting in a tissue construct with high similarity to the human skin tissue regarding the morphology and the biological activity. The 3D bioprinting technology applied in skin engineering and regeneration enhances the ability to control the geometry and architecture of the stratified human skin and have bioprinted skin with the human skin characteristics.[318] The printed skin was observed to retain its structural network shape during in vitro cultures.[148,319]

Cardiac tissue: Cardiovascular diseases are the leading cause of death worldwide, resulting in 19.9 million deaths (32.1%) in 2015.[320,321] Once the myocytes have been differentiated and mature, they stop to proliferate, which limits the ability of the myocardium to be regenerated.[322] Even though, tissue engineering approaches have aimed to fabricate this complex tissue structure exhibiting similar functionality when compared with the native cardiac tissue. Heart valves have been already bioprinted[323] and human vascular endothelial cells (HUVECs) along with cardiac cells have been bioprinted in order to form tissue spheroids.[324] It is very interesting and promising at the same time that these tissue spheroids exhibit the ability to be fused after about 70 h to form a cardiac patch able to beat synchronously. Furthermore, a scientific team achieved to bioprint an aortic valve with the appropriate mechanical heterogeneity and high cell viability for up to 21 days.[111] Likewise, Duan and his colleagues printed heterogenous aortic valve conduits with the use of hydrogels consisted of alginate and gelatin where they encapsulated SMCs in the valve root and aortic valve (leaflet) interstitial cells in the leaflet.[325] Both type of cells showed high cell viability, satisfactory spreading, and good phenotype retention in vitro. In addition, scientists managed to print a trileaflet aortic valve using methacrylated hyaluronan and GelMA hydrogels and human aortic valve interstitial cells with high cell viability and remodeling ability.[266] However, it is still triggering the biofabrication of cardiac tissues with the similar geometry, mechanical, and spatial heterogeneity of the native tissue. 3D bioprinting technology should contribute to this direction and plenty of studies have been conducted. However, the currently bioprinted tissues are still far from implantation.[325] It is very interesting to mention that for the first time, Israeli scientists using the 3D bioprinting technology created functional vascularized cardiac patches for small-scale human hearts.[326] In a recent study, scientists achieved to bioprint full-scale human heart components such as cardiomyocytes, heart valves, and ventricles making significant progress toward the engineering of functional tissues and organs.[327]

Bionic ear: The idea of 3D printing of living cells along with electronic components and growing them into functional organs inspired Manoor and his colleagues to form bionic ears.[328] Hydrogels containing alginate seeding with chondrocytes were printed in an architecture and geometry of the human ear. After the printing process, a coil antenna was embedded in order to detect wireless signals by using silver nanoparticles. Around the coil antenna, cartilage formation was observed with excellent the morphology and high tissue-level viability. The printed ear was able to maintain its shape during the in vitro culture and to receive electromagnetic signals and listen to stereo audio music.

Liver, kidney, and bladder: The Organovo company, a San Diego-based biotech company, has developed 3D printed human liver tissues that exhibit ful functionality and stability for up to 28 days applied for drug testing.[329,330] However, most of the liver tissues bioprinted so far fail to mimic the physiologic microstructure of the native liver tissue and lack vascularization, and 3D bioprinting tools might overcome the barriers and lead to the development of functional liver. Recently, another scientific team demonstrated that 3D bioprinting of liver spheroids derived from human iPSCs contributes significantly in enhanced liver function and prolonged tissue survival over a long period of time in vitro.[331] Scientists have also printed kidney tissue constructs with high similarity with natives. These bioprinted kidney constructs dispose an apical layer of polarized primary renal proximal tubule epithelial cells in a configuration supported by a collagen IV-rich tubulointerstitial interface of primary renal fibroblasts and endothelial cells.[332] Atala and his team, representing the Wake Forest Institute for Regenerative Medicine, bioprinted a bladder-shaped scaffold with human cells and collagen as bioink, in the contex of autologous bladder regeneration.[333,334] After the maturation of the structure into a bioreactor for about 7 weeks, it was sutured in the patient in order to restore some of the normal function.

3D microchannels: A major limitation of 3D bioprinting methodology is the vascularization of thick tissues.[335] Despite the great advances in engineering 3D structures with adequate cell density and specific design, similar to the properties of the native tissues, the difficulty of vascularization needs to be overcome in order to ensure the cell viability. It is expected that the tissues requiring minimal or no vascularization (such as skin and cartilage) would be the first tissues to be transplanted compared with those (such as the liver, pancreas, heart), which have more complex architecture. Although the development of a vascular network can be achieved by treatment with biochemical factors, the angiogenesis it is a time-consuming process of 1−2 weeks. The vascular network must be incorporated as soon as possible so as to ensure the necessary transport of nutrients, oxygen, and growth factors, and waste removal, which is critical for preventing cell death.[335-337] Bioprinting microchannels is a promising technique to achieve the appropriate vascular perfusion.

In several studies, scientists developed parallel channels in tissue constructs through printing a tubular structure within the hydrogels. According to Huang and his colleagues, a template-free method was developed and printed gelatin-alginate-fibrinogen hydrogels along with adipose-derived stem cells with internal microchannels of ~3 mm diameter.[338] However, the channel's size is bigger than the native vascular tissues, and they failed to replicate the complex hierarchical structure of native vascular network.

Multicellular tissue spheroids or cylinders were used as well for printing vascular tissue constructs. In a study performed, the scientists printed vascular tissue construct by dispensing of multicellular spheroids or cylinders around sacrificial templates in order to form tubular structures.[21] They introduced the use of scaffold-free vascular tissue spheroids as a method for assembling vascular tubes since it is possible to avoid the undesirable rejection or inflammation of biomaterials.[22,324] Inspired by this work, another scientific team formed vessel-like constructs hyaluronan hydrogels with encapsulated cells around sacrificial agarose templates.[339] As it was mentioned earlier, the rheological properties and mechanical strength of hyaluronan hydrogel was enhanced by cross-linking them with PEG derivatives. Recently, microvascular aortic tissues were developed with the use of hydrogels and embryonic fibroblast cell aggregates that were printed having a tubular structure. High cell viability and robust tissue conformation were observed.[340]

Sacrificial materials have contributed to the formation of microchannels. Dextran, sucrose, and glucose have been printed into interconnected microchannels.[341] In cell culture media, these interconnected microchannels could be dissolved resulting in the fabrication of vascular channels, which could be perfused by exerting high-pressure pulsatile flow. The channels were then lined with endothelial cells in order to create an endothelium. Likewise, agarose have been used for printing microchannel networks[342] and gelatin mixed with endothelial cells[343] has been used for the development of perfused vascular channels. Furthermore, a gel of fibrin consisted of endothelial cells and fibroblasts was printed in the space between vascular channels aiming to promote angiogenesis.[184]

Despite the great advances in the creation of microvascular network, the current approaches result in perfusable channels, which do not dispose the anatomy of human vessels.[273] In addition to that, the resolution of the printed microchannels range between a few hundred micrometers. Recently, a novel method has been developed and comprises the use of fugitive ink in order to achieve omnidirectional printing of biomimetic microvascular structures.[104] Regarding the regeneration of thick tissues, cell-laden perfusable vascular conduits have been printed.[344]

The angiogenesis is a process that requires a variety of different types of cells and chemical stimulation as well, and there is a wide range of factors that promote the angiogenesis including VEGF, FGF, platelet-derived growth factor, and transforming growth factor. It is assumed that the incorporation of these factors could promote new vascular development.[345]

According to a study, VEGF can be incorporated during printing by mixing gelatin microparticles (GMPs) with bioinks. The prolonged release of VEGF from GMPs resulted in enhanced vascularization of the scaffold.[346] A wide variety of cell can be used for vascularization including human umbilical vein endothelial cells (HUVECs), while recently vascular progenitor cells have been used to promote angiogenesis.[347]

Clinical applications of bioprinted tissues and organs

Despite of the advances described above, the bioprinting of fully functional organs still remains a challenge. The applications and potentials of bioprinted tissues and/or organs could be realized only after successful clinical trials. Until today, the clinical applications of 3D bioprinted tissue constructs are in their infacy and a variety of scientists aim to bioprint volumetric composite tissues.

The bioprinted tissues and/or organs could serve as models for testing drugs, examining drug toxicity, validation studies, or investigating the pathophysiology of a disease, instead of using animal models. The perspective of using bioprinted organoids in order to examine the pathophysiology of a disease or for drug testing instead of animal models results not only in reducing the need for animal testing but also could be proved more reliable and effective. The bioprinted models could put the bases for the establishment of personalized medicine by biofabricating tissue or organs on demand. For instance, the human liver tissues printed by Organovo could possibly be implanted into patients with liver damage. Alternatively, bioprinted constructs could be very useful as training tools not only to improve the education of the residents and of the new surgeons but also to plan a surgery by determining the specific features of each patient's anatomy. Finally, it will be very useful for the patient to understand the planned intervention through his own bioprinted construct and to become aware of the expected outcome and possible associated complications.

Conclusion and future perspectives

In the United States, approximately 20 people die daily while waiting for an organ transplant and more than 113,000 people, including men, women, and children, are reported in the national waiting list requiring transplantation until July 2019.[348] However, only 36,528 transplant operations were performed in 2018.[348] Thus, the fabrication of 3D bioprinted organs seems to offer the expectations in order to eliminate this ever-increasing organ shortage crisis. This potential requires the optimal understanding of the anatomy, the cellular functionality, and the molecular pathways of the organs that are going to be replaced and the ability to translate this knowledge to the bioprinting methodologies.

Bioprinting will enable the creation of customized tissues/tissue components/organs from the patient's own cells (that reduces the risk of rejection) and with geometry (size and shape) that matches perfectly to the patient's requirements and thus poses the principals of personalized medicine. Even though the technology of 3D bioprinting is not yet "ready" to bioprint an entire functional and transplantable organ, it is possible that in the future, designed biological structures will become as available as the text in modern literate societies.[349]

Even though bioprinting can avoid the ethical dilemmas associated with xeno-transplantation and/or clinical organ transplantation, it has its own challenges which are needed to be addressed. It is extremely important to define the role of bioprinting human organs in medicine, the parameters of its function, its limitations, and the ethical perspectives. Furthermore, it is a new method applied in the field of medicine, which means that ethical oversight, regulation, and further consideration are mandatory. A very interesting paper entitled "3D bioprint me: a socioethical view of bioprinting human organs and tissues" sets the bases for the beginning of a constructive debate.[349]

Further optimization of the components is crucial so as to develop more complex and personalized 3D structures. The formation of the ideal bioink is still under development, and there is the need for researching bioprintable, biocompatible, and affordable biomaterials that can direct the cells to a specific lineage, support cell adhesion, ensure the cellular proliferation, and regulate the differentiation. In addition to that, the operation parameters of the bioprinting modalities and the development of advanced bioprinters should be enhanced in order to facilitate the in vitro biofabrication of constructs containing cells by mimicking as much as possible the native tissue microenvironment. This means that the conditions should optimized for reducing the cell damage and/or the research should be directed in exploring the possible mechanisms that endanger the cell viability and integrity. It is crucial for all components of the bioprinting process to be "cell-friendly" in order to secure and protect the complex cellular functions, and it is pivotal to overcome the limitation of generating functional vascular network in the bioprinted structures so as to obtain bioprinted tissues and/or organs ready for transplantation.

Although bioprinting technology is far from entering the clinical practice, the great advances performed in the last decade fill the scientific community with great expectations that in the future this technology will provide structures with enhanced functional quality, high resolution, and advanced 3D design.

Co-financed by the European Union and Greek national funds through the Operational Program Competitiveness, Entrepreneurship and Innovation, under the call RESEARCH? CREATE - INNOVATE (project code:T1EDK-03599).

References

1. Langer R, Vacanti JP. Tissue engineering. *Science*. 1993;260(5110):920−926.
2. Ozbolat IT, Yu Y. Bioprinting toward organ fabrication: challenges and future trends. *IEEE Trans Biomed Eng*. 2013;60(3):691−699.
3. Tarik Arafat M, Gibson I, Li X. State of the art and future direction of additive manufactured scaffolds-based bone tissue engineering. *Rapid Prototyp J*. 2014;20(1):13−26.
4. Bose S, Vahabzadeh S, Bandyopadhyay A. Bone tissue engineering usind 3D printing. *Matter Today*. 2013;16(12):496−504.
5. Singh D, Thomas D. Advances in medical polymer technology towards the panacea of complex 3D tissue and organ manufacture. *Am J Surg*. 2019;217(4):807−808.
6. Sum M, Liu A, Shao H, Yang X, Ma C, Yan S, Liu Y, He Y, Gou Z. Systematical evaluation of mechanically strong 3D printed diluted magnesium dopping wollastonite scaffolds on osteogenic capacity in rabbit calvarial defects. *Sci Rep*. 2016;6:34029.
7. Liu A, Sun M, Shao H, Yang X, Ma C, He D, et al. The outstanding mechanical response and bone regeneration capacity of robocast dilute magnesium-doped wollastonite scaffolds in critical size bone defects. *J Mater Chem B*. 2016;4(22):3945−3958.
8. Liu A, Xue G, Sun M, Shao H, Ma C, Gao Q, et al. 3D printing surgical implants at the clinic: an experimental study on anterior cruciate ligament reconstruction. *Sci Rep*. 2016;6:21704.
9. Yan Y, Wang X, Pan Y, Liu H, Cheng J, Xiong Z, et al. Fabrication of viable tissue-engineered constructs with 3D cell-assembly technique. *Biomaterials*. 2005;26(29): 5864−5871.
10. Hull CW. *Apparatus for Production of Three-Dimensional Objects by Stereolithography*. United States Patent US 4,575,330. 1986:1−16.
11. Ozbolat IT, Peng W, Ozbolat V. Appliccation areas of 3D bioprinting. *Drug Discov Today*. 2016;21(8):1257−1271.
12. Lee H, Cho DW. One step fabrication of an organ-on-a-chip with spatial heterogeneity using a 3D bioprinting technology. *Lab Chip*. 2016;16(14):2618−2625.
13. Klebe RJ. Cytoscribing: a method for micropositioning cells and the construction of two- and three- dimensional synthetic tissues. *Exp Cell Res*. 1988;179(2):362−373.
14. Roth EA, Xu T, Das M, Gregory C, Hickman JJ, Boland T. Inkjet printing for high-throughput cell patterning. *Biomaterials*. 2004;25(17):3707−3715.
15. Xu T, Jin J, Gregory C, Hickman JJ, Boland T. Inkjet printing of viable mammalian cells. *Biomaterials*. 2005;26(1):93−99.
16. Boland T, Wilson Jr WC, Xu T. *Ink-Jet Printing of Viable Cells*. United States Patent US 20067051654. 2006.
17. Mironov V, Boland T, Trusk T, Forgacs G, Markwald RR. Organ printing: computer-aided jet-based 3D tissue engineering. *Trends Biotechnol*. 2003;21(4):157−161.
18. Forgacs G, Jakab K, Neagu A, Mironov V. *Self-Assembling Cell Aggregates and Methods of Making Engineered Tissue Using the Same*. United States Patent US 20128241905. 2012.
19. Robbins JB, Gorgen V, Min P, Shepherd BR, Presnell SC. A novel in vitro three-dimensional bioprinted liver tissue system for drug development. *FASEB J*. 2013; 27(872):812.

20. Olsen TR, Alexis F. Bioprocessing of tissues using cellular spheroids. *J Bioprocess Biotech.* 2014;4:1−4.
21. Norotte C, Marga FS, Niklason LE, Forgacs G. Scaffold-free vascular tissue engineering using bioprinting. *Biomaterials.* 2009;30(30):5910−5917.
22. Mironov V, Visconti RP, Kasyanov V, Forgacs G, Drake CJ, Markwald RR. Organ printing: tissue spheroids as building blocks. *Biomaterials.* 2009;30(12):2164−2174.
23. Dababneh AB, Ozbolat IT. Bioprinting technology: A current state-of-the-art review. *J Manuf Sci Eng.* 2014;136(6):061016.
24. Gudapati H, Dey M, Ozbolat I. A comprehensive review on droplet-based bioprinting: Past, present and future. *Biomaterials.* 2016;102:20−42.
25. Derby B. Bioprinting: Inkjet printing proteins and hybrid cell-containing materials and structures. *J Mater Chem.* 2008;18(47):5717−5721.
26. Nishiyama Y, Nakamura M, Henmi C, Yamaguchi K, Mochizuki S, Nakagawa H, et al. Fabrication of 3D cell supporting structures with multi materials using the bio-printer. In: *ASME 2007 International Manufacturing Science and Engineering Conference. Proceeding of American Society of Mechanical Engineers. 2007 Oct 15−18; Atlanda, GA: Solid Freeform Fabr Biomed Tissue Eng.* 2008:97−102.
27. Saunders RE, Gough JE, Derby B. Delivery of human fibroblast cells by piezoelectric drop-on-demand inkjet printing. *Biomaterials.* 2008;29(2):193−203.
28. Khalil S, Sun W. Bioprinting endothelial cells with alginate for 3D tissue constructs. *J Biomech Eng.* 2009;131(11):111002.
29. Tuan RS, Boland G, Tuli R. Adult mesenchymal stem cells and cell-based tissue engineering. *Arthritis Res Ther.* 2003;5(1):32−45.
30. Cui X, Dean D, Ruggeri ZM, Boland T. Cell damage evaluation of thermal inkjet printed Chinese hamster ovary cells. *Biotechnol Bioeng.* 2010;106(6):963−969.
31. Cui X, Boland T. Human microvasculator fabrication using thermal inkjet printing technology. *Biomaterials.* 2009;30(31):6221−6227.
32. Norman J, Madurawe RD, Moore CMV, Khan MA, Khairuzzaman A. A new chapter in pharmaceutical manufacturing: 3D printed drug products. *Adv Drug Deliv Rev.* 2017; 108:39−50.
33. Zhang X, Zhang Y. Tissue engineering applications of three-dimensional bioprinting. *Cell Biochem Biophys.* 2015;72(3):777−782.
34. Cui X, Boland T, D'Lima DD, Lotz MK. Thermal inkjet printing in tissue engineering and regenerative medicine. *Recent Pat Drug Deliv Formulation.* 2012;6(2):149−155.
35. Xu C, Christensen K, Zhang Z, Huang Y, Fu J, Markwald RR. Predictive compensation-enabled horizontal inkjet printing of alginate tubular constructs. *Manuf Lett.* 2013;1(1): 28−32.
36. Xu C, Chai W, Huang Y, Markwald RR. Scaffold-free inkjet printing of three-dimensional zigzag cellular tubes. *Biotechnol Bioeng.* 2012;109(12):3152−3160.
37. Ferris CJ, Gilmore KJ, Beirne S, McCallum D, Wallace GG, in het Panhuis M. Bio-ink for on demand printing of living cells. *Biomater Sci.* 2013;1(2):224−230.
38. Demirci U, Montesano G. Cell encapsulating droplet vitrification. *Lab Chip.* 2007; 7(11):1428−1433.
39. Shim JH, Lee JS, Kim JY, Cho DW. Bioprinting of a mechanically enhanced three-dimensional dual cell-laden construct for osteochondral tissue engineering using a multi-head tissue/organ building system. *J Micromech Microeng.* 2012;22:085014.
40. Khalil S, Nam J, Sun W. Multi-nozzle deposition for construction of 3D biopolymer tissue scaffolds. *Rapid Prototyp J.* 2005;11(1):9−17.

41. Smith CM, Stone AL, Parkhill RL, Stewart RL, Simpikins MW, Kachurin AM, et al. Three-dimensional bioassembly tool for generating viable tissue-engineered constructs. *Tissue Eng.* 2004;10:1566−1576.

42. Cohen DL, Malone E, Lipson H, Bonassar LJ. Direct freeform fabrication of seeded hydrogels in arbitrary geometries. *Tissue Eng.* 2006;12(5):1325−1335.

43. Tabriz AG, Hermida MA, Leslie NR, Shu W. Three-dimensional bioprinting of complex cell laden alginate hydrogel structures. *Biofabrication.* 2015;7(4):045012.

44. El-Ayoubi R, DeGrandpré C, DiRaddo R, Yousefi AM, Lavigne P. Design and dynamic culture of 3D-scaffolds for cartilage tissue engineering. *J Biomater Appl.* 2011;25(5):429−444.

45. Ozbolat IT, Hospodiuk M. Gurrent advances and future perspectives in extrusion-based bioprinting. *Biomaterials.* 2016;76:321−343.

46. Colosi C, Shin SR, Manoharan V, Massa S, Constantini M, Barbetta A, et al. Microfluidic bioprinting of heterogeneous 3D tissue constructs using low-viscocity bioink. *Adv Mater.* 2016;28(4):677−684.

47. Trachtenberg JE, Placone JK, Smith BT, Piard CM, Santoro M, Scott DW, et al. Extrusion-based 3D printing of poly (propylene fumarate) in a full-factional design. *ACS Biomater Sci Eng.* 2016;2(10):1771−1780.

48. Faulkner Jones A, Fyfe C, Cornelissen DJ, Gardner J, King J, Courtney A, Shu W. Bioprinting of human pluripotent stem cells and their directed differentiation into hepatocyte-like cells for the generation of mini-livers in 3D. *Biofabrication.* 2015;7(4):044102.

49. Zhao Y, Yao R, Ouyang L, Ding H, Zhang T, Zhang K, et al. Three-dimensional printing of Hela cells for cervical tumor model in vitro. *Biofabrication.* 2014;6(3):035001.

50. Khaled SA, Burley JC, Alexander MR, Jing Y, Roberts CJ. 3D printing of tablets containing multiple drugs with defined release profiles. *Int J Pharm.* 2015;494(2):643−650.

51. Genina N, Holländer J, Jukarainen H, Mälikä E, Salonen J, Sandler N. Ethylene vinyl acetate (EVA) as a new drug carrier for 3D printed medical drug delivery devices. *Eur J Pharmaceut Sci.* 2016;90:53−63.

52. Melchels FPW, Domingos MAN, Klein TJ, Malda J, Bartolo PJ, Hutmacher DW. Additive manufacturing of tissues and organs. *Prog Polym Sci.* 2012;37(8):1079−1104.

53. Malda J, Visser J, Melchels FP, Jüngst T, Hennink WE, Dhert WJ, et al. 25th Anniversary article: Engineering hydrogels for biofabrication. *Adv Mater.* 2013;25(36):5011−5028.

54. Tirella A, Ahluwalia A. The impact of fabrication parameters and substrate stiffness in direct writing of living constructs. *Biotechnol Prog.* 2012;28(5):1315−1320.

55. Jose RR, Rodriguez MJ, Dixon TA, Omenetto F, Kaplan DL. Evolution of bioinks and additive manufacturing technologies for 3D bioprinting. *ACS Biomater Sci Eng.* 2016;2(10):1662−1678.

56. Jose RR, Raja WK, Ibrahim AM, Koolen PG, Kim K, Abdurrob A, Kluge JA, Lin SJ, Beamer G, Kaplan DL. Rapid prototyped sutureless anastomosis device from self-curing silk-bioink. *J Biomed Mater Res B.* 2015;103(7):1333−1343.

57. He Y, Hue GH, Fu JZ. Fabrication of low cost soft tissue prostheses with the desktop 3D printer. *Sci Rep.* 2014;4:6973.

58. Odde DJ, Renn MJ. Laser-guided direct writing for applications in biotechnology. *Trends Biotechnol.* 1999;17(10):385−389.

59. Odde DJ, Renn MJ. Laser-guided direct writing of living cells. *Biotechnol Bioeng.* 2000;67(3):312−318.

60. Koch L, Deiwick A, Schlie S, Michael S, Gruene M, Coger V, et al. Skin tissue generation by laser cell printing. *Biotechnol Bioeng*. 2012;109(7):1855−1863.

61. Ringeisen BR, Kim H, Barron JA, Krizman DB, Chrisey DB, Jackman S, et al. Laser printing of pluripotent embryonal carcinoma cells. *Tissue Eng*. 2004;10(3-4):483−491.

62. Schiel NR, Corr DT, Huang Y, Raof NA, Xie Y, Chrisey DB. Laser-based direct-write techniques for cell printing. *Biofabrication*. 2010;2(3):032001.

63. Barron JA, Wu P, Ladouceur HD, Ringeisen BR. Biological laser printing: a novel technique for creating heterogeneous 3-dimensional cell-patterns. *Biomed Microdevices*. 2004;6(2):139−147.

64. Barron JA, Krizman DB, Ringeisen BR. Laser printing of single cells: statistical analysis, cell viability, and stress. *Ann Biomed Eng*. 2005;33(2):121−130.

65. Guillemot F, Souquet A, Catros S, Guillotin B, Lopez J, Faucon M, et al. High-throughput laser printing of cells and biomaterials for tissue engineering. *Acta Biomater*. 2010;6(7):2494−2500.

66. Gruene M, Pflaum M, Hess C, Diamantouros S, Schlie S, Deiwick A, et al. Laser printing of three-dimensional multicellular arrays for studies of cell-cell and cell-environment interactions. *Tissue Eng C Methods*. 2011;17(10):973−982.

67. Skardal A, Atala A. Biomaterials for integration with 3-D bioprinting. *Ann Biomed Eng*. 2015;43(3):730−746.

68. Peng W, Datta P, Ayan B, Ozbolat V, Sosnoski D, Ozbolat IT. 3D bioprinting for drug discovery and development in pharmaceutics. *Acta Biomater*. 2017;57:26−46.

69. Guillotin A, Souquet AS, Duocastella M, Pippenger B, Bellance S, Bareille R, et al. Laser assisted bioprinting of engineered tissue with high cell density and microscale organization. *Biomaterials*. 2010;31(28):7250−7256.

70. Dinka V, Kasotakis E, Cathrerine J, Mourka A, Ranella A, Ovsianikov A, et al. Directed three-dimensional patterning of self-assembled peptide fibrils. *Nano Lett*. 2008;8(2):538−543.

71. Guillotin B, Catros S, Keriquel V, Souquet A, Fontaine A, Remy M. Rapid prototyping complex tissues laser assisted bioprint (LAB). *Woodhead Publ Ser Biomater*. 2014;70:156−175.

72. Raof NA, Schiele NR, Xie Y, Chrisey DB, Corr DT. The maintenance of pluripotency following laser direct-write of mouse embryonic stem cells. *Biomaterials*. 2011;32(7):1802−1808.

73. Kawecki F, Clafshenkel WP, Auger FA, Bourhet JM, Fradette J, Devillard R. Self-assembled human osseous cell sheet as living biopapers for the laser-assisted bioprinting of human endothelial cells. *Biofabrication*. 2018;10(3):035006.

74. Catros S, Guillemot F, Nandakumar A, Ziane S, Moroni L, Habibovic P, et al. Layer-by-layer tissue microfabrication supports cell proliferation in vitro and in vivo. *Tissue Eng C Methods*. 2012;18(1):62−70.

75. Wang Z, Abdulla R, Parker B, Samanipour R, Ghosh S, Kim K. A simple and high-resolution stereolithography-based 3D bioprinting system using visible light crosslinkable bioinks. *Biofabrication*. 2015;7(4):045009.

76. Lin H, Zhang D, Alexander PG, Yang G, Tan J, Cheng AW, Tuan RS. Application of visible light-based projection stereolithography for live cell-scaffold fabrication with designed architecture. *Biomaterials*. 2013;34(2):331−339.

77. Thomas D, Jessop Z, Whitaker I. *3D bioprinting for reconstructive surgery*. Duxford: Woodhead Publishing, an imprint of Elsevier; 2018.

78. Nikol J, Khademhosseini A. Modular tissue engineering: Engineering biological tissues from the bottom-up. *Soft Mater.* 2009;5(7):1312−1319.

79. Jakab K, Norotte C, Marga F, Murphy K, Vunjak-Novakovic G, Forgacs G. Tissue engineering by self-assembly and bioprinting of living cells. *Biofabrication.* 2010;2(2): 022001.

80. Marga F, Jakab K, Khatiwala C, Shepherd B, Dorfman S, Hubbard B, Colbert S, Gabor F. Toward engineering functional organ modules by additive manufacturing. *Biofabrication.* 2012;4(2):022001.

81. Kaushik SN, Kim B, Walma A, Choi SC, Wu H, Mao JJ, et al. Biomimetic microenvironments for regenerative endodontics. *Biomater Res.* 2016;20:14.

82. Hospodiuk M, Dey M, Sosnoski D, Ozbolat IT. The bioink: a comprehensive review on bioprintable materials. *Biotechnol Adv.* 2017;35(2):217−239.

83. Billiet T, Vandenhaute M, Schelfhout J, Van Vlierberghe S, Dubruel P. A review of trends and limitations in hydrogel-rapid prototyping for tissue engineering. *Biomaterials.* 2012;33(26):6020−6041.

84. Murphy SV, Skardal A, Atala A. Evaluation of hydrogels for bio-printing applications. *J Biomed Mater Res.* 2013;101(1):272−284.

85. Tirrella A, Vozzi F, De Maria C, Vozzi G, Sandri T, Sassano D, et al. Substrate stiffness influences high resolution printing of living cells with an inkjet system. *J Biosci Bioeng.* 2011;112(1):79−85.

86. Fedorovich NE, Swennen I, Girones J, Moroni L, van Blitterswijk CA, Schacht E, et al. Evaluation of photocrosslinked Lutrol hydrogel for tissue printing applications. *Biomacromolecules.* 2009;10(7):1689−1696.

87. Arealis G, Nikolaou VS. Bone printing: new frontiers in the treatment of bone defects. *Injury.* 2015;46(8):20−22.

88. Thiele J, Ma Y, Bruekers SM, Ma S, Huck WT. 25th anniversary article: designer hydrogels for cell cultures: a meterials selection guide. *Adv Mater.* 2014;26(1):125−147.

89. Chen C, Bang S, Cho Y, Lee S, Zhang S, Noh I. Research trends in biomimetic medical materials for tissue engineering: 3D bioprinting, surface modification, nano/micro technology and clinical aspects in tissue engineering of cartilage and bone. *Biomater Res.* 2016;20(1):10.

90. Gopinathan J, Noh I. Recent trends in bioinks for 3D printing. *Biomater Res.* 2018;22: 11.

91. Collins SF. Bioprinting is changing regenerative medicine forever. *Stem Cell Dev.* 2014; 23(1):79−82.

92. Calo E, Khutoryanski VV. Biomedical applications of hydrogels: a review of patents and commercial products. *Eur Polym J.* 2015;65:252−267.

93. Datta P, Barui A, Wu Y, Ozbolat V, Moncal KK, Ozbolat IT. Essential steps in bioprinting: From pre- to post-bioprinting. *Biotechnol Adv.* 2018;36(5):1481−1504.

94. Chimene D, Lennox KK, Kaunas RR, Gaharwar AK. Advanced bioinks for 3D printing: a materials science perspective. *Ann Biomed Eng.* 2016;44(6):2090−2102.

95. Kirchmajer DM, Gorkin III R, in het Panhuis M. An overview of the suitability of hydrogel-forming polymers for extrusion-based 3D-printing. *J Mater Chem B.* 2015; 3:4105−4117.

96. Wang Z, Jin X, Dai R, Holzman JF, Kim K. An ultrafast hydrogel photocrosslinking method for direct laser bioprinting. *RSC Adv.* 2016;6:21099−21104.

97. Rodriguez MJ, Brown J, Giordano J, Lin SJ, Omenetto FG, Kaplan DL. Silk based bio-inks for soft tissue reconstruction using 3-dimensional (3D) printing with in vitro and in vivo assessments. *Biomaterials*. 2017;117:105—115.

98. Rodríguez-Salvador M, Rio-Belver RM, Garechana-Anacabe G. Scientometric and patentometric analyses to determine the knowledge landscape in innovative technologies: The case of 3D bioprinting. *PLoS One*. 2017;12(6):e0180375.

99. Peppas NA, Hilt JZ, Khademhosseini A, Langer R. Hydrogels in biology and medicine: from molecular principles to bionanotechnology. *Adv Mater*. 2006;18(11):1345—1360.

100. Guvendiner M, Burdick JA. Engineering synthetic hydrogel microenvironments to instruct stem cells. *Curr Opin Biotechnol*. 2013;24(5):841—846.

101. Dimas LS, Buehler MJ. Modeling and additive manufacturing of bio-inspired composites with tunable fracture mechanical properties. *Soft Matter*. 2014;10(25):4436—4442.

102. Batrakova EV, Kabanov AV. Pluronic block copolymers: evolution for drug delivery concept from inert nanocarriers to biological response modifiers. *J Contr Release*. 2008;130(2):98—106.

103. Kang HW, Lee SL, Ko IK, Kengla C, Yoo JJ, Atala A. A 3D bioprinting system to produce human-scale tissue constructs with structural integrity. *Nat Biotechnol*. 2016; 34(3):312—319.

104. Wu W, DeConick A, Lewis JA. Omnidirectional printing of 3D microvascular networks. *Adv Mater*. 2011;23(24):H178—H183.

105. Müller M, Becher J, Schnabelrauch M, Zenobi-Wong M. Nanostructured pluronic hydrogels as bioinks for 3D bioprinting. *Biofabrication*. 2015;7(3):035006.

106. Hersel U, Dahmen C, Kessler H. RGD modified polymers: biomaterials for stimulated cell adhesion and beyond. *Biomaterials*. 2003;24(24):4385—4415.

107. Cui X, Breitenkamp K, Lotz M, D'Lima D. Synergistic action of fibroblast growth factor-2 and transforming growth factor-beta 1 enhances bioprinted human neocartilage formation. *Biotechnol Bioeng*. 2012;109(9):2357—2368.

108. Lee AG, Arena CP, Beebe DJ, Palecek SP. Development of macroporous poly(ethylene glycol) hydrogel arrays within microfluidic channels. *Biomacromolecules*. 2010; 11(12):3316—3324.

109. Hribar KC, Soman P, Warner J, Chung P, Chen S. Light-assisted direct write of 3D functional biomaterials. *Lab Chip*. 2014;14(2):268—275.

110. Wüst S, Müller R, Hofman S. 3D bioprinting of complex channels —effects of material, orientation, geometry and cell embedding. *J Biomed Mater Res*. 2015;103(8): 2558—2570.

111. Hockaday LA, Kang KH, Colangelo NW, Cheung PY, Duan B, Malone E, et al. Rapid 3D printing of anatomically acurate and mechanically heterogenous aortic valve hydrogel scaffolds. *Biofabrication*. 2012;4(3):035005.

112. Chen G, Tanaka J, Tateishi T. Osteochondral tissue engineering using a PLGA-collagen hybrid mesh. *Mater Sci Eng C*. 2006;26(1):124—129.

113. Censi R, Schuurman W, Malda J, di Dato G, Burgisser PE, Dhert WJA. Printable photopolymerizable thermosensitive p(HPMAm-lactate)-PEG hydrogel for tissue engineering. *Adv Funct Mater*. 2011;21(10):1833—1842.

114. Burdick JA, Prestwich GD. Hyaluronic acid hydrogels for biomedical applications. *Adv Mater*. 2011;23(12):H41—H56.

115. Hong S, Sycks D, Chan HF, Lin S, Lopez GP, Guilak F, et al. 3D printing of highly stretchable and tough hydrogels into complex, cellularized structures. *Adv Mater*. 2015;27(27):4035—4040.

116. Rutz AL, Hyland KE, Jakus AE, Burghardt WR, Shah RN. A multimaterial bioink method for 3D printing tunable, cell-compatible hydrogels. *Adv Mater.* 2015;27(9): 1607−1614.

117. Ji S, Guvendiren M. Recent advances in bioink design for 3D bioprinting of tissues and organs. *Front Bioeng Biotechnol.* 2017;5:23.

118. Mozetic P, Maria Giannitelli S, Gori M, Trombetta M, Rainer A. Engineering muscle cell alignment through 3D bioprinting. *J Biomed Mater Res A.* 2017;105(9): 2582−2588.

119. Xiong JY, Narayanan J, Liu XY, Chong TK, Chen SB, Chung TS. Topology evolution and gelation mechanism of agarose gel. *J Phys Chem B.* 2005;109(12):5638−5643.

120. Jepson JO, Laurell CB, Franzen B. Agarose gel electrophoresis. *Clin Chem.* 1979; 25(4):629−638.

121. Mao D, Divoux T, Snabre P. Impact of saccharides on the drying kinetics of agarose gels measured by in-situ interferometry. *Sci Rep.* 2017;7:41185.

122. Zucca P, Fernandez-Lafuente R, Sanjust E. Agarose and its derivatives as supports for enzyme immobilization. *Molecules.* 2016;21(11):1577.

123. Garrido T, Etxabide A, Guerrero P, de la Gaba K. Characterization of agar/soy protein biocomposite films: effect of agar on the extruded pellets and compression moulded films. *Carbonhydr Polym.* 2016;151:408−416.

124. Fedorovich NE, De wijn JR, Verbout AJ, Alblas J, Dhert WJ. Three-dimensional fiber deposition of cell-laden, viable, patterned constructs for bone tissue engineering. *Tissue Eng A.* 2008;14(1):127−133.

125. Jakus AE, Rutz AL, Shah RM. Advancing the field of 3D biomaterial printing. *Biomed Mater.* 2016;11:014102.

126. Kreimendahl F, Köpf M, Thiebes AL, Duarte Campos DF, Blaezer A, Schmitz-Rode T, et al. Three-dimensional printing and angiogenesis: tailored agarose-type I collagen blends comprise three-dimensional printability and angiogenesi potential for tissue-engineered substitutes. *Tissue Eng C Methods.* 2017;23(10):604−615.

127. Yang X, Lu Z, Wu H, Li W, Zheng L, Zhao J. Collagen-alginate as bioink for three-dimensional (3D) cell printing based cartilage tissue engineering. *Mater Sci Eng C.* 2018;83:195−201.

128. Gu Q, Tomaskovic-Crook E, Kapsa R, Cook M, Zhou Q, Wallace G, Crook J. Bio-printing 3D functional neural tissue using human neural and induced pluripotent stem cells. In: *Front Bioeng Biotechnol Conference Abstact: 10th World Biomaterials Congress.* 2016.

129. Gu Q, Tomaskovic-Crook E, Lozano R, Chen Y, Kapsa RM, Zhou Q, et al. Functional 3D neural mini-tissues from printed gel-based bioink and human neural stem cells. *Adv Healthc Mater.* 2016;5(12):1429−1438.

130. Forget A, Blaeser A, Miesmer F, Köpf M, Campos DF, Voelker NH, et al. Mechanically tunable bioink for 3D bioprinting of human cells. *Adv Healthc Mater.* 2017;6(20).

131. Daly AC, Critchley SE, Rencsok EM, Kelly DJ. A comparison of different bioinks for 3D bioprinting of fibrocartilage and hyaline cartilage. *Biofabrication.* 2016;8(4): 045002.

132. Daly AC, Cunniffe GM, Sathy BM, Jeon O, Alsberg E, Kelly DJ. 3D bioprinting of developmentally inspired templates for whole bone organ engineering. *Adv Healthc Mater.* 2016;5(18):2353−2362.

133. Ozler SB, Bakirci E, Kucukgul C, Koc B. Three-dimensional direct cell bioprinting for tissue engineering. *J Biomed Mater Res B Appl Biomater.* 2017;105(8):2530−2544.

134. Jia J, Richards DJ, Pollard S, Tan Y, Rodriguez J, Visconti RP, et al. Engineering alginate as bioink for bioprinting. *Acta Biomater.* 2014;10(10):4323−4331.

135. Kulseng B, Skjåk-Braek G, Ryan L, Andersson A, King A, Faxvaag A, Espevik T. Transplantation of alginate microcapsules: generation of antibodies against alginates and encapsulated porcine islet-like cell clusters. *Transplantation.* 1999;67(7):978−984.

136. Chang JH, Naficy S, Yue Z, Kapsa R, Quigley A, Moulton SE, et al. Bio-ink properties and printability for extrusion printing living cells. *Biomater Sci.* 2013;1(7):763−773.

137. Cohen J, Zaleski KL, Nourissat G, Julien TP, Randolph MA, Yaremchuk MJ. Survival of porcine mesenchymal stem cells over the alginate recovered cellular method. *J Biomed Mater Res A.* 2011;96(1):93−99.

138. Song SJ, Choi J, Park YD, Hong S, Lee JJ, Ahn CB, et al. Sodium alginate hydrogel-based bioprinting using a novel multinozzle bioprinting system. *Artif Organs.* 2011;35(11):1132−1136.

139. Axpe E, Oyen ML. Applications of alginate-based bioinks in 3D bioprinting. *Int J Mol Sci.* 2016;17(12):E1976.

140. Zhang Y, Yu Y, Chen H, Ozbolat IT. Characterization of printable cellular micro-fluidic channels for tissue engineering. *Biofabrication.* 2013;5(2):025004.

141. Yu Y, Zhang Y, Martin JA, Ozbolat IT. Evaluation of cell viability and functionality in vessel-like bioprintable cell-laden tubular channels. *J Biomech Eng.* 2013;135(9):091011.

142. Gao Q, He Y, Fu JZ, Liu A, Ma L. Coaxial nozzle-assisted 3D bioprinting with built-in microchannels for nutrients delivery. *Biomaterials.* 2015;61:203−215.

143. Wang X, Tolba E, Schröder HC, Neufurth M, Feng Q, Diehl-Seifert B, Müller WE. Effect of bioglass on growth and biomineralization of SaOS-2 cells in hydrogel after 3D cell bioprinting. *PLoS One.* 2014;9(11):e112497.

144. Jang CH, Ahn SH, Yang GH, Kim GH. A MSCs-laden polycaprolactone/collagen scaffold for bone tissue regeneration. *RSC Adv.* 2016;6(8):6259−6265.

145. Armstrong JP, Burke M, Carter BM, Davis SA, Perriman AW. 3D bioprinting using a templated porous bioink. *Adv Healthc Mater.* 2016;5(14):1724−1730.

146. Ning L, Xu Y, Chen X, Schreyer DJ. Influence of mechanical properties of alginate-based substrates on the performance of Schwann cells in culture. *J Biomater Sci Polym Ed.* 2016;27(9):898−915.

147. Geiger M. Collagen sponges for bone regeneration with rhBMP-2. *Adv Drug Deliv Rev.* 2003;55(12):1613−1629.

148. Lee V, Singh G, Trasatti JP, Bjornsson C, Xu X, Tran TN, et al. Design and fabrication of human skin by three-dimensional bioprinting. *Tissue Eng Part C Methods.* 2014;20(6):473−484.

149. Wang W, Jin S, Ye K. Development of islet organoids from H9 human embryonic stem cells in biomimetic 3D scaffolds. *Stem Cell Dev.* 2017;26(6):394−404.

150. Wang X, Ye K. Three-dimensional differentiation of embryonic stem-cells into islet-like insulin-producing clusters. *Tissue Eng Part A.* 2009;15(8):1941−1952.

151. Rodriguez-Pascual F, Slatter DA. Collagen cross-linking: insights on the evolution of metazoan extracellular matrix. *Sci Rep.* 2016;6:37374.

152. van Uden S, Silva-Correia J, Oliveira JM, Reis RL. Current strategies for treatment of intervertebral disc degeneration: substitution and regeneration possibilities. *Biomater Res.* 2017;21(1):22.

153. Ahn HJ, Khalmuratova R, Park SA, Chung EJ, Shin HW, Kwon SK. Serial analysis of tracheal restenosis after 3D-printed scaffold implantation: recruited inflammatory cells and associated tissue changes. *Tissue Eng Regen Med*. 2017;14(5):631−639.

154. Wollensak G. Crosslinking treatment of progressive keratoconus: new hope. *Curr Opin Ophthalmol*. 2006;17(4):356−360.

155. Mrochen M. Current status of accelarated corneal cross-linking. *Indian J Ophthalmol*. 2013;61(8):428.

156. Ferreira AM, Gentile P, Chiono V, Ciarfelli G. Collagen for bone tissue regeneration. *Acta Biomater*. 2012;8(9):3191−3200.

157. Mori H, Shimizu K, Hara M. Dynamic viscoelastic properties of collagen gells with high mechanical srtength. *Mater Sci Eng C*. 2013;33(6):3230−3236.

158. Stratesteffen H, Köpf M, Kreimendahl F, Blaeser A, Jockenhoevel S, Fischer H. GelMA-collagen blends enable drop-on-demand 3D printability and promote angiogenesis. *Biofabrication*. 2017;9(4):045002.

159. Yeo M, Lee JS, Chun W, Kim GH. An innovative collagen-based cell-printing method for obtaining human adipose stem cell-laden structures consisting of core-sheath structures for tissue engineering. *Biomacromolecules*. 2016;17(4):1365−1375.

160. Yeo MG, Kim GH. A cell-printing approach for obtaining hASC-laden scaffolds by using a collagen/polyphenol bioink. *Biofabrication*. 2017;9(2):025004.

161. Irvin SA, Agrawal A, Lee BH, Chua HY, Low KY, Lau BC, et al. Printing cell-laden gelatin constructs by free-form fabrication and enzymatic protein crosslinking. *Biomed Microdevices*. 2015;17(1):16.

162. Hoch E, Hirth T, Tovar GEM, Borchers K. Chemical tailoring of gelatin to adjust its chemical and physical properties for functional bioprinting. *J Mater Chem B*. 2013; 1(41):5675−5685.

163. Melchels FPW, Dhert WJA, Hutmacher DW, Malda J. Development and characterization of a new bioink for additive tissue manufacturing. *J Mater Chem B*. 2014;2(16): 2282−2289.

164. Boere KW, Visser J, Seyednejab H, Rahimian S, Gawlitta D, van Steenbergen MJ, et al. Covalent attachement of a three-dimensionally printed thermoplast to a gelatin hydrogel for mechanically enhanced cartilage constructs. *Acta Biomater*. 2014;10(6): 2602−2611.

165. Nichol JW, Koshy ST, Bae H, Hwang CM, Yamanlar S, Khademhosseini A. Cell-laden microengineered gelatin methacrylate hydrogels. *Biomaterials*. 2010;31(21): 5536−5544.

166. Billiet T, Gevaert E, De Schryver T, Cornelissen M, Dubruel P. The 3D printing of gelatin methacrylamide cell-laden tissue engineered constructs with high cell viability. *Biomaterials*. 2014;35(1):49−62.

167. Pimentel R, Ko SK, Caviglia C, Wolff A, Emnéus J, Keller SS, Dufva M. Three-dimensional fabrication of thick and densely populated soft constructs with complex and actively perfused channel network. *Acta Biomater*. 2018;65:174−184.

168. Fraser JR, Laurent TC, Laurent UB. Hyaluronan: its nature, distribution, function and turnover. *J Intern Med*. 1997;242(1):27−33.

169. Pescosolido L, Schuurman W, Malda J, Matricardi P, Alhaique F, Coviello T, et al. Hyaluronic acid and dextran-based semi-IPN hydrogels as biomaterials for bioprinting. *Biomacromolecules*. 2011;12(5):1831−1838.

170. Highley CB, Prestwich GD, Burdick JA. Recent advances in hyaluronic acid hydrogels for biomedical applications. *Curr Opin Biotechnol*. 2016;40:35−40.

171. Skardal A, Zhang J, McCoard L, Xu X, Oottamasathien S, Prestwich GD. Photocros-slinkable hyaluronan-gelatin hydrogels for two-step bioprinting. *Tissue Eng A*. 2010; 16(8):2675−2685.

172. Ouyang L, Highley CB, Rodell CB, Sun W, Burdick JA. 3D printing of shear-thinning hyaluronic acid hydrogels with secondary cross-linking. *ACS Biomater Sci Eng*. 2016; 2(10):1743−1751.

173. Poldervaart MT, Goversen B, de Ruijter M, Abbadessa A, Melchels FP, Öner FC, et al. 3D bioprinting of methacrylated hyaluronic acid (MeHA) hydrogel with intrinsic osteogenecity. *PLos One*. 2017;12(6):e0177628.

174. Stichler S, Böck T, Paxton N, Bertlein S, Levato R, Schill V, et al. Double printing of hyaluronic acid/poly(glycidol) hybrid hydrogels with poly(ε-caprolactone) for MSC chondrogenesis. *Biofabrication*. 2017;9(4):044108.

175. Sakai S, Ohi H, Hotta T, Kamei H, Taya M. Differentiation potential of human adipose stem cells bioprinted with hyaluronic acid/gelatin-based bioink through microextrusion and visible light-initiated crosslinking. *Biopolymers*. 2018;109(2).

176. Updegraff DM. Semimicro determination of cellulose in biological materials. *Anal Biochem*. 1969;32(3):420−424.

177. Kobayashi K, Huang CI, Lodge TP. Thermoreversible gelation of aqueous methylcel-lulose solutions. *Macromolecules*. 1999;32(21):7070−7077.

178. Nguyen D, Hägg DA, Forsman A, Ekholm J, Nimkingratana P, Brantsing C, et al. Carti-lage tissue engineering by the 3D bioprinting of iPS cells in a nanocelluloselginate bioink. *Sci Rep*. 2017;7(1):658.

179. Law N, Doney B, Glover H, Qin Y, Aman ZM, Sercombe TB, et al. Characterization of hyaluronic acid methylcellulose hydrogels for 3D bioprinting. *J Mech Behav Biomed Mater*. 2018;77:389−399.

180. Wu C, Luo Y, Cuniberti C, Xiao Y, Gelinsky M. Three-dimensional prinitng of hierar-chical and tough mesoporous bioactive glass scaffolds with a controlable pore architec-ture, excellent mechanical strength and mineralization ability. *Acta Biomater*. 2011; 7(6):2644−2650.

181. Markstedt K, Mantas A, Tournier I, Ávila HM, Hägg D, Gatenholm P. 3D bioprinting human chondrocytes with nanocellulose-alginate bioink for cartilage tissue engineering applications. *Biomacromolecules*. 2015;16(5):1489−1496.

182. Ávila HM, Schwarz S, Rotter N, Gatenholm P. 3D bioprinting of human chondrocyte-laden nanocellulose hydrogels for patient-specific auricular cartilage regeneration. *Bio-printing*. 2016;1:22−35.

183. Zhang K, Fu Q, Yoo J, Chen X, Chandra P, Mo X, et al. 3D bioprinting of urethra with PCL/PLCL blend and dual dual autologous cells in fibrin hydrogel: an in vitro evolution of biomimetic mechanical property and cell growth environment. *Acta Biomater*. 2017; 50:154−164.

184. Lee VK, Lanzi AM, Haygan N, Yoo SS, Vincent PA, Dai G. Generation of multi-scale vascular network system within 3D hydrogel using 3D bio-printing technology. *Cell Mol Bioeng*. 2014;7(3):460−472.

185. Lee YB, Polio S, Lee W, Dai G, Menon L, Carroll RS, Yoo SS. Bio-printing of collagen and VEGF-releasing fibrin gel scaffolds for neural stem cell culture. *Exp Neurol*. 2010; 223(2):645−652.

186. Kolesky DB, Homan KA, Skylar-Scott MA, Lewis JA. Three-dimensional bioprinting of thick vascularized tissues. *Proc Natl Acad Sci USA*. 2016;113(12):3179−3184.

187. Homan KA, Kolesky DB, Skylar-Scott MA, Herrmann J, Obuobi H, Moisan A, et al. Bioprinting of 3D convulated renal proximal tubules on perfusable chips. *Sci Rep.* 2016;6:34845.
188. England S, Rajaram A, Schreyer DJ, Chen X. Bioprinted fibrin-factor XIII-hyaluronate hydrogel scaffolds with encapsulated Schwann cells and their in vitro characterization for use in nerve regeneration. *Bioprinting.* 2017;5:1−9.
189. Floren M, Bonani W, Dharmarajan A, Motta A, Migliaresi C, Tan W. Human mesenchymal stem cells cultured on silk hydrogels with variable stiffness and growth factor differentiate into mature smooth muscle cell phenotype. *Acta Biomater.* 2016;31: 156−166.
190. Das S, Pati F, Choi YJ, Rijal G, Shim JH, Kim SW, et al. Bioprintable, cell-laden silk fibroin-gelatin hydrogel supporting multilineage differentiation of stem cells for fabrication of three-dimensional tissue constructs. *Acta Biomater.* 2015;11:233−246.
191. Compaan AM, Christensen K, Huang Y. Inkjet bioprinting of 3D silk fibroin cellular constructs using sacrificial alginate. *ACS Biomater Sci Eng.* 2017;3(8):1519−1526.
192. Xiong S, Zhang X, Lu P, Wu Y, Wang Q, Sun H, et al. A gelatin-sulfonated silk composite scaffold based on 3D printing technology enhances skin regeneration by stimulating epidermal growth and dermal neovascularization. *Sci Rep.* 2017;7(1):4288.
193. Zheng Z, Wu J, Liu M, Wang H, Li C, Rodriguez MJ, et al. 3D bioprinting of self-standing silk-based bioink. *Adv Healthc Mater.* 2018;7(6):e1701026.
194. DeSimone E, Schacht K, Pellert A, Scheibel T. Recombinant spider silk-based bioinks. *Biofabrication.* 2017;9(4):044104.
195. Theocharis AD, Skandalis SS, Gialeli C, Karamanos NK. Extracellular matrix structure. *Adv Drug Deliv Rev.* 2016;97:4−27.
196. Jung JP, Bhuiyan DB, Ogle BM. Solid organ fabrication: comparison of decellularization to 3D bioprinting. *Biomater Res.* 2016;20(1):27.
197. Crapo PM, Gilbert TW, Badylak SF. An overview of tissue and whole organ decellularization processes. *Biomaterials.* 2011;32(12):3233−3243.
198. Pati F, Jang J, Ha DH, Kim SW, Rhie JW, Shim JH, et al. Printing three-dimensional tissue analogues with decellularized extracellular matrix bioink. *Nat Commun.* 2014; 5:3935.
199. Anh G, Min KH, Kim C, Lee JS, Kang D, Won JY, et al. Precise stacking of decellularized extracellular matrix based 3D cell-laden constructs by a 3D cell printing system equipped with heating modules. *Sci Rep.* 2017;7(1):8624.
200. Jang J, Park HJ, Kim SW, Kim H, Park JY, Na SJ, et al. 3D printed complex tissue construct using stem cell-laden decellularized extracellular matrix bioinks for cardiac repair. *Biomaterials.* 2017;112:264−274.
201. Khati V. *Development of a Robust Decellularized Extracellular Matrix Bioink for 3D Bioprinting.* Tampere University of Technology; 2016.
202. Fennema E, Rivron N, Rouwkema J, van Blitterswijk C, de Boer J. Spheroid culture as a tool for creating 3D complex tissues. *Trends Biotechnol.* 2013;31(2):108−115.
203. Yu Y, Moncal KK, Li J, Peng W, Rivero I, Martin JA, Ozbolat IT. Three-dimensional bioprinting using self-assembling scalable scaffold-free "tissue strands" as a new bioink. *Sci Rep.* 2016;6:28714.
204. Bakirci E, Toprakhisar B, Zeybek MC, Ince GO, Koc B. Cell sheet based bioink for 3D bioprinting applications. *Biofabrication.* 2017;9(2):024105.
205. Mironov V, Kasyanov V, Markwald RR. Organ printing: from bioprinter to organ biofabrication line. *Curr Opin Biotechnol.* 2011;22(5):667−673.

206. Wang Y, Zhang Z, Chi Y, Zhang Q, Xu F, Yang Z, et al. Long-term cultured mesenchymal stem cells frequently develop genomic mutations but do not undergo malignant transformation. *Cell Death Dis*. 2013;4:e950.

207. Leberfinger AN, Ranvic DJ, Dhawan A, Ozbolat IT. Consise review: bioprinting of stem cells for transplantable tissue fabrication. *Stem Cells Transl Med*. 2017;6(10): 1940−1948.

208. Irvine SA, Venkatraman SS. Bioprinting and differentiation of stem cells. *Molecules*. 2016;21(9):E1188.

209. Plusa B, Hadjantonakis AK. Embryonic stem cell identity grounded in the embryo. *Nat Cell Biol*. 2014;16(6):502−504.

210. Yamanaka S. Induced pluripotent stem cells: Past, present, and future. *Cell Stem Cell*. 2012;10(6):678−684.

211. *The Nobel Prize in Physiology or Medicine − 2012 Press Release"Nobel Media AB*. October 2012.

212. Yoshihara M, Hayashizaki Y, Murakawa Y. Genomic instability of iPSCs: challenges towards their clinical applications. *Stem Cell Rev Rep*. 2017;13(1):7−16.

213. Miura K, Okada Y, Aoi T, Okada A, Takahashi K, Okita K, et al. Variation in the safety of induced pluripotent stem cell lines. *Nat Biotechnol*. 2009;27(8):743−745.

214. Puri MC, Nagy A. Concise review: Embryonic stem cells versus induced pluripotent stem cells: The game is on. *Stem Cell*. 2012;30(1):10−14.

215. Singh VK, Kalsan M, Kumar N, Saini A, Chandra R. Induced pluripotent stem cells: Applications in regenerative medicine, disease modeling, and drug discovery. *Front Cell Dev Biol*. 2015;3:2.

216. Nombela-Arrieta C, Ritz J, Silberstein LE. The elusive nature and function of mesenchymal stem cells. *Nat Rev Mol Cell Biol*. 2011;12(2):126−131.

217. Skardal A. Bioprinting essentials of cell and protein viability. In: Atala A, Yoo JJ, eds. *Essentials of 3D Biofabrication Translation*. Boston, MA, USA: Academic Press; 2015: 1−17.

218. Huang NF, Li S. Mesenchymal stem cells for vascular regeneration. *Regen Med*. 2008; 3(6):877−892.

219. Huang NF, Li S. Mesenchymal stem cells for tissue regeneration. In: Li S, L'Heureux N, Elisseeff J, eds. *Stem Cell Tissue Engineering*. Singapore: World Scientific; 2012:49−70.

220. Kariminekoo S, Movassaghpour A, Rahimzadeh A, Talebi M, Shamsasenjan K, Akbarzadeh A. Implications of mesenchymal stem cells in regenerative medicine. *Artif Cells Nanomed Biotechnol*. 2016;44(3):749−757.

221. Lindroos B, Suuronen R, Miettinen S. The potential of adipose stem cells in regenerative medicine. *Stem Cell Rev Rep*. 2011;7(2):269−291.

222. Si JW, Wang XD, Shen SGF. Perinatal stem cells: A promising cell resource for tissue engineering of craniofacial bone. *World J Stem Cell*. 2015;7(1):149−159.

223. Skardal A, Mack D, Kapetanovic E, Atala A, Jackson JD, Yoo J, et al. Bioprinted amniotic fluid-derived stem cells accelerate healing of large skin wounds. *Stem Cells Transl Med*. 2012;1(11):792−802.

224. De Coppi P, Bartsch Jr G, Siddiqui MM, Xu T, Santos CC, Perin L, et al. Isolation of amniotic stem cell lines with potential for therapy. *Nat Biotechnol*. 2007;25(1): 100−106.

225. Ozbolat IT. *3D Bioprinting: Fundementals, Principles and Applications*. Academiv Press is an imprint of Elsevier; 2016.

226. Jakobs SA, Roobrouck VD, Verfaille CM, Van Gool SW. Immunological characteristics of human mesenchymal stem cells and multipotent adult progenitor cells. *Immunol Cell Biol.* 2013;91(1):32–39.

227. Gu LH, Zhang TT, Li Y, Yan HJ, Qi H, Li FR. Immunogenicity of allogenic mesenchymal stem cells transplanted via different routes in diabetic rats. *Cell Mol Immunol.* 2015;12(4):444–455.

228. Barry FP, Murphy JM, English K, Mahon BP. Immunogenicity of adult mesenchymal stem cells: lessons from the fetal allograft. *Stem Cell Dev.* 2005;14(3):252–265.

229. Ren ML, Peng W, Yang ZL, Sun XJ, Zhang SC, Wang ZG, et al. Allogeneic adipose-derived stem cells with low immunogenicity constructing tissue-engineered bone for repairing bone defects in pigs. *Cell Transplant.* 2012;21(12):2711–2721.

230. Larocca RA, Moraes-Vieira PM, Bassi EJ, Semedo P, de Almeida DC, de Silva MB, et al. Adipose tissue-derived mesenchymal stem cells increase skin allograft survival and inhibit Th-17 immune response. *PLoS One.* 2013;8(10)::e76396.

231. Gao B, Yang Q, Zhao X, Jin G, Ma Y, Xu F. 4D bioprinting for biomedical applications. *Trends Biotechnol.* 2016;34(9):746–756.

232. Gao F, Chiu SM, Motan DAL, Zhang Z, Chen L, Ji HL, et al. Mesenchymal stem cells and immunomodulation: current status and future prospects. *Cell Death Dis.* 2016;7: e2062.

233. Madrigal M, Rao KS, Riordan NH. A review of therapeutic effects of mesenchymal stem cell secretions and induction of secretory modification by different culture methods. *J Transl Med.* 2014;12:260.

234. Shav D, Einav S. The effect of mechanical loads in the differentiation of precursor cells into mature cells. *Ann NY Acad Sci.* 2010;1188:25–31.

235. Stolberg S, McCloskey KE. Can shear stress direct stem cell fate? *Biotechnol Prog.* 2009;25(1):10–19.

236. Gruene M, Deiwick A, Koch L, Schlie S, Unger C, Hofmann N, et al. Laser printing of stem cells for biofabrication of scaffold-free autologous grafts. *Tissue Eng C Methods.* 2011;17(1):79–87.

237. Peerani R, Rao BM, Bauwens C, Yin T, Wood GA, Nagy A, et al. Niche-mediated control of human embryonic stem cell selfrenewal and differentiation. *EMBO J.* 2007; 26(22):4744–4755.

238. Bianco P, Robey PG. Stem cells in tissue engineering. *Nature.* 2001;414(6859): 118–121.

239. Phillippi JA, Miller E, Weiss L, Huard J, Waggoner A, Campbell P. Microenvironments engineered by inkjet bioprinting spatially direct adult stem cells toward muscle- and bone-like subpopulations. *Stem Cell.* 2008;26(1):127–134.

240. Miller ED, Li K, Kanade T, Weiss LE, Walker LM, Campbell PG. Spatially directed guidance of stem cell population migration by immobilized patterns of growth factors. *Biomaterials.* 2011;32(11):2775–2785.

241. Habib SJ, Chen BC, Tsai FC, Anastassiadis K, Meyer T, Betzig E, et al. A localized Wnt signal orients asymmetric stem cell division in vitro. *Science.* 2013;339(6126): 1445–1448.

242. Brafman DA. Constructing stem cell microenvironments using bioengineering approaches. *Physiol Genom.* 2013;45(23):1123–1135.

243. Chen G, Deng C, Li YP. TGF-β and BMP signaling in osteoblast differentiation and bone formation. *Int J Biol Sci.* 2012;8(2):272–288.

244. Sekiya I, Colter DC, Prockop DJ. BMP-6 enhances chondrogenesis in a subpopulation of human marrow stromal cells. *Biochem Biophys Res Commun.* 2001;284(2): 411−418.

245. Diekman BO, Estes BT, Guilak F. The effects of BMP6 overexpression on adipose stem cell chondrogenesis: Interactions with dexamethasone and exogenous growth factors. *J Biomed Mater Res A.* 2010;93(3):994−1003.

246. Ding S, Schultz PG. A role for chemistry in stem cell biology. *Nat Biotechnol.* 2004; 22(7):833−840.

247. Phadke A, Chang CW, Varghese S. Functional biomaterials for controlling stem cell differentiation. In: Roy K, ed. *Biomaterials as Stem Cell Niche.* Berlin, Germany; Heidelberg, Germany: Springer; 2010:19−44.

248. Ninomiya Y, Sugahara-Yamashita Y, Nakachi Y, Tokuzawa Y, Okazaki Y, Nishiyama M. Development of a rapid culture method to induce adipocyte differentiation of human bone marrow-derived mesenchymal stem cells. *Biochem Biophys Res Commun.* 2010;394(2):303−308.

249. Scott MA, Nguyen VT, Levi B, James AW. Current methods of adipogenic differentiation of mesenchymal stem cells. *Stem Cell Dev.* 2011;20(10):1793−1804.

250. Xu W, Zhang X, Qian H, Zhu W, Sun X, Hu J, et al. Mesenchymal stem cells from adult human bone marrow differentiate into a cardiomyocyte phenotype in vitro. *Exp Biol Med.* 2004;229(7):623−631.

251. Levato R, Visser J, Planell JA Engel E, Malda J, Mateos-Timoneda MA. Biofabrication of tissue constructs by 3D bioprinting of cell-laden microcarriers. *Biofabrication.* 2014; 6(3):035020.

252. Levato R, Mateos-Timoneda MA, Planell JA. Preparation of biodegradable polylactide microparticles via a biocompatible procedure. *Macromol Biosci.* 2012;12(4):557−566.

253. Sart S, Agathos SN, Li Y. Engineering stem cell fate with biochemical and biomechanical properties of microcarriers. *Biotechnol Prog.* 2013;29(6):1354−1366.

254. Ayyildiz-Tamis D, Avci K, Deliloglu-Gurhan SI. Comparative investigation of the use of various commercial microcarriers as a substrate for culturing mammalian cells. *In Vitro Cell Dev Biol Anim.* 2014;50(3):221−231.

255. Frauenschuh S, Reichmann E, Ibold Y, Goetz PM, Sittinger M, Ringe J. A microcarrier-based cultivation system for expansion of primary mesenchymal stem cells. *Biotechnol Prog.* 2007;23(1):187−193.

256. Frondoza C, Sohrabi A, Hungerford D. Human chondrocytes proliferate and produce matrix components in microcarrier suspension culture. *Biomaterials.* 1996;17(9): 879−888.

257. Malda J, Kreijveld E, Temenoff JS, van Blitterswijk CA, Riesle J. Expansion of human nasal chondrocytes on macroporous microcarriers enhances redifferentiation. *Biomaterials.* 2003;24(28):53−61.

258. Shikani AH, Fink DJ, Sohrabi A, Phan P, Polotsky A, Hungerford DS, et al. Propagation of human nasal chondrocytes in microcarrier spinner culture. *Am J Rhinol.* 2004;18(2): 105−112.

259. Perez RA, El-Fiqi A, Park JH, Kim TH, Kim JH, Kim HW. Therapeutic bioactive microcarriers: co-delivery of growth factors and stem cells for bone tissue engineering. *Acta Biomater.* 2014;10(1):520−530.

260. Malda J, van Blitterswijk CA, Grojec M, Martens DE, Tramper J, Riesle J. Expansion of bovine chondrocytes on microcarriers enhances redifferentiation. *Tissue Eng.* 2003; 9(5):939−948.

261. Nair K, Gandhi M, Khalil S, Yan KC, Marcolongo M, Barbee K, et al. Characterization of cell viability during bioprinting processes. *Biotechnol J*. 2009;4(8):1168−1177.

262. Ouyang L, Yao R, Chen X, Na J, Sun W. 3D printing of HEK 293FT cell-laden hydrogel into macroporous constructs with high cell viability and normal biological functions. *Biofabrication*. 2015;7(1):015010.

263. Zhao Y, Li Y, Mao S, Sun W, Yao R. The influence of printing parameters on cell survival rate and printability in microextrusion-based 3D cell printing technology. *Biofabrication*. 2015;7(4):045002.

264. Blaeser A, Duarte Campos DF, Puster U, Richtering W, Stevens MM, Fischer H. Controlling shear stress in 3D bioprinting is a key factor to balance printing resolution and stem cell integrity. *Adv Healthc Mater*. 2016;5(3):326−333.

265. Ng WL, Yeong WY, Naing MW. Polyvinylpyrrolidone-based bio-ink improves cell viability and homogeneity during drop-on-demand printing. *Materials*. 2017;10(2): E190.

266. Duan B, Kapetanovic E, Hockaday LA, Butcher JT. Three-dimensional printed trileaflet valve conduits using biological hydrogels and human valve interstitial cells. *Acta Biomater*. 2014;10(5):1836−1846.

267. Chang R, Nam J, Sun W. Effects of dispensing pressure and nozzle diameter on cell survival from solid freeform fabrication−based direct cell writing. *Tissue Eng A*. 2008;14(1):41−48.

268. Huang Y, Zhang X, Gao G, Yonezawa T, Cui X. 3D bioprinting and the current applications in tissue engineering. *Biotechnol J*. 2017;12(8).

269. Derby B. Printing and prototyping of tissues and scaffolds. *Science*. 2012;338(6109): 921−926.

270. Murphy SV, Atala A. 3D Bioprinting of tissues and organs. *Nat Biotechnol*. 2014;32(8): 773−785.

271. Horváth L, Umehara Y, Jud C, Blank F, Petrifink A, Rothen-Rutishauser B. Engineering: an in vitro air-blood barrier by 3D bioprinting. *Sci Rep*. 2015;5:7974.

272. Sfafiee A, Atala A. Printing technologies for medical applications. *Trends Mol Med*. 2016;22(3):254−265.

273. Ozbolat IT. Bioprinting scale-up tissue and organ constructs for transplantation. *Trends Biotechnol*. 2015;33(7):395−400.

274. Ballyns JJ, Bonassar LJ. Image-giuded tissue engineering. *J Cell Mol*. 2009;13(8a): 1428−1436.

275. Reiffel AJ, Kafka C, Hernandez KA, Popa S, Perez JL, Zhou S, et al. High-fidelity tissue engineering of patient-specific auricles for reconstruction of pediatric microtia and other auricular deformities. *PLoS One*. 2013;8(2):e56506.

276. Mycek MA. Clinical translation of optical molecular imaging to tissue engineering: opportunities and challenges.In: *Optics in the Life Sciences, OSA Technical Digest*. Optical Society of America, Vancouver (p. OT1C.1). Bio-Optics: Design and Application 2015 Vancouver Canada, ISBN: 978-1-55752-954-1, 12−15 April 2015.

277. McCormick M, Liu X, Jomier J, Marion C, Ibanez L. ITK: enabling reproducible research and open science. *Front Neuroinf*. 2014;8:13.

278. Sun W, Starly B, Darling A, Gomez C. Computer-aided tissue engineering: application to biomimetic modelling and design of tissue scaffolds. *Biotechnol Appl Biochem*. 2004;39(Pt 1):49−58.

279. Khoda AKM, Ozbolat IT, Koc B. Designing heterogeneous porous tissue scaffolds for additive manufacturing processes. *Comput Des*. 2013;45:1507−1523.

280. Coakley MF, Hurt DE, Weber N, Mtingwa M, Fincher EC, Alekseyev V, et al. The NIH 3D print exchange: a public resource for bioscientific and biomedical 3D Prints. *3D Print Addit Manuf*. 2014;1(3):137—140.

281. Ozbolat IT, Gudapati H. A review on design for bioprinting. *Bioprinting*. 2016;3:1—14.

282. Li YC, Zhang YS, Akpek A, Shin SR, Khademhosseini A. 4D bioprinting: the next-generation technology for biofabrication enabled by stimuli-responsive materials. *Biofabrication*. 2016;9(1):012001.

283. Margaliot M. Biomimicry and fuzzy modeling: a match made in heaven. *IEEE Comput Intell Mag*. 2008:38—48.

284. Nicodemus GD, Bryant SJ. Cell encapsulation in biodegradable hydrogels for tissue engineering applications. *Tissue Eng Part B Rev*. 2008;14(2):149—165.

285. Derakhshanfar S, Mbeleck R, Xu K, Zhang X, Zhong W, Xing M. 3D bioprinting for biomedical devices and tissue engineering: A review of recent trends and advances. *Bioact Mater*. 2018;3(2):144—156.

286. Lee HY, Kim HW, Lee JH, Oh SH. Controlling oxygen release from hollow microparticles for prolonged cell survival under hypoxic environment. *Biomaterials*. 2015;53: 583—591.

287. Möller T, Amoroso M, Hägg D, Brantsing C, Rotter N, Apelgren P, et al. In Vivo Chondrogenesis in 3D Bioprinted Human Cell-laden Hydrogel Constructs. *Plast Reconstr Surg Glob Open*. 2017;5(2):e1227.

288. Seidel J, Ahlfeld T, Adolph M, Kümmritz S, Steingroewer J, Krujatz F, et al. Green bioprinting: extrusion-based fabrication of plant cell-laden biopolymer hydrogel scaffolds. *Biofabrication*. 2017;9(4):045011.

289. Clarke B. Normal bone anatomy and physiology. *Clin J Am Soc Nephrol*. 2008;3(Suppl 3):S131—S139.

290. Bianconi E, Piovesan A, Facchin F, Beraudi A, Casadei R, Frabetti F, et al. An estimation of the number of cells in the human body. *Ann Hum Biol*. 2013;40(6):463—471.

291. Hölzl K, Lin S, Tytgat L, Van Vlierberghe S, Gu L, Ovsianikov A. Bioink properties before, during and after 3D bioprinting. *Biofabrication*. 2016;8(3):032002.

292. Ouyang L, Yao R, Zhao Y, Sun W. Effect of bioink properties on printability and cell viability for 3D bioplotting of embryonic stem cells. *Biofabrication*. 2016;8(3):035020.

293. Kim JD, Choi JS, Kim BS, Chan Choi Y, Cho YW. Piezoelectric inkjet printing of polymers: stem cell patterning on polymer substrates. *Polymer*. 2010;51:2147—2154.

294. Peltola SM, Melchels FPW, Grijpma DW, Kellomäki M. A review of rapid prototyping techniques for tissue engineering purposes. *Ann Med*. 2008;40:268—280.

295. Mauck RL, Wang CB, Oswald ES, Ateshian GA, Hung CT. The role of cell seeding density and nutrient supply for articular cartilage tissue engineering with deformational loading. *Osteoarthritis Cartilage*. 2003;11:879—890.

296. He Y, Yang F, Zhao H, Gao Q, Xia B, Fu J. Research on the printability of hydrogels in 3D bioprinting. *Sci Rep*. 2016;6:29977.

297. Xing Q, Yates K, Vogt C, Qian Z, Frost MC, Zhao F. Increasing mechanical strength ofgelatin hydrogelsby divalent metalion removal. *Sci Rep*. 2014;4:4706.

298. Martin I, Wendt D, Heberer M. The role of bioreactors in tissue engineering. *Trends Biotechnol*. 2004;22:80—86.

299. Plunkett N, O'Brien FJ. Bioreactors in tissue engineering. *Stud Health Technol*. 2011; 19(1):55—69.

300. Bhuthalingam R, Lim PQ, Irvine SA, Venkatraman SS. Automated robotic dispensing technique for surface guidance and bioprinting of cells. *J Vis Exp*. 2016;117.

301. Correira C, Pereira AL, Duarte ARC, Frias AM, Pedro AJ, Oliveira JT, et al. Dynamic culturing of cartilage tissue: the significance of hydrostatic pressure. *Tissue Eng A*. 2012;18(19-20):1979−1991.

302. Wernik E, Li Z, Alini M, Grad S. Effect of reduced oxygen tension and long-term mechanical stimulation on chondrocyte-polymer constructs. *Cell Tissue Res*. 2008;331(2): 473−483.

303. Trumbull A, Subramanian G, Yildirim-Ayan E. Mechanoresponsive musculoskeletal tissue differantiation of adipose-derived stem cells. *Biomed Eng Online*. 2016;15:43.

304. Zhang HB, Xing TL, Yin RX, Shi Y, Yang SM, Zhang WJ. Three-dimensional bioprinting is not only about cell-laden structures. *Chin J Traumatol*. 2016;19(4):187−192.

305. Zhang YS, Arneri A, Bersini S, Shin SR, Zhu K, Goli-Malekabadi Z, et al. Bioprinting 3D microfibrous scaffolds for engineering endothelialized myocardium and heart-ona-chip. *Biomaterials*. 2016;110:45−59.

306. Detsch R, Boccaccini AR. The role of osteoclasts in bone tissue engineering. *J Tissue Eng Regen Med*. 2015;9(10):1133−1149.

307. Converse GL, Buse EE, Hopkins RA. Bioreactors and operating room centric protocols for clinical heart valve tissue engineering. *Prog Pediatr Cardiol*. 2013;35:95−100.

308. Moffat KL, Neal RA, Freed LE, Guilak F. Engineering functional tissues: in vitro culture parameters. In: *Princ Tissue Eng Fourth Edition*. Academic Press; 2003:237−259.

309. Fedorovich NE, Alblas J, Hennink WE, Oner FC, Dhert WJ. Organ printing: the future of bone regenaration? *Trends Biotechnol*. 2011;29(12):601−606.

310. Zhu W, Holmes B, Glazer RI, Zhang LG. 3D printed nanocomposite matrix for the study of breast cancer bone metastasis. *Nanomedicine*. 2016;12(1):69−79.

311. Rajaram A, Schreyer D, Chen D. Bioplotting alginate/hyaluronic acid hydrogel scaffold with structural integrity and preserved Schwann cell viability. *3D Print*. 2014;1(4): 194−203.

312. Xu T, Zhao W, Zhu JM. Complex heterogeneous tissue constructs containing multiple cell types prepared by inkjet printing technology. *Biomaterials*. 2013;34(1):130−139.

313. Cui X, Gao G, Yonezawa T, Dai G. Human cartilage tissue fabrication using threedimensional inkjet printing technology. *J Visualised Exp*. 2014;88.

314. Kundu J, Shim JH, Jang J, Kim SW, Cho DW. An additive manufacturing-based PCLalginate-chondrocyte bioprinted scaffold for cartilage tissue engineering. *J Tissue Eng Regen Med*. 2015;9(11):1286−1297.

315. Martínez-Santamaría L, Guerrero-Aspizua S, Del Río M. Skin bioengineering: preclinical and clinical applications. *Actas Dermosifiliogr*. 2012;103(1):5−11.

316. Michael S, Sorg H, Peck CT, Koch L, Deiwick A, Chichkov B, et al. Tissue engineered skin substitutes created by laser-assisted bioprinting form skin-line structures in the dorsal skin fold chamber in mice. *PLoS One*. 2013;8(3):e57741.

317. Yannas IV, Burke JF, Orgill DP, Skrabut EM. Wound tissue can utilize a polymeric template to synthesize a functional extension of skin. *Science*. 1982;215(4529):174−176.

318. Pourchet LJ, Thepot A, Albouy M, Courtial EJ, Boher A, Blum LJ, et al. Human skin 3D bioprinting using scaffold-free approach. *Adv Healthc Master*. 2017;6(4).

319. Lee W, Debasitis JC, Lee VK, Lee JH, Fischer K, Edminster K, et al. Multi-layered culture of human skin fibroblasts and karetinocytes through three-dimensional freeform fabrication. *Biomaterials*. 2009;30(8):1587−1595.

320. Mendis S, Puska P, Norrving B. *Global Atlas on Cardiovascular Disease Prevention and Control (PDF)*. World Health Organization in collaboration with the World Heart Federation and the World Stroke Organization. 2011:3−18.

321. Wang H, Naghavi M, Allen C, Barber RM, Bhutta ZA, Carter A, GBD 2015 Mortality and Causes of Death Collaborators, et al. Global, regional, and national life expectancy, all-cause mortality, and cause-specific mortality for 249 causes of death, 1980-2015: a systematic analysis for the Global Burden of Disease Study 2015. *Lancet.* 2016; 388(10053):1459−1544.

322. Hirt MN, Hansen A, Eschenhagen T. Cardiac tissue engineering: state of the art. *Circ Res.* 2014;114(2):354−367.

323. Jana S, Tefft BJ, Spoon DB, Simari RD. Scaffolds for tissue engineering of cardiac valves. *Acta Biomater.* 2014;10(7):2877−2893.

324. Jakab K, Norotte C, Damon B, Marga F, Neagu A, Besch-Williford CL, et al. Tissue engineering by self-assembly of cells printed into topologically defined structures. *Tissue Eng A.* 2008;14(3):413−421.

325. Duan B, Hockaday LA, Kang KH, Butcher JT. 3D bioprinting of heterogenous aortic valve conduits with alginate/galetin hydrogels. *J Biomed Mater Res A.* 2013;101(5): 1255−1264.

326. Nadav N, Assaf S, Reuven E, Idan G, Lior W, Tal D. Tissue engineering: 3D printing of personalized thich and perfusable cardiac patches and hearts. *Adv Sci.* 2019;6(11): 1970066.

327. Lee A, Hudson AR, Shiwarski DJ, Tashman JW, Hinton TJ, Yerneni S, et al. 3D bio-printing of collagen to rebuild components of the human heart. *Science.* 2019; 365(6452):482−487.

328. Manoor MS, Jiang Z, James T, Kong YL, Malatesta KA, Soboyejo WO, et al. 3D printed bionic ears. *Nano Lett.* 2013;13(6):2634−2639.

329. Nguyen DG, Funk J, Robbins JB, Crogan-Grundy C, Presnell SC, Singer T, et al. Bio-printed 3D primary liver tissues allow assessment of organ-level response to clinical drug induced toxicity in vitro. *PLoS One.* 2016;11(7):e0158674.

330. Norona LM, Nguyen DG, Gerber DA, Presnell SC, LeCluyse EL. Editor's highlight: modeling compound-induced fibrogenesis in vitro using three-dimensional bioprinted human liver tissues. *Toxicol Sci.* 2016;154(2):354−367.

331. Goulart E, de Caires-Junior LC, Telles-Silva KA, Araujo BHS, Rocco SA, Sforca M, et al. 3D bioprinting of liver spheroids derived from human induced pluripotent stem cells sustain liver function and viability in vitro. *Biofabrication.* 2019;12(1):015010.

332. King SM, Higgins JW, Nino CR, Smith TR, Paffenroth EH, Fairbairn CE, et al. 3D proximal tubule tissues recapitulate key aspects of renal physiology to enable nephro-toxicity testing. *Front Physiol.* 2017;8:123.

333. Atala A. Tissue engineering of human bladder. *Br Med Bull.* 2011;97:81−104.

334. Atala A, Bauer SB, Soker S, Yoo JJ, Retik AB. Tissue-engineered autologous bladders for patients needing cystoplasty. *Lancet.* 2006;367:1241−1246.

335. Muehleder S, Ovsianikov A, Zipperle J, Redl H, Holnthoner W. Connections matter: channeled hydrogels to improve vascularization. *Front Bioeng Biotechnol.* 2014;2:52.

336. Kim S, Lee H, Chung M, Jeon NL. Engineering of functional perfusable networks on a chip. *Lab Chip.* 2013;13(8):1489−1500.

337. Bishop ES, Mostafa S, Pakvasa M, Luu HH, Lee MJ, Wolf JM, et al. 3D bioprinting technologies in tissue engineering and regenerative medicine: current and future trends. *Genes Dis.* 2017;4(4):185−195.

338. Huang Y, He K, Wang X. Rapid prototyping of a hybrid hierarchical polyurethane-cell/ hydrogel construct for regenerative medicine. *Mater Sci Eng C Mater Biol Appl.* 2013; 33(6):3220−3229.

339. Skardal A, Zhang J, Prestwich GD. Bioprinting vessel-like constructs using hyaluronan hydrogels crosslinked with polythylene glycol tetracrylates. *Biomaterials*. 2010;31(24): 6173−6181.

340. Kucukgul C, Ozler SB, Inci I, Karakas E, Irmak S, Gozuacik D, et al. 3D bioprinting of biomimetic aortic vascular constructs with self-supporting cells. *Biotechnol Bioeng*. 2015;4:811−821.

341. Miller JS, Stevens KR, Yang MT, Baker BM, Nguyen DH, Cohen DM, et al. Rapid casting of patterned vascular networks for perfusable engineered three-dimensional tissues. *Nat Mater*. 2012;11(9):768−774.

342. Bertassoni LE, Cecconi M, Manoharan V, Nikkhah M, Hjortnaes J, Cristino AL, et al. Hydrogel bioprinted microchannel networks for vascularization of tissue engineering constructs. *Lab Chip*. 2014;14(13):2202−2211.

343. Mironov V, Prestwich G, Forgacs G. Bioprinting living structures. *J Mater Chem*. 2007; 17(20):2054−2060.

344. Zhang Y, Yu Y, Akkouch A, Dababneh A, Dolati F, Ozbolat IT. In vitro study of directly bioprinted perfusable vasculature conduits. *Biomater Sci*. 2015;3(1):134−143.

345. Ucuzian AA, Gassman AA, East AT, Greisler HP. Molecular mediators of angiogenesis. *J Burn Care Res*. 2010;31:158−175.

346. Poldervaart MT, Gremmels H, van Deventer K, Fledderus JO, Oner FC, Verhaar MC, et al. Prolonged presence of VEGF promotes vascularization in 3D bioprinted scaffolds with defined architecture. *J Contr Release*. 2014;184:58−66.

347. Romanazzo S, Vedicherla S, Moran C, Kelly DJ. Meniscus ECM-functionalized hydrogels containing infrapatellar fat pat-derived stem cells for bioprinting of regionally defined meniscal tissue. *J Tissue Eng Regen Med*. 2018;12:1826−1835.

348. *Health resources and services administration*. U.S. Government Information on Organ Donation and Tranplantation; 2020. https://www.organdonor.gov/statistics-stories/statistics.html. Accessed January 19, 2020. Date last reviewed: February 2019.

349. Vermeulen N, Haddow G, Seymour T, Faulkner-Jones A, Shu W. 3D bioprint me: a socioethical view of bioprinting human organs and tissues. *J Med Ethics*. 2017;43: 618−624.

3D printing and virtual and augmented reality in medicine and surgery: tackling the content development barrier through co-creative approaches

Panagiotis E. Antoniou[1], Panagiotis D. Bamidis[2]

[1]*Senior Postdoctoral Researcher on Medical Physics, Biomedical Engineering and Digital Healthcare Innovations, Lab of Medical Physics and Digital Innovation, Department of Medicine, School of Health Sciences, Aristotle University of Thessaloniki, Thessaloniki, Greece;* [2]*Professor of Medical Physics, Medical Informatics and Medical Education, Lab of Medical Physics and Digital Innovation, Department of Medicine, School of Health Sciences, Aristotle University of Thessaloniki, Thessaloniki, Greece*

Introduction

Information and Communication Technologies (ICT) defined healthcare interventions from their inception. Reduced costs, increased efficacy toward growth, social equality, diagnostic efficacy, and treatment effectiveness were the outcomes of these interventions. Contemporary education for healthcare, in particular, has greatly advanced toward widely varying educational resources and activities in the ICT area.[1] The incentive behind this lies in the need for unconstrained time and place to access clinical skills worldwide.[2] The incorporation of virtual, augmented, and, recently, mixed reality (VR/AR/MR) technologies was an approach that has greatly impacted the immersive medical education field. Defining these immersive technologies sometimes is difficult as there are, at points, overlaps. Nevertheless, a viable description of VR is the replacement of external sensory inputs (mainly visual and audio) with those generated by computers using a headset device. AR, instead, is the overlap of digital content over the real world using either 2D or 3D markers in the real-world environment. Finally, MR is similar to AR with one key difference. Instead of the real-world marker being a preprogrammed static item or image, the content overlay is done after completing a 3D mapping of the current environment. This way features can be used in intuitive ways such as table-positioned 3D models or 2D images and "hanging" notes on walls. There is evidence that such technologies significantly increase the educational impact of an episode of learning and subsequently can have a significant impact on educational outcomes.[3] Realized examples include experiential world exploration,[4] visualizations of high-impact physics and chemistry concepts,[5−7] and even the incorporation of such modalities for VPs.[8] It is this immediate capacity of engagement of these modalities that not only motivates the student but also allows the educational material to be internalized, thus avoiding conceptual errors.[9]

Specifically in the field of surgery, there is a significant body of literature for both the efficacy and the specific technologies implemented for VR/AR visualizations. Additional features such as haptic technologies and suites of sensors (e.g., hand and finger tracking) have been implemented for all aspects of surgical training and education. Preoperative training, surgical anatomy, 3D visualizations for new approaches, and incision paths are the first and obvious ones. Real-time augmentation of the surgical field with MR content, or even the use of VR for relaxing the patient prior to surgery, is the less obvious ones. Preoperative patient VR presentations for better understanding of the specific surgical process have even impacted the overall litigation cost of healthcare institutions, since the visualizations prevented frivolous lawsuits against them by uneducated patients or relatives. These really exciting contemporary developments are mentioned here, only in passing since they are very well documented in the literature. For example, a contemporary, at the time of writing of this work, and rather succinct review of the overall applications and impact of VR/AR in the field of surgery is the one by Desselle et al.[10]

Recent advances in technology have also moved the field of application for ICT technologies from the intangible (AR/VR/MR) to the realm of the tangible with easily accessible 3D print capabilities and applications.[11−13]

This work aims to present the state of the art of the newly emergent 3D print technology in medical/surgical applications while moving past a simple description of the technologies for the maturing AR/VR/MR field and presenting a viable roadmap for participatory immersive content creation and standardized workflows and implementation pipelines. As such, it aims to become a useful tool for the medical/surgical educator and technologist in order to incorporate faster and easier immersive content in their curricula.

3D printing in surgery

The development of 3D printing (3DP) technology, also referred to as rapid prototyping (RP), has produced a more sophisticated method for an intuitive and realistic 3D-manufactured model that goes beyond basic 3D-shaped simulation on a flat screen.[14] For its usage in medical fields, the immediacy between concept and final development is the most significant of the many benefits of 3DP technology. In a clinical environment, the prospect of one-stop development from medical imaging to 3DP intensified the current medical movement toward personalized, patient-specific care. Second, 3DP, as an additive manufacturing technique,[15] demonstrates the characteristics of "zero constraint—zero skill" for 3D manufacturing, which are suitable for medical applications, since the form of 3D models produced from patient-specific medical photographs is typically too complicated to be created utilizing traditional manufacturing methods. In comparison to industrial approaches, 3D model architecture for 3DP medical applications is simpler since most can be obtained utilizing 3D surface reconstruction of medical images with the aid of postprocessed images. Thus, 3DP computers have been used in a number of medical applications since the early 2000s. The technique has been used primarily for rough tissue applications owing to the strength of most 3D-printable products.[16] The advantage of such manufactures derives from the improved sensory perception that the sense of contact conveys to the user.[17]

Technically, to achieve these goals, high-quality images must be collected from multidetector computed tomography (MDCT) or magnetic resonance imaging scans in order to create a valuable 3D virtual (3DV) reconstruction. The slicing width of the obtained photographs should not reach 2 mm, with an optimum value of less than 1 mm.[16,18] Picture preparation for 3DP begins with a segmentation process, the purpose of which is to reduce the complexity of the original image by choosing the anatomy to be printed, which is then extrapolated from the rest of the image.[16]

The 3DV model is then exported as a surface triangulation language (STL) file that defines the spatial geometry of the object via a set of oriented triangular facets named mesh[16,18] software. The smaller the scale of these triangles, the more detailed is the surface of the 3DV model.[16] At this point, surface smoothing is used to fix defects or sharp edges; in addition, further preparation of the STL file should be carried out in conjunction with the final purpose of the printed item, such as the production of interlocking parts to allow the assembly/disassembly of the model, which is then ready for 3DP.

The core idea in the actual 3DP production phase is the development of artifacts by a layer process: the 3DV model is broken down into a sequence of 2D layers that are deployed one after the other by a 3D printer. This "additive" method is the perfect way for 3D printers to handle extremely complicated geometries, such as anatomical templates.[16,18,19]

3DP technology

3D printers may be differentiated by the method of deposition and curing method (e.g., content jetting, material extrusion), each requiring a broad variety of functional materials of various characteristics, such as clarity, stiffness or deformity, mechanical power, chromatic performance, and so on[16,20,21] (Figs. 4.2 and 4.3). In certain instances, a support frame or dedicated support content can be used to help the building and may be discarded or dissolved until the printing phase has been completed.[16,21] In rare instances, owing to the difficulties of cleaning and postprocessing complex anatomies, each configuration may be printed separately and then stuck together to reconstruct the final object; however, this technique is avoided due to potential misalignments during the assembly of 3D-printed components.[18]

3DP technology used in medicine[22] can be categorized according to the technique, substrate, or planned deposition process used. Scientific grouping covers stereolithography (SLA), polyjet printing, multijet printing (MJP), digital light processing (DLP), direct metal laser sintering (DMLS), selective laser sintering (SLS), color-jet printing (CJP or binder-jet), fused deposition modeling (FDM), laminated object manufacturing, and electron beam melting. Material classification covers titanium alloys, metal powder, eutectic metals, alloy metals, ceramic powder, photopolymer, paper, foil, plastic film, and thermoplastic.

SLA apparatus

The SLA device consists of a photosensitive resin tank, a model-building frame, and an ultraviolet (UV) laser for curing the resin (Fig. 4.2). A computer-controlled mirror is used to concentrate the UV laser on the resin surface and to cure the resin on a slice-by-slice basis. This slice data are fed to the RP unit, which guides the exposure direction of the UV laser to the resin surface. The layers are cured sequentially and tie together to create a strong object, starting from the bottom of the model and building upward. Each fresh layer of resin is cleaned through the surface of the previous layer using a wiper blade until it is revealed and cured. The model is then extracted from the bath and cured for a longer time in the UV compartment.[22] Generally, stereolithography (SL) is known to have the maximum precision and the best surface finish in any RP technology. The content of the model is durable, mildly brittle, and comparatively lightweight.[23,24]

Polyjet printing

Polyjet printing is achieved utilizing state-of-the-art, layer-by-layer, extrusion of photopolymer materials in ultrathin layers of 16 μm on a built-in tray before the model is finished. Each photopolymer layer is cured by UV light directly after it has been injected, providing completely cured versions that can be treated and used immediately without postcuring. A gel-like support layer that is specifically formulated to preserve intricate geometries and that is quickly withdrawn by hand and water jetting is used.[22] Polyjet printing may take advantage of a range of materials, like rubberlike content, and the postprocessing period is short and easy. At present, this procedure is excessively time intensive and thus too costly to use in surgical applications.

Multijet printing

MJP's liquid-based 3DP technology uses a print head to spread acrylic photopolymer (part) and wax (support) simultaneously. Injected products are treated with UV light. MJP is the most accurate 3DP method. The opaqueness of the key acrylic photopolymer resins can be managed, but its intensity is relatively poor. In addition, the shape deformation arises at 65 degrees or higher.

Digital light processing

DLP's liquid-based 3DP approach uses the traditional method of a DLP projector as a light source. In principle, a 2D image is projected onto a light-curable resin in a vat sculpting the print. This system demonstrates an outstanding surface finish and the quickest printing operation. The mechanical properties of the material used are fine, but the form and color of the material are limited. In addition, the content and printing device are costly.

Direct metal laser sintering

Using a solid-state Yb fiber laser beam, the powder-based 3DP process of the DMLS methodology selectively produces several variants.[25] Through SLS of various metal powders (e.g., aluminum, cobalt, brass, nickel alloy, stainless steel, and titanium) by the laser, guided through each layer of the 3D model, a variety of materials can be constructed. Since the metal powder used plays the role of a support in the model, postprocessing, including support removal, is not needed. Moreover, the printing efficiency is usually outstanding.

Selective sintering laser

SLS's powder-based 3DP processing utilizes the CO_2 laser beam to selectively produce materials. 2D slice data are fed into the SLS unit, which guides the exposure direction of the laser over a thin layer of powder already accumulated on the baking tray and leveled with a roller. The laser heats the powder particles, fuses them to create a dense sheet, and then travels along the X- and Y-axes to design the structures according to the computer-aided design (CAD) results. After the first layer fuses, the create tray moves down, where a fresh layer of powder is placed and sintered. The method is replicated before the item is done. The prototype surface is postprocessed with sandblasting.[22] The SLS prototype is opaque and has an abrasive surface. The production period of the prototype is long, spanning sometimes 15 h. The precision of the SLS model is reasonably high, with an overall standard error of 0.1–0.6 mm. Owing to the high cost of the components, multiple pieces are assembled concurrently.[26] The equipment is costly, but, due to patent expiry, low-cost SLS devices are starting to emerge.

Color-jet printing

The CJP approach uses the print head to selectively spread the binder onto the powder sheet. Next, a thin film of powder is applied over a tray using a roller, identical to the one used in the SLS method. The print head scans the powder tray and delivers a continuous jet of solution, which fuses the powder particles when it touches them. No support systems are needed when the prototype is being assembled, as the surrounding powder supports the unconnected components. The leftover underlying powder is sucked until the process is complete. In the finishing process, the surfaces of the prototype are infiltrated with a cyanoacrylate-based substance to harden the framework.[26] The printing technique allows the construction of complex geometric constructs, such as hanging partitions within cavities, without artificial support structures.[22] Since it uses a CMYK color ink cartridge, as used in traditional 2D printers, a 3D molded model may be printed in about the same color spectrum. Printing and infiltration procedures take ~4–6 h. The 3D printers used in this method are reasonably inexpensive, have short construction times, and are simple to manage. In addition, these 3D printers are cost efficient, produce minimal waste, and are precise (± 0.1 mm in the Z-axis, ± 0.2 mm in the X- and Y-planes). They are also compact in scale and capable of manufacturing hard, soft, and versatile versions. This technology has lower costs than related methods.[26]

Modeling of fused deposition

FDM's solid-based 3DP technology uses a similar concept to SL in that it creates models on a layer-by-layer basis. The key distinction is that the layers are dispersed as a thermoplastic, which is extruded from a fine nozzle. Acrylonitrile butadiene styrene is a widely used substance for this treatment. The 3D model is built by extrusion of the heated thermoplastic material onto the foam surface along the direction shown by the model details. When the coating has been deposited, the nozzle is lifted from 0.278 to 0.356 mm and the next layer is put at the top of the previous layer. This step is replicated until completion.[22] As with SL, support systems for FDM models are necessary because time is needed for the thermoplastic to harden and the layers to fuse together.[27] Supports may be extracted using simple mechanical tools, or dissolved with specific acidic solutions. While it is the most common 3D printer technology, the surface finish is reasonably poor. To improve that, several postprocessing options, including acetone fumigation, may also be used.

Surgical applications for 3DP

Preoperational training

3D-printed anatomical representations are exceptionally precise reproductions of the target anatomy. When they are observed and manipulated, they can assist visual and tactile input to fuse and transfer vital information to the surgeon.[18,28] Surgery measures may be mapped or checked directly on the blueprint, identifying possible technical difficulties owing to adverse anatomy or disease-related changes, if any.[18,28,29] Several studies from various specialties have demonstrated the effectiveness of this application in presurgical decision-making, such as head, spinal, maxillofacial, transplantation, general surgery, and orthopedics.[29–31] Here, 3DP has helped to identify vital at-risk structures, describe resection lines or dissection planes, and determine the magnitude of the disease to be ablated, in short, thoroughly familiarize the surgeon with anatomy prior to surgery.[18,29–31] The degree of precision was verified in several experiments by the incredibly low margin of error in terms of mm when users were requested to approximate measurements (i.e., distances, lengths, or volumes) on both 3D-printed models and other picture platforms such as MDCT or 3DV.[28,32] In other analyses, the volume of resection of the liver was completely compatible with that expected with 3DP prior to surgery in a series of studies.[28,32]

Intraoperative navigation

There is a very fine distinction in the usage of 3D-printed anatomical fabricates for preoperative or intraoperative navigation. One of their benefits is that they are lightweight items that the surgeon is able to carry into the operating room for intraoperative reassessment in the event of complicated orientation.[18,28,29] In robotic surgery, where the operator is stationary at the console, this usage is readily accessible without restrictions; for other environments, there are a number of printing materials appropriate for sterilization, thereby expanding the use to the operational field.[30,31]

Education and training

The ability of 3DP for educational purposes has been largely evaluated at several stages.[16,29–31,33–38] The study of human anatomy by medical students is traditionally focused on simple pictures or sketches drawn from books or atlases with low understanding of information and spatial relation, as dissection opportunities are limited. Surgical residents and inexperienced surgeons are subjected to everyday in-room surgery, but profound anatomical expertise requires time to acquire, given the interindividual differences and pathological distortions that are frequently experienced. The 3D-printed versions, based on patient-specific imaging details, enable accurate identification of anatomical landmarks independent of any divergence from the standard. They have been shown to be successful in a variety of evaluation studies, including a few randomized controlled trials, in which participants of varying experience (medical students, interns, junior or senior surgeons, radiologists) were asked to test a given anatomy on 3D-printed model and other platforms (CT scans, 3DV reconstructions, or cadavers according to particular criteria). The 3D-printed versions received higher scores than the 2D or 3DV formats and were not comparable to those of the cadaveric materials in the accurate recognition of main anatomical components. In addition, participants greatly appreciated the added benefit of 3D-printed models in the learning phase, as seen by the average high rates provided in specific studies.[18,35,36]

The 3DP replication of a certain anatomical area or configuration can be shared by doctors of various specialties in order to enhance the comprehension of a particular treatment, or the handling of a particular patient. A 3D stable, tangible entity with special features such as transparency or detachable sections that render internal components transparent will easily cross differences between practitioners in the evaluation of traditional 2D imaging.

Patient therapy

3D-printed models have proven to be valuable methods for preoperative therapy with patients and relatives, allowing doctors to clarify problems linked to the illness or the surgery.[18,28] Patients and their families were extremely satisfied when guidance was given on a tangible anatomical model that they could see and treat as they wished; indeed, the model prompted more questions on their part, thereby facilitating consideration of technical information and alternative alternatives, if any.[18] Patients have been seen to have a far better comprehension about how the operation is conducted, what kind of results can be anticipated, what difficulties might be met intraoperatively, or what problems can emerge thereafter, if these issues are addressed in their own 3D-printed platform. When this complete agreement is obtained, the approval of the suggested therapy is likely to rise, while the incidence of future medical–legal conflicts will decrease accordingly.

Simulation of surgery

Reproduction of hollow structures, such as hearts or vessels of different sizes, from aorta to tiny divisions of arteries and veins, may be made of soft, deformable photopolymer resins that imitate the mechanical properties of real human tissue.[16,39] These mark the advent of a modern age of surgical simulation. Surgeons, with every sort of experience, from trainees to professionally qualified operators, may train themselves in as many activities as these models can reproduce. Objectives of the simulation may be to refine a certain ability by several repetitions of the same exercise, to evaluate experimental surgical devices outside the operating room, or to plan for a specific operation until it takes place on the patient. Preoperative simulation of complex procedures has recently been attempted on patient-specific 3D-printed models where vascular anatomy was made of deformed material that enabled vessel clamping, stapling, and anastomosis.[40] The subsequent experience was evaluated by the surgeon to be sufficiently realistic, in terms of the technical efficiency of the material, and successful in supporting the tasks. Also, instruction on the same realistic anatomy improved confidence for the actual operation. Overall, 3DP is currently enabling for customized instruction that users with every sort of experience may adapt to their own needs of expertise and caters to the specific anatomical structure of the patient, thanks to the precision of the printed manufacturers.

Production of anatomical phantoms

A 3D phantom reconstruction of an anatomical region of concern (i.e., the abdominal cavity, the cranium, the thorax or a tiny portion of it) may be printed from the same patient's radiological imaging data set to match the corresponding 3D-printed model.[19,41] This kind of platform allows additional activities to be carried out, rather than those linked to the goal of the operation, for example, access to the target itself. In certain cases, it can be a question of how to access a deep anatomical location, particularly if it is limited to a small space or surrounded by delicate structures. In others, the restrictions placed by the procedure or the complexion of the patient may pose challenges in deciding the most simple, less painful, and most efficient access to surgery. For example, the use of these 3D-printed architectures in minimally invasive surgery can help to decide the optimal configuration of the trocars or to formulate technological solutions to improve the exposure of the area of interest even in a simulation setting.

Surgical equipment

Printing in 3D has almost no restrictions, a fact which paves the way for an infinite range of applications. This is especially the case for reconstructive skeletal surgery, not just because the solidity of bone tissue can be readily replicated with 3DP but also because many of the methods and equipment that are routinely utilized (such as implants, prostheses, or surgical instruments) are ideal for 3DP. These, in addition to the patient-specific form, are able to be used instead of the corresponding standard models. To date, many forms of models, maps, jigs, and other contour-shaped instruments have been printed in 3D to support basic procedure steps: bone drilling at predetermined depths and positions, length estimation of screws or other fixing mechanisms, trajectories and angles, placing in the proper place, and so on.[16,30,42] Other devices are intentionally printed for use as implantable materials and remain in place indefinitely.[30,31] In comparison to traditional prosthesis, 3DP technology allows for a patient-specific configuration of manufactures that suit seamlessly the anatomy to be substituted. Exact curvatures or symmetries will ensure absolute conformity to the needs of the situation, not least of them, aesthetic concerns. In reality, such highly personalized implants allow possible precise, lifelike reconstructions of recognizable sections such as the skull, face, or limbs, the social effect which is indispensable for patients.[30,31] However, the better an implant suits an anatomical structure, the stronger the practical results would be regarding potential adverse effects. Poor suitability could lead to persistent postoperative pain, or motor disfunction in joint replaced or reconstructive surgery.

In addition, when not specifically inserted to replace weakened structures, these customized instruments may be used as precise prototypes or scaffolds from which other forms of prosthetic material may be molded before being grafted to the patient.[30,31] The use of 3D-printed scaffolds has also been explored for the development of biological tissue implants generated by stromal cell migration and distributed inside the 3D scaffolding architecture.[30,31,43] This novel boundary of the printing of 3D tissues, as well as the 3DP of cells (bioprinting) with the final goal of specifically constructing living tissues, is still at its early stage of study, while encouraging findings can be anticipated from the preliminary evidence available in the literature.[16,30,31,43] The same refers to whole organ printing that has already been proposed by several scholars, but whose actualization appears much more far-reaching due to the difficulty of numerous cell types employed during the bioprinting process and the complicated vasculature needed to preserve tissue viability.

Intangible immersive media in medical/surgical training and education

All applications of eXtended reality (XR) (AR/VR/MR) in the field of surgery, or medicine in general, are aimed at presenting the surgeon/doctor with information necessary for them to complete their objectives. This information aims to improve their manual, decision-making, or theoretical skills, thus enabling them in their tasks. Thus, in one way or another, XR is intrinsically a training/educational tool in the healthcare field. For that reason, in this chapter, XR will be explored in the context of surgery education and training. In this outline, we will move away from the description of technologies and means to present (a) an overview of the challenges that medical/surgical technology enhanced learning face, (b) the current way for implementing XR in surgical or medical cases, and (c) an overview of the emerging approach for XR digital content, that of participatory design and development.

Case- or problem-based instruction and other small group training frameworks are currently used extensively in medical education.[44,45] Simulations, examples of future cases, and other task-based episodes of learning are also included. A special advantage of scenario narratives nominated as virtual patients (VPs) in the health-care field is that they are expressly designed to facilitate the learning goals, while simultaneously fulfilling students' standards and skill sets to create a gaming-informed, media-saturated learning environment. A case can be explored across several channels, allowing students to practice their decision-making skills, and the effects of their decisions can be uncovered in a comfortable and interesting at-mosphere.[46] VPs are defined as "interactive computer simulations of real-life clin-ical scenarios for the purpose of healthcare and medical training, education, or assessment."[47] Web-based VPs, unlike actual patients, are repeatable because they are applied as branching narratives,[48] with little time, location, and failure con-straints during clinical competence practice. Medical students have the ability to read about and practice a wide range of even unusual and complicated diseases that they can experience later in their clinical careers. Due to the reproducibility of case outcomes and the structured validated appraisal provisions that occur in most VP platforms, VP positions have been recognized as an effective and essential teaching method for contemporary medical education. There is a global movement toward VP growth, due to which there are many academic institutions working to-ward that aim. The long-term effect of VPs on medical education was recognized early on,[47] and standardization solutions for repurposing, reuse, and transferability were introduced as early as 2010,[49,50] with a formal standard, the MedBiquitous VP standard. A series of modifications, such as semantic annotations, have been intro-duced so that VP content can be reused, while other projects have also devoted them-selves to a range of areas, including elderly care[51] and still more intensified techniques, such as virtual environments,[52,53] or VR and AR.

There are several ideas that have been applied on this experiential front. One of them is the immersive laboratory. Virtual laboratories use simulations and computer models in addition to a multitude of other tools, such as film, to help replace real-life laboratory experiences. A virtual laboratory can include several interactive simula-tions that are sponsored by discussion boards and video demonstrations, or even so-phisticated simulations that are meant to be used collaboratively. They encourage self-directed, self-paced learning (e.g., repetitive content, off-hour access). This en-sures that learners can retain their initiative and expanded participation in the learning process, while interactivity allows students to acquire more advanced lab-oratory skills beyond merely learning content. Such laboratory methods mask the fundamental shortcomings of modern medical school curricula. Most commonly, laboratory hands-on procedures are inaccessible to student training due to cost, time, or safety issues. With theoretical understanding but without clinical and labo-ratory knowledge in the real world, this leaves medical students to train for their clinical and laboratory rotations.

The focus of this work, as previously outlined, is not to describe the state of the art for the relevant technologies. A far more interesting, albeit more challenging topic for the medical/surgical educator and/or technologist is that of AR/VR content availability. Immersive content is expensive and time consuming in its production as reflected by its financial projections circa 2021.[54] Costs in the span of tens or hundreds of millions are acceptable in the entertainment industry where there can be a sustainable return on such investments. In the medical education sector, this is not always the case regarding return on investment; however, the cost, based on market size, is still substantial.[55] Expensive, state-of-the-art solutions are usually available for specific use cases, but these incur significant overheads not so much for the initial purchase, but for updating and maintaining a significant, relevant amount of content for such bespoke solutions.

A different, currently emerging solution involves a participatory approach for content design and development. It involves a standardized use case based on the VP template of interactive medical content. The core of this template is the navigation in a tree of narrative, or exploratory nodes through user-selectable links. This use case, being tried and true in a web-based format, has a number of requirements for transferring effectively in MR or VR:

a) It requires a standardized pipeline for design and implementation in MR or VR.
b) It needs a rather specific co-creative user-centric workflow for collaboration between technologists and educators.
c) Greatly benefits from the use of tangible, 3D-printed anatomical props for additional immediacy and accessibility to the learners.

In the following sections of this chapter, we will explore the standard implementation pipeline as it has been applied in a previous work. Pickering et al.[56–58] present a roadmap for integrating the aforementioned components into a cohesive medical and surgical education content development approach for immersive, tangible, or intangible media.

Implementing a standardized pipeline for MR medical spaces

An MR space that could run simulated environments in a minimally equipped room was a reasonably common use case that has been introduced in previous works.[52] The only thing that needed to be done was to add any printed pictures. To explore the space, a user would use their mobile device. The interface provided the consumer with a narrative medical event that checked their decision-making capabilities as it scanned the specific augmented image objectives in the room. In such instances, time-sensitive procedures or even object encounters can be involved. As visualized from a mobile screen, digital objects that augment real ones can communicate, overlap, or recognize one another. Since digital assets displayed in the real world will radically change due to user interaction, digital content has developed into a very strong storytelling tool in that capacity. For example, in a cardiology case, a person will be able to communicate with a simulated electrocardiogram on their mobile device and gain real-time updates about a particular patient case that would be apparent in the actual space.

In terms of execution, such a case follows a stateful solution that has been used in other platforms.[53] In brief, as the VP episode unfolds in the MR world, the game logic keeps track of the progress through the nodes and shows content and feedback as the player moves across the VP nodes. The instructional goals of this material determined the production platform for this implementation. Since the overall approach must be reuseable and transferable, custom game engines or standalone 3D solutions are not suitable. For deployment, a solution incorporating Unity 3D and the Vuforia AR/digital eyewear interface was chosen. This production environment blends the ease of use needed for accelerated development with the flexibility required for the form and amount of content intended to be required within the scope of this project.

The back end of this program uses an efficient database scheme with a VP repurposing environment to accommodate such a use case. There are three sections of the schema. The VP component helps you to save connections, nodes, and cases that identify entire VPs. The environment portion helps you to save details about the configuration of 3D assets and ecosystems. These components come together in the 3D case component to store a meaningful representation of a simulated case as it appears in a 3D world. This schema is listed in more detail elsewhere.[53]

A simple, low-cost VR setup with a mobile device and a low-cost headset, such as a Google Cardboard, is used in this solution. The use case capacities are compounded and converted as the platform is updated to a more powerful MR platform, such as the MS HoloLens.

Storyboarding the educational resource

The HoloLens MR program, code-named "HoloAnatomy," was developed as a teaching aid for the lecturer. With that, we hoped to construct a holographic "Mannequin" that would serve as an anatomical cadaver and show the central nervous system's ascending and descending pathways. The scenario was developed using the lecture's narration as a reference. Following the lecturer's initial introduction to the subject, the MR application will be launched and projected for all users to see. The introduction opened with a brief graphic representation of the human body, accompanied by a color-coded identification of the somatomes (defined as a field of somatic and autonomic innervation based on embryologic segmental origin of the somatic tissues[59]).

Following that, a clear representation of a human body was seen, with the spinal cord being the only visible structure. The app allowed the user to pick particular parts of the spinal cord, pons, medulla, or midbrain. There the lecturer could pick one of four ascending or descending neural pathways to be represented in each segment, either independently or collectively with different color coding.

Finally, the lecturer may illustrate where each pathway leads to the cerebral cortex using a divided vision of the two hemispheres of the brain. A demonstration panel was also mounted so that chosen structures could be viewed at all times. Fig. 4.1 displays the graphical storyboarding for the HoloAnatomy app.

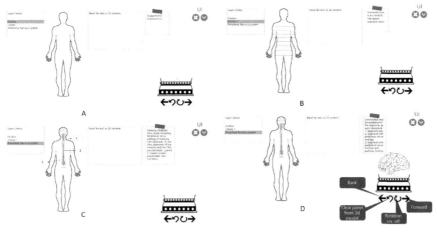

FIGURE 4.1

Storyboarding of the HoloAnatomy mixed reality application. (A) Introductory stage, (B) somatome view, (C) central nervous system (CNS) view, and (D) detailed CNS section with relevant pathways demonstrated.

Development methodology

The fulcrum of the educentric approach to "HoloAnatomy's" growth deviated from the traditional software development phase of specification elicitation, design, and development. Instead, it was an iterative cross-disciplinary approach that immersed developers in medical subjects and medical professionals in the digital resource's design processes. Several sessions were conducted, during which medical experts trained the development team on medical issues so that the engineering team could foresee potential points of implementation when expert intervention would be needed. Additionally, the engineering team reciprocated by familiarizing the medical educators with the medium's and implementation platform's technical shortcomings and possibilities such that they could make better design decisions in their iterative function requests. The HoloAnatomy application was built in an iterative, incrementally optimized manner, thanks to this participatory design method. Furthermore, this process provided the lecturer and participating medical experts with valuable, realistic digital knowledge, allowing them to be as effective as possible when using the resource in the classroom.

Description of the final application and its presentation

The application was built in Unity 3D, Microsoft's chosen environment for HoloLens deployment. The "HoloAnatomy" application was produced after an iterative educationally centric design process with only slight improvements to the presentation. Fig. 4.2 provides a representative snapshot of the development environment.

With two exceptions, the storyboarded central flow was retained. The lecturer considered the original requirement for a panel in which each part of the spinal cord would be presented to be disorienting. Both the instructor and probably the students

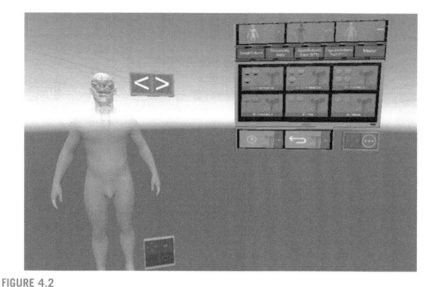

FIGURE 4.2

Screenshot of the HoloAnatomy application.

were puzzled by the transition from the whole anatomical body to the panel. As a result, it was decided to delete it and present chosen parts of the CNS in midair in front of the entire human depiction. Aside from that, the lecturer demanded that we have two presentation modes in the app. There are two modes: "lecturer" and "exploratory." The first would be linear, with arrows to pass forward and backward in the application's narrative so that the lecturer could concentrate on presenting the content (Fig. 4.3).

The second will be for questions and debate, with the lecturer being able to quickly switch from one subject to the next and illustrate things as needed (Fig. 4.4).

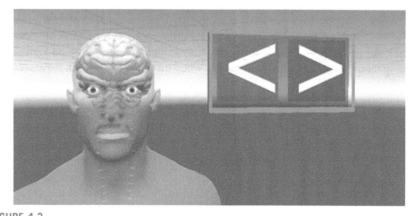

FIGURE 4.3

Lecturer mode.

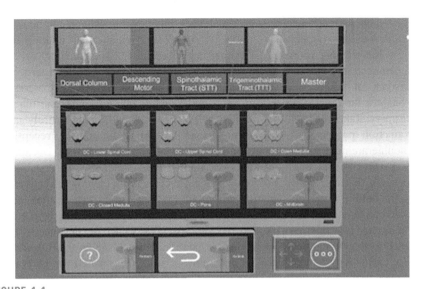

FIGURE 4.4

Exploratory mode.

Proposing a co-creative digital content development pipeline

The idea of co-creation was born out of marketing, primarily product design. The method of assessing an item's value bid through client involvement rather than conventional statistical surveying avenues was originally known as value co-creation (VCC).[60,61] Clients/users played a dynamic role in VCC, working with the central stakeholder (firm, developers, etc.) to create product value.[60,62] The core components of the joint effort for forming added value were defined as self-reliance, contact, commitment, and experience.[63] When it comes to problems like commodity use and the whole value distribution chain, VCC is more than the sum of these components.[60,64] According to marketing analysis,[65] the two elements of VCC, referred to as benefit in use and co-creation, have over 27 different meanings. VCC is reiterated in earlier literature as a combining factor of buyer skills and actual cooperative firm—client product co-creation.[64,66,67]The numbers at the end should link to the references of the same number.

In the context of coproduction, co-creation provides dynamic input for new item changes to the product design phase.[68,69] Coproduction requires actual or indirect "collaboration with customers,"[70,71] as well as constructive involvement in the product/service configuration process.[72,73] Client investment can take the form of a passive component on the edges of a company's workflows[72] or a dynamic, central component focused on the sharing and learning of the firm's skills and data.[74,75] Client association, rather than illustrating mutual physical, behavioral, and exchange practices, as well as access to traditional masteries, has been used to characterize co-creation.[76] Cogeneration[77,78] has been described as an arrangement of acts completed by actors (financial, social, and others) engaged in value chain networks. It is carried out by cooperation,[79] trade,[80,81] and the participation of common assets in the value-creating process.[82] The primary stakeholder (firm, creator) achieves both demonstrated client request fulfillment and leveraging client expertise for firm expansion when clients invest assets by co-creation forms.[83,84] Co-creation also enables the artistic process to be dispersed while staying under the reach of the primary stakeholder.[85] This method helps clients to participate entirely in the coproduction process,[86,87] with some research defining mutualism, receptivity, and nonhierarchical partnerships as components of coproduction.[75,83] Because of this expansive understanding of the co-creation process, research[61] has established information sharing as one of the most critical factors in co-creation effectiveness.

In the field of medical education, this exact exchange of expertise is tapped for the co-creative endeavor. The medical sector is the focus group for medical education material, and this section also has the specialist expertise that needs to be included in the development of medical education content. Given this inspiration, the aim of this research is to explain the architecture of a co-creative digital content production pipeline for medical education, allowing digital medical content creation to keep up with increasingly expanding medical awareness.

The above methodologies and tools are streamlined into a content creation pipeline. Flexible scheduling of program and 3D model resource iterations based on multiple Scrum pushes as described in the Scrum and Agile development system[88,89] will be the basis of the technique in this endeavor. The particulars are described below. Professionals who specialize in technological resource creation (coders, 3D designers, etc.) are referred to as "the development team," "developers," or "the engineering team" in this section. Topical professionals and co-creators, such as physicians, teachers, and other healthcare educators, would be referred to as "co-creating consumers," "co-creators," and "domain experts," respectively.

Preparation and planning stage

The co-creating users' acclimation and exposure to the pipeline's technique and tools take place in this point. This will be in the form of a short workshop that would get all of the participants up to date on how to use the co-creative infrastructure. Planning would likely require the assigning of specifically defined positions. Domain experts would be identified not only as a co-creator in the pipeline but also as a structured product owner in the SCRUM position scheme[89] for each resource or community of resources. The production team will be able to offer concentrated feedback across familiar positions as a result of this.

Co-creation stage

Participants are granted access to the co-creative infrastructure and are given a deadline for finishing their content. Users will have access to professional support from the technical staff in the co-creation period, which is still assembling the appropriate material that must be created from scratch.

Technical facilitation stage

The technical team creates the appropriate content, which is then accepted by the co-creating customers. This stage would see the construction of entirely new, essential capital. This means that medical 3D designers can produce multiple versions of the 3D models online, and programming technological facilitators will create interaction templates that are not protected by current tools. Until agreeing to launching a resource for integration in a particular instructional episode, the respective product owner will review it.

Prototyping stage

The resource has been deployed and is being investigated. The tools' instructional alignment will be checked by trial runs and tested by focus group sessions with customers. For the next move of the resource through the pipeline, bugs, problems, and material issues are found.

Components for implementing the pipeline

A ubiquitous use case

The part of an experiential resource for healthcare education that is provided is rather well defined. It is a simulated space that is superimposed over every real space (room, auditorium, etc.). Modern headsets, such as Microsoft's HoloLens,[90] support spatial visualization of the external world for this purpose, enabling ubiquitous application of visual information in any environment. Furthermore, the introduction of game development frameworks such as Unity 3D[91] makes for a single development—multiple platform implementation. Customizability of such environments with visual data structures (e.g., Unity 3D's scriptable objects[92]) is a key factor in making their transition into an editing tool that even nontechnical users can use for such unique use cases and data models.

Linking medical data repositories with the user experience

A structured information level modeling is required to connect particular healthcare issues to applicable technology enhanced learning (TEL) services. This method of modeling necessitates the use of existing relevant taxonomies that succinctly define relevant medical environments, as well as the development of user experience (UX) taxonomies to include hierarchies connecting user interface and 3D environment features with UXs (collision, button click, etc.). The MeSH.A and MeSH.E04 taxonomies of the Medical Subject Headings systematic taxonomy[93] include examples of taxonomic distinctions between systemic and practical realms for healthcare. Healthcare learning goals and contextual fields would be able to easily correlate with assets used in AR/MR services if semantic connections are used. Such experiential elements would be codified in a more ad hoc yet self-consistent data level modeling way to promote a semantically enriched back end where no formal taxonomies exist.

A semantically annotated visual data structures

The data modeling for such a project will be based on a method that has previously been used in other platforms. A story scenario can be applied[94] in any 3DV world using a basic state-full, node-link branching strategy (display based, AR, VR, MR). An exploratory educational environment may be generated with the same method, with the nodes acting as basic stages of the discovery and the connections serving as switches (e.g., through buttons or position triggers) between each stage of the learning process. The VDS is an entity that includes many attributes that can be manipulated programmatically. A 3D model with or without animation, a text narration, or explanations are examples of these. It will also provide data modeling details such as the asset's function in a particular educational resource, complete with connections to and from other related tools, as well as the 3D resource's graphical points of contact (colliders, keys, and so on). When annotated with custom or current taxonomies, this VDS is easy to use even by nonexperts (they can easily search through a repository of such resources, find, explore them, and finally edit the narrative details to fit their new purpose). It is also clear enough for a nontechnical person to grasp how to do it. The user will drag and drop these visual tools together and convey narrative or exploratory connections between them directly in the 3D context using preprogrammed provisions. As a consequence, a full resource can be prototyped solely by the co-creating user without the need for technological assistance. When preexisting solutions are inadequate, the technical experts' task would be to promote the process by developing brand new 3D assets and coding unforeseen interaction specifications from the co-creating customer.

Conclusions

This brief overview of 3D print and virtual resources coalesces to a rather emergent and ambitious vision. 3D prints have advanced to the point where they can be a viable solution for rapid creation of bespoke, customized models for training, implants, or tool development. However, VR/AR is becoming prolific enough to move from the purely technical audience to the tech-savvy educated enthusiast. Technologies such as object scanning and CAD identification, available commercially for developers (at the time of the chapter's writing a widespread implementation of such use cases was available through the Vuforia AR platform[95]), are making complex 3D objects targets for AR and provide an unprecedented level of flexibility for digital augmentation of complex 3D objects. This level of maturity can support a vision for merging tangible with intangible resources in order to create a simple holistic, tangible, digitally augmented, immersive educational resource. This technological integration can lead to accessible highly versatile resources, reusable, repurposable, and highly available for education, training, and surgical assistance on the field, in the classroom, or in accessible laboratories.

References

1. Fry H, Ketteridge S, Marshall S. *A Handbook for Teaching and Learning in Higher Education: Enhancing Academic Practice*. New York: Routledge; 2009.

2. Downes S. *Distance Educators Before the River Styx Learning*; 2001. URL: http://technologysource.org/article/distance_educators_before_the_river_styx/.

3. Chiu JL, DeJaegher CJ, Chao J. The effects of augmented virtual science laboratories on middle school students' understanding of gas properties. *Comput Educ*. 2015;85:59—73.

4. Dede C. Immersive interfaces for engagement and learning. *Science*. 2009;323(5910): 66—69.

5. Klopfer E, Squire K. Environmental detectives—the development of an augmented reality platform for environmental simulations. *Educ Technol Res Dev*. 2008;56(2):203—228.

6. Dunleavy M, Dede C, Mitchell R. Affordances and limitations of immersive participatory augmented reality simulations for teaching and learning. *J Sci Educ Technol*. 2009;18(1): 7—22.

7. Wu H-K, Wen S, Lee -Yu, Chang H-Y, Liang J-C. Current status, opportunities and challenges of augmented reality in education. *Computer and Education*. 2013;62.

8. Antoniou PE, Dafli E, Arfaras G, Bamidis PD. Versatile mixed reality medical educational spaces; requirement analysis from expert users. In: *Personal and Ubiquitous Computing*, 2017.

9. Olympiou G, Zacharia ZC. Blending physical and virtual manipulatives: An effort to improve students' conceptual understanding through science laboratory experimentation. *Sci Educ*. 2012;96(1):21—47.

10. Desselle MR, Brown RA, James AR, Midwinter MJ, Powell SK, Woodruff MA. Augmented and virtual reality in surgery. *Comput Sci Eng*. 2020;22(3):18—26. https://doi.org/10.1109/MCSE.2020.2972822.

11. Michalski MH, Ross JS. The shape of things to come: 3D printing in medicine. *JAMA*. 2014;312(21):2213—2214.

12. Liaw CY, Guvendiren M. Current and emerging applications of 3D printing in medicine. *Biofabrication*. 2017;9(2):024102.

13. Pugliese L, Marconi S, Negrello E, Mauri V, Peri A, Gallo V, Auricchio F, Pietrabissa A. The clinical use of 3D printing in surgery. In: *Updates in Surgery*. Vol. 70, 3. Springer-Verlag Italia s.r.l; 2018:381—388. https://doi.org/10.1007/s13304-018-0586-5.

14. McGurk M, Amis AA, Potamianos P, Goodger NM. Rapid prototyping techniques for anatomical modelling in medicine. *Ann R Coll Surg Engl*. 1997;79:169—174.

15. Wong KV, Hernandez A. A review of additive manufacturing. *ISRN Mech Eng*. 2012. https://doi.org/10.5402/2012/208760.

16. Rengier F, Mehndiratta A, von Tengg-Kobligk H, Zechmann CM, Unterhinninghofen R, Kauczor HU, et al. 3D printing based on imaging data: review of medical applications. *Int J Comput Assist Radiol Surg*. 2010;5:335—341.

17. Kappers AM. Human perception of shape from touch. *Philos Trans R Soc Lond B Biol Sci*. 2011;366:31063114.

18. Pietrabissa A, Marconi S, Peri A, Pugliese L, Auricchio F. From CT scanning to 3-D printing technology for the pre- operative planning in laparoscopic splenectomy. *Surg Endosc*. 2015;30(1):366—371.

19. Kim GB, et al. Three-dimensional printing: basic principles and applications in medicine and radiology. *Korean J Radiol*. 2016;17(2):182—197.

20. Lorensen WE, Cline HE. Marching cubes: a high resolution 3D surface construction algorithm. *SIGGRAPH Comput Graphics.* 1987;21:163–169.
21. Tiede U, Höehne KH, Bomans M, Pommert A, Riemer M, Wiebecke G. Investigation of medical 3D-rendering algorithms. *Comput Graphics Appl.* 1990;10:41–53.
22. Raphael O, Hervé R. Clinical applications of rapid prototyping models in cranio-maxillofacial surgery. In: Hoque M, ed. *Advanced Applications of Rapid Prototyping Technology in Modern Engineering.* Rijeka, Croatia: InTech; 2011.
23. Choi JY, Choi JH, Kim NK, Kim Y, Lee JK, Kim MK, et al. Analysis of errors in medical rapid prototyping models. *Int J Oral Maxillofac Surg.* 2002;31:23–32.
24. Chang PS, Parker TH, Patrick Jr CW, Miller MJ. The accuracy of stereolithography in planning craniofacial bone replacement. *J Craniofac Surg.* 2003;14:164–170.
25. Shellabear M, Nyrhilä O. DMLS-Development history and state of the art. In: *Proceedings of the 4th LANE; 2004 Sep 21–24.* Erlangen, Germany. Bamberg: Meisenbach-Verlag; 2004.
26. Silva DN, Gerhardt de Oliveira M, Meurer E, Meurer MI, Lopes da Silva JV, Santa-Bárbara A. Dimensional error in selective laser sintering and 3D-printing of models for craniomaxillary anatomy reconstruction. *J Cranio-Maxillo-Fac Surg.* 2008;36: 443–449.
27. Ohtani T, Kusumoto N, Wakabayashi K, Yamada S, Nakamura T, Kumazawa Y, et al. Application of haptic device to implant dentistry–accuracy verification of drilling into a pig bone. *Dent Mater J.* 2009;28:75–81.
28. Marconi S, Pugliese L, Botti M, et al. Value of 3D-printing for the comprehension of surgical anatomy. *Surg Endosc.* 2017;31(10):4102–4110.
29. Martelli N, Serrano C, van den Brink H, et al. Advantages and disadvantages of 3-dimensional printing in surgery: a systematic review. *Surgery.* 2016;159(6):1485–1500.
30. Malik HH, Darwood ARJ, Shaunak S, Kulatilake P, El-Hilly AA, Mulki O, Baskaradas A. Three-dimensional printing in surgery: a review of current surgical applications. *J Surg Res.* 2015;199:512–522.
31. Li C, Cheung F, Fan VC, Ka Kit Leung G. Application of three-dimensional printing in surgery. *Surg Innovat.* 2017;24(1):82–88.
32. Olivieri LJ, Krieger A, Loke YH, Nath DS, Kim PCW, Sable CA. Three-dimensional printing of intracardiac defects from three-dimensional echocardiographic images: feasibility and relative accuracy. *J Am Soc Echocardiogr.* 2015;28:392–397.
33. Kong X, Nie L, Zhang H, et al. Do three-dimensional visualization and three-dimensional printing improve hepatic segment anatomy teaching? A randomized controlled study. *J Surg Educ.* 2016;73:264–269.
34. Lim KH, Loo ZY, Goldie SJ, Adams JW, McMenamin PG. Use of 3D printed models in medical education: a randomized control trial comparing 3D prints versus cadaveric materials for learning external cardiac anatomy. *Anat Sci Educ.* 2016;9:213–221.
35. Fasel JH, Aguiar D, Kiss-Bodolay D, et al. Adapting anatomy teaching to surgical trends: a combination of classical dissec- tion, medical imaging, and 3D-printing technologies. *Surg Radiol Anat.* 2016;38:361–367.
36. Jones DB, Sung R, Weinberg C, Korelitz T, Andrews R. Three-dimensional modeling may improve surgical education and clinical practice. *Surg Innovat.* 2016;23:189–195.
37. Garcia J, Yang Z, Mongrain R. Lachapelle K (2018) 3D printing materials and their use in medical education: a review of current technology and trends for the future. *BMJ Stel.* 2018;4:27–40.

38. Langridge B, Mamin S, Coumbe B, et al. Systematic review of the use of 3 dimensional printing in surgical teaching assess- ment. *J Surg Educ*. 2018;75:209−221.

39. Rasheed K, Mix D, Chandra A. Numerous applications of 3D printing in vascular surgery. *Ann Vasc Surg*. 2015;29(4):643−644.

40. Pugliese L, Marconi S, Negrello E, Mauri V, Peri A, … & Gallo V, Pietrabissa A. The clinical use of 3D printing in surgery. *Updates in surgery*. 2018;70(3):381−388.

41. Tack P, Victor J, Annemans L. 3D-printing techniques in a medical setting: a systematic literature review. *Biomed Eng Online*. 2016;15:115.

42. Diment E, Thompson M, Begmann J. Clinical efficacy and effectiveness of 3D printing: a systematic review. *BMJ Open*. 2017;7:e016891.

43. Gross BC, Erkal JL, Lockwood SY, Chen C, Spence DM. Evaluation of 3D printing and its potential impact on biotechnology and the chemical sciences. *Anal Chem*. 2014;86: 3240−3253.

44. Williams B. Case based learning–a review of the literature: is there scope for this educational paradigm in prehospital education? *Emerg Med J*. 2005;22(8):577−581. https://doi.org/10.1136/emj.2004.022707 [Medline: 16046764].

45. Larson JR. *In Search of Synergy in Small Group Performance*. New York: Psychology Press; 2010.

46. Poulton T, Ellaway RH, Round J, Jivram T, Kavia S, Hilton S. Exploring the efficacy of replacing linear paper-based patient cases in problem-based learning with dynamic web-based virtual patients: randomized controlled trial. *J Med Internet Res*. 2014;16(11).

47. Ellaway R, Poulton T, Fors U, McGee JB, Albright S. Building a virtual patient commons. *Med Teach*. 2008;30(2):170−174. https://doi.org/10.1080/01421590701874074 [Medline: 18464142].

48. Cook DA, Erwin PJ, Triola MM. Computerized virtual patients in health professions education: a systematic review and meta-analysis. *Acad Med*. 2010;85(10):1589−1602. https://doi.org/10.1097/ACM.0b013e3181edfe13 [Medline: 20703150].

49. *MedBiquitous. Standards*. URL: http://www.medbiq.org/std_specs/standards/index.html.

50. *MedBiquitous Virtual Patient Summary*; 2010. URL: http://www.medbiq.org/working_groups/virtual_patient/MedBiquitousVirtualPatientSummary.pdf.

51. Antoniou PE, Sidiropoulos EA, Bamidis PD. DISCOVER-ing beyond openSim; immersive learning for carers of the elderly in the VR/AR era". In: *Communications in Computer and Information Science*. Cham: Springer; 2017:189−200 [cited 2018 May 8]. Available from: http://link.springer.com/10.1007/978-3-319-60633-0_16.

52. Antoniou PE, Athanasopoulou CA, Dafli E, Bamidis PD. Exploring design requirements for repurposing dental virtual patients from the web to second life: A focus group study. *J Med Internet Res*. 2014;16(6):1−19.

53. Antoniou PE, Ioannidis L, Bamidis PD. OSCase: Data schemes, architecture and implementation details of virtual patient repurposing in multi user virtual environments. *EAI Endorsed Trans Futur Intell Educ Environ*. 2016;2(6):151523. Available from: http://eudl.eu/doi/10.4108/eai.27-6-2016.151523.

54. *"Virtual Reality Market Share" Fortune Business Insights VR Market Trends*. [Online]. Available: https://www.fortunebusinessinsights.com/industry-reports/virtual-reality-market-101378. Accessed 15 Feb 2021.

55. *"Virtual Reality Healthcare Market Size" Fortune Business Insights VR Health*. [Online]. Available: https://www.fortunebusinessinsights.com/industry-reports/virtual-reality-vr-in-healthcare-market-101679. Accessed 15 Feb 2021.

56. Pickering J, Bamidis PD, Antoniou PE. Workshop: developing and integrating a neuro-anatomy virtual reality tool for medical education. In: *Proceedings of the Annual Conference of the Association of Medical Education in Europe, AMEE 2018, 25−29 August, 2018, Basel, Switzerland*. 2018.

57. Antoniou PE, Arfaras G, Pandria N, Athanasiou A, Ntakakis G, Babatsikos E, Bamidis P. Biosensor real-time affective analytics in virtual and mixed reality medical education serious games: cohort study. *JMIR Serious Games*. 2020;8(3):e17823. https://doi.org/10.2196/17823.

58. Antoniou P, Arfaras G, Pandria N, Ntakakis G, Bambatsikos E, Athanasiou A. Real-time affective measurements in medical education, using virtual and mixed reality. In: Frasson C, Bamidis P, Vlamos P, eds. *Brain Function Assessment in Learning. BFAL 2020*. Cham: Springer; 2020:. Lecture Notes in Computer Science; vol. 12462.

59. Inman VT, Saunders JBDEC. Referred Pain from skeletal structures. *J Nerv Ment Dis*. 1944;99:660−667.

60. Prahalad CK, Ramaswamy V. Co-creating unique value with customers. *Strat Leader*. 2004;32(3):4−9.

61. Ranjan KR, Read S. Value co-creation: concept and measurement. *J Acad Mark Sci*. 2016;44(3):290−315. Available from: http://link.springer.com/10.1007/s11747-014-0397-2.

62. Kohler T, Fueller J, Matzler K, Stieger D. Co-creation relation in virtual worlds: the design of the user experience. *MIS Q*. 2011;35(3):773−788.

63. Bendapudi N, Leone RP. Psychological implications of customer participation in co-production. *J Market*. 2003;67(1):14−28.

64. Kristensson P, Matthing J, Johansson N. Key strategies for the successful involvement of customers in the co-creation of new technology-based services. *Int J Serv Ind Manag*. 2008;19(4):474−491.

65. McColl-Kennedy JR, Vargo SL, Dagger TS, Sweeney JC, van Kasteren Y. Health care customer value cocreation practice styles. *J Serv Res*. 2012;15(4):370−389.

66. Lusch RF, Vargo SL. Service-dominant logic: reactions, reflections and refinements. *Market Theor*. 2006;6(3):281−288.

67. Grönroos C, Voima P. Critical service logic:making sense of value creation and co-creation. *J Acad Market Sci*. 2013;41(2):133−150.

68. Chien S-H, Chen J-J. Supplier involvement and customer involvement effect on new product development success in the financial service industry. *Serv Ind J*. 2010;30(2):185−201.

69. Droge C, Stanko MA, Pollitte WA. Lead users and early adopters on the web: the role of new technology product blogs. *J Prod Innovat Manag*. 2010;27(1):66−82.

70. Hu Y, McLoughlin D. Creating new market for industrial services in nascent fields. *J Serv Market*. 2012;26(5):322−331.

71. Nuttavuthisit K. If you can't beat them, let them join: the development of strategies to foster consumers' co-creative practices. *Bus Horiz*. 2010;53(3):315−324.

72. Auh S, Bell SJ, McLeod CS, Shih E. Co-production and customer loyalty in financial services. *J Retailing*. 2007;83(3):359−370.

73. Lemke F, Clark M, Wilson H. Customer experience quality: an exploration in business and consumer contexts using repertory grid technique. *J Acad Market Sci*. 2011;39(6):846−869.

74. Boselli R, Cesarini M, Mezzanzanica M. Customer knowledge and service development, the web 2.0 role in co-production. *Proc World Acad Sci Eng Technol*. 2008;30.

75. Ordanini A, Pasini P. Service co-production and value co- creation: the case for a service-oriented architecture (SOA). *Eur Manag J.* 2008;26(5):289−297.

76. Ertimur B, Venkatesh A. Opportunism in co-production: implications for value co-creation. *Australas Market J.* 2010;18(4):256−263.

77. Vargo SL, Lusch RF. Service-dominant logic: continuing the evolution. *J Acad Market Sci.* 2008;36(1):1−10.

78. Achrol R, Kotler P. Frontiers of the marketing paradigm in the third millennium. *J Acad Market Sci.* 2012;40(1):35−52.

79. Lusch RF, Vargo SL, O'Brien M. Competing through service: Insights from service-dominant logic. *J Retailing.* 2007;83(1):5−18.

80. Aarikka-Stenroos L, Jaakkola E. Value co-creation in knowledge intensive business services: a dyadic perspective on the joint problem solving process. *Ind Market Manag.* 2012;41(1):15−26.

81. Grönroos C. Conceptualising value co-creation: a journey to the 1970s and back to the future. *J Market Manag.* 2012;28(13/14):1520−1534.

82. Ballantyne D, Varey RJ. The service-dominant logic and the future of marketing. *J Acad Market Sci.* 2008;36(1):11−14.

83. Arvidsson A. Ethics and value in customer co-production. *Market Theor.* 2011;11(3):261−278.

84. Chen JS, Tsou HT, Ching RKH. Co-production and its effects on service innovation. *Ind Market Manag.* 2011;40(8):1331−1346.

85. Vargo SL, Lusch RF. Evolving to a new dominant logic for marketing. *J Market.* 2004;68(January):1−17.

86. Krishna A, Morrin M. Does touch affect taste? The perceptual transfer of product container haptic cues. *J Consum Res.* 2008;34(6):807−818.

87. Troye SV, Supphellen M. Consumer participation in coproduction: "I made it myself" effects on consumers' sensory perceptions and evaluations of outcome and input product. *J Market.* 2012;76(2):33−46.

88. Schwaber K. *AGILE Project Management with SCRUM, Microsoft.* 2004.

89. https://www.scrumalliance.org.

90. https://www.microsoft.com/en-us/hololens.

91. https://unity3d.com/.

92. https://docs.unity3d.com/Manual/class-ScriptableObject.html.

93. https://meshb.nlm.nih.gov.

94. Antoniou PE, Ioannidis L, Bamidis PD. OSCase : A data scheme for transfer of web based virtual patients to OpenSim. In: Prauveneers D, ed. *Op Pro Ernatio Ent En.* 2015:228.

95. https://www.ptc.com/en/products/vuforia.

3D printing and pancreatic surgery

Kleanthis E. Giannoulis, MD, FRCS, FEBS

Associate Professor of Surgery, Aristotle University of Thessaloniki, Thessaloniki, Greece

Introduction

The first and foremost rule every general surgical trainee is taught early in their apprenticeship is to "Eat when you can, sleep when you can, and do not mess with the pancreas!" Indeed, even in modern-day surgical training, a combination of high commitment, exhaustive effort, and extreme level of stress causes trainees to neglect their personal health and risk burning out, at the beginning of their aspired career in surgery. But why the pancreas out of all organs? What makes it so dangerous to treat with surgery?

In the following pages, we will briefly review the topography and chronology of the pancreas, obstacles, and breakthroughs in the field of pancreatic surgery. Evolution of multidetector computer tomography, 3D imaging, and 3D printing has contributed to the improvement of many surgical subspecialties. As their impact in modern-day medicine expands, hope for upgraded training, effectiveness, and reduced complications in pancreatic surgery is also growing. Perhaps, God created the pancreas and placed it in such a rough neighborhood, waiting for surgeons to train until they had enough simulated experience with personalized 3D printed models. The time has arrived when additive manufacturing could bring about advances in pancreatic surgery. Along with significant victories in the field of diagnosis and systemic treatment of pancreatic disease, this would supplementarily improve the lives of millions of sufferers around the world.

Anatomy

The pancreas is situated deep into the retroperitoneal space and is notorious for the difficulty to access surgically. It crosses the lumbar vertebrae anteriorly, roughly at level with the transpyloric plane. It can be divided into four parts: head, neck, body, and tail. The head is surrounded by the duodenal loop and gives out the uncinate process, extending posteriorly and below the superior mesenteric vessels as they emerge from behind the neck. The body tapers into the tail that extends to the splenic hilum.

3D Printing: Applications in Medical Surgery. https://doi.org/10.1016/B978-0-323-66193-5.00005-8

Situated behind the pancreas lies the inferior vena cava, the portal vein formed by the confluence of the superior mesenteric and splenic veins behind the neck, the aorta, superior mesenteric vessels, diaphragmatic crura, celiac plexus, the left kidney, and suprarenal gland. In front of the pancreas lies the stomach forming part of the anterior wall of the lesser sac. The splenic artery undulates along the upper border of the pancreas, whereas the splenic vein travels behind it and receives the inferior mesenteric vein under the paraduodenal recess, laterally to the ligament of Treitz.

The common bile duct courses behind the pancreatic head, usually forming a groove in its lateral aspect. However, it can occasionally run through it to join with the main pancreatic duct of Wirsung and confluently drain into the medial aspect of the second part of the duodenum.

The arterial supply to the pancreatic head is common with the duodenum, derived from the superior (from the gastroduodenal artery) and inferior (from the superior mesenteric) pancreaticoduodenal arteries. The rest of the gland is perfused by branches of the splenic artery. Venous blood from the head and uncinate process drains to the right gastroepiploic and anterior-inferior pancreaticoduodenal veins. Together they form the gastrocolic trunk, which opens into the superior mesenteric vein on the right lateral side. Venous outflow from the body and tail ends into the splenic vein through short and fragile tributaries.

Lymph drains into peripancreatic lymph nodes along its upper and lower border, infra pyloric, portal, mesenteric, mesocolic, and aortocaval nodes. There are also lymph nodes around the splenic hilum, splenic artery, and tail of the pancreas.

Innervation of the pancreas is abundant. Pancreatic nerves carry nociceptive and visceral signals to the celiac plexus. Preganglionic efferent fibers of the greater, lesser, and least splanchnic nerves pass through the sympathetic chain and form the celiac ganglia, providing preganglionic input to the celiac plexus. Parasympathetic supply is derived from the left and right vagal trunks. The celiac plexus forms around the origin of the celiac axis and superior mesenteric artery.

Macroscopically, the gland is lobulated and covered by a fine capsule. The lobules consist of acini of epithelial secretory cells whose ductules drain into principal ducts. Between the pancreatic acini lie the hormone-secreting islets of Langerhans. The main duct occasionally drains separately into the duodenum and does not join with the common bile duct at the ampulla of Vater. The accessory duct (of Santorini) arises from the lower part of the head and crosses anterior to the main duct to drain into the duodenum proximal to it. It usually communicates with it, and sometimes it is absent.

Development of pancreatic surgery

Globally, there were 460,000 new cases of pancreatic cancer in 2018, making it the 12th most common cancer in men and the 11th most common cancer in women. In the United States, about 56,770 people (29,940 men and 26,830 women) will be diagnosed and 45,750 people (23,800 men and 21,950 women) will die from pancreatic cancer in 2019. By 2030, pancreatic cancer is expected to be the second commonest cause of cancer-related death.[1] Despite progress in diagnosis and treatment, mortality from pancreatic cancer is expected to rise steeply in the following decades.

Surgery at an early stage represents the only hope for cure but only 15%−20% of patients are candidates for an operation at the time of diagnosis. Median postoperative survival is smaller than 20 months,[2] 5-year survival is about 20%, and approximately 10% of patients are still alive after 10 years.[3] Despite recent advances, long-term survival is uncommon even among patients eligible for surgical resection.

However, some decades ago, pancreatic resections were considered to be impossible owing to their deadly outcomes. Later, when mortality rates finally improved, they still were near 30%. Today, pancreaticoduodenectomy is the commonest type of pancreatic procedure and is safely carried out in high-volume centers (more than 19 cases per year) with mortality less than 2%.[4]

The evolution of pancreaticoduodenectomy to its present form has been made possible by the efforts of several giants of the surgical legacy. This formidable type of surgery demands excellent surgical training and skills. Some of the important surgeons, operations, and dates in the evolution of pancreatic resections are listed below.

Alessandro Codivilla performed the first reported pancreaticoduodenectomy for carcinoma of the pancreas in 1898. He removed part of the pancreas, duodenum, distal stomach, and common bile duct. Reconstruction was achieved by Roux-en-Y gastrojejunostomy and cholecystojejunostomy. No anastomosis or closure of the pancreatic stump was performed. The patient died 18 days later from cachexia and diarrhea.[5]

William Halsted performed the first successful resection of ampullary carcinoma by excising parts of the duodenum and pancreas in 1899.[6]

Walther Kausch resected the bigger part of the duodenum en bloc with a significant part of the pancreas in 1912. Owing to the established ideas at the time, he did not complete the duodenectomy and restored continuity with a pancreaticoduodenostomy.[7]

Allen Whipple published the first cases of a two-stage resection of the duodenum and greater part of the pancreatic head for ampullary cancer in 1935.[8] Of the three operated patients, the first died the following day from anastomotic failure and the last survived for 2 years to finally succumb to liver metastases. Whipple is also credited with the first report of complete one-stage resection of the head of the pancreas and duodenum.[9] While operating on a patient for pyloric ulcer, he observed that he also had a tumor in the pancreatic head. He continued to accomplish a distal gastrectomy, resection of the mass and choledochoduodenostomy. Pancreatic reconstruction was not performed in this patient but in later ones.

William Longmire reintroduced the concept of pylorus-preserving pancreatoduodenectomy in 1977, to control postgastrectomy syndrome.[10] It was originally described by Kenneth Watson 30 years earlier. Despite early criticism on the radicality and oncological safety of the procedure, it proved to be equally effective with the traditional pancreaticoduodenectomy with the added advantages of shorter operative time, smaller blood loss. and better quality of life for long-term survivors.[11]

Michel Gagner performed the first laparoscopic pylorus-preserving pancreatoduodenectomy in 1994. It was reported on a patient with pancreas divisum and chronic pancreatitis confined to the pancreatic head.[12] In following years, many publications of successful distal pancreatectomy and pancreatoduodenectomy for neoplastic disease emerged from centers around the world.

Adoption of laparoscopic pancreatic surgery has been slow owing to the technical complexity, long learning curve, higher cost, and concerns about late complications and oncologic safety of the approach. The general advantages of laparoscopy over open surgery, such as diminished tissue trauma and blood loss, less requirement for analgesics, faster patient mobilization, and decreased length of stay, have been confirmed for laparoscopic pancreatic resections. Compared to open surgery, complications as pancreatic fistula and delayed gastric emptying have not been excessive, while abortion of the procedure after the initial inspection of the abdominal cavity spares the morbidity of an unnecessary laparotomy for patients with undiagnosed metastatic disease. Furthermore, similarly to the laparoscopic extirpation of other gastrointestinal malignancies, overall patient survival and incidence of positive resection margins after laparoscopic pancreatoduodenectomy for pancreatic head and periampullary cancer is comparable to open surgery.[13]

Pier Giulianotti performed the first robotic pancreatectomy and reported his personal series of 13 robotic pancreatic resections 3 years later.[14] Robotic surgery represents the latest development in the field of minimally invasive surgery. It was first used in the 1990s in military and major catastrophe applications and called telepresence surgery. It shares advantages of laparoscopic surgery such as small incisions, diminished blood loss, short length of stay, and faster recovery. Additionally, the robotic platform offers a better viewing experience in full high-definition 3D vision, improving hand-eye coordination. Compared to laparoscopy, it also reduces instrument tremor and abolishes the fulcrum effect, permitting 7° of mechanical freedom and allowing for easier and precise intracorporal maneuverability. Improvements in ergonomics provide a comfortable sitting for the surgeon who can perform longer operations with less fatigue and higher precision.

The prevailing commercially available system is the Da Vinci Surgical System (Intuitive Surgical, Sunnyvale, CA, USA). It consists of three fundamental elements: the surgeon's console where the surgeon seats wearing a 3D visor and using an interface for instrument control (Endowrist technology, Sunnyvale, CA, USA), the patient-side cart with four articulated arms (reproducing surgical manipulations in the operative field), and a vision control unit.

To date, the largest published series consisted of 250 consecutive robotic pancreatectomies, the majority of which for pancreatic adenocarcinoma. The reported rate of 30- and 90-day mortality was 0.8% and 2.0%, respectively, and overall postoperative morbidity was equivalent to open and laparoscopic operations in specialized high-volume centers. Conversion to open surgery was necessary in 6% of cases.[15] There have also been reports of better oncologic results compared to laparoscopic resections, characterized by higher rates of negative resection margins and higher lymph node yields.[16]

However, there is lack of evidence from multicentre randomized controlled trials, difficult to conduct because of high costs and limited availability of the robotic platform, surgical training, and patient consent issues. Level of evidence of the reported robotic pancreatic surgery studies is low and based mainly on single institution (and frequently single surgeon) series, with biased patient selection. This is likely to improve in the future with robotic technology improving continuously and becoming more affordable and accessible to healthcare applications.

Earlier diagnosis and evolution of neoadjuvant therapy are also expected to further improve the outcomes in pancreatic cancer treatment. Developments in surgical training and technique are similarly anticipated, possibly with the implementation of 3D printing, enabling surgeons to safely practice the operation in training facilities, on case-specific, exact anatomic models, before embarking on live surgery.

Technical considerations in pancreatic surgery

Pancreatic surgery is mainly performed to address pancreatic adenocarcinoma and periampullary tumors. In a recently published nationwide audit from the Netherlands, all patients who underwent pancreatic surgery during 2014 and 2015 were prospectively studied to assess outcomes. From a total of 2107 patients undergoing surgery for pancreatic disease, about 85% had a pancreatic resection. Of these, approximately 46% were female and 54% male. Nearly 21% were older than 75 years. Among patients undergoing pancreatic resections, almost 76% had a pancreatoduodenectomy and 18% a distal pancreatectomy. Most of them suffered from pancreatic adenocarcinomas (39%) and periampullary (distal bile duct, duodenum, ampulla) cancers (25%). Other indications for surgery included pancreatic neuroendocrine tumors (9%), intraductal papillary mucinous neoplasms (8%), and chronic pancreatitis (3%).[17] Similar results from population-based pancreatic surgery registries originate mainly from the United States. These include the Surveillance, Epidemiology, and End Results Program and the American College of Surgeons National Surgical Quality Improvement Program. Despite individually studying substantially larger numbers of patients and hospitals, national coverage is lower than 100% and published results are invariably older.[18]

Apart from pancreatoduodenectomy, distal, and total pancreatectomy, pancreatic operations also encompass pancreatic drainage procedures for chronic pancreatitis, central pancreatic resections, duodenum-preserving resections of the pancreatic head, necrosectomy for acute pancreatitis, localized resections for endocrine tumors of the pancreas, ampullary resections for ampullary tumors, operations for pancreatic trauma, and pancreatic transplantation. Pancreatic surgery should ideally be performed in high-volume centers by experienced surgeons. This way short- and long-term outcomes are optimal.[19] As most of the operations are performed on patients with cancer, equally important aspects of care are multidisciplinary assessment and follow-up, to ensure the correct application of surgical and other treatments tailored for the individual patients and their disease. Pancreatic surgery is technically challenging and excellent results are hard to obtain, mainly because of the physiologic role, anatomic structure, and close relation of the pancreas to the celiac and superior mesenteric vascular arcades. Particularly in pancreatoduodenectomy, the combination of pancreatic consistency and enzymatic secretions jeopardize the integrity of reconstruction by pancreatojejunostomy or pancreatogastrostomy, making it prone to failure and source of life-threatening complications.

Pancreaticoduodenectomy modifies the anatomic arrangement of the pancreas, upper gastrointestinal tract, and extrahepatic biliary tree allowing for untimely interaction between the exocrine pancreatic secretions and intestinal enterokinase. This represents a significant hazard, as activated pancreatic enzymes leaking from the pancreatic stump may cause serious complications. Additionally, the soft consistency of normal pancreatic parenchyma and small size of the main pancreatic duct makes intraoperative manipulation difficult and can lead to dehiscence of the sutured anastomosis between the pancreas and the jejunum or stomach.[20] In the worst-case scenario, activated enzymes could digest the surrounding structures, causing severe inflammation and liquefaction of the pancreatic remnant and peripancreatic tissue. This can lead to breakdown of the anastomotic reconstruction and to formation of fistulas, as well as inflammatory collections and abscesses almost anywhere in the abdominal cavity. Postoperative pancreatic fistulas (POPFs) are the main cause of major morbidity and mortality after pancreatic surgery. Soft pancreas consistency, pancreatic duct diameter <3 mm, nonpancreatic cancer or chronic pancreatitis pathology, and excessive intraoperative blood loss (transfusion with more than two units of blood), are consistently shown to be predictive of POPF. The above criteria can be used to determine the "Fistula Risk Score," a validated scoring system predictive of POPF after pancreatoduodenectomy.[21] Other predisposing factors for POPF development include age and male gender, poor preoperative nutrition, central obesity, and excessive intraoperative fluid administration.[22] Surgeon-related causes include long operating time, increased pancreatic parenchymal remnant volume,[23] vascular or multiorgan resections, type of the anastomosis or otherwise management of the pancreatic stump, and preoperative use of use stents.

POPFs can have consequences ranging from light like delayed gastric emptying to grave ones such as septic shock, severe hemorrhage, multiorgan failure, and postoperative death. The incidence of POPF ranges between 13% and 41%.[24] It is smaller for pancreatoduodenectomies (13%), high for distal pancreatectomies (30%), and peaks after central pancreatectomies (41%). POPF represent the major cause of postoperative morbidity and mortality following pancreatic surgery. The first widely accepted definition of POPF was "drain output of any measurable volume of fluid on or after postoperative day 3 with an amylase content greater than 3 times the serum amylase activity." This was established in 2005 by an International Working Group of 375 surgeons.[25] A grading system was also proposed and later revised, to classify patients into those with a relatively benign clinical syndrome (biochemical leak), and others with a POPF "associated with a clinically relevant development/condition related directly to the postoperative pancreatic fistula" (grades B and C). Patients with grade B POPF generally require medical or minimally invasive intervention, and those with grade C POPF are critically ill with sepsis and organ failure, requiring reoperation and often succumbing to complications.[26] This grading system has been successfully evaluated in association with other non-POPF complications, cost, length of hospitalization, and stay in the intensive care unit.[27]

Improvement of outcomes in patients with diseases treatable by pancreatic surgery can be facilitated by early diagnosis, prompt referral to surgery, and reduction of perioperative mortality brought about by meticulous surgical technique. Equally important is the prevention of complications, combined with early diagnosis and efficient management when these occur. A high rate of complete tumor extirpation and appropriate neoadjuvant and adjuvant treatment further improves long-term survival in patients with cancer. Mortality after pancreatoduodenectomy for cancer is reported to be low in Asian countries. Nationwide studies from South Korea and Japan have reported in-hospital mortality rates of 2.1% and 3.3%, respectively.[19,28] In Europe and the United States, recent studies report mortality of 4.1% in the Netherlands,[17] 7.7% in Germany,[29] and 2.9% in the United States.[18] Mortality rate has generally declined over the last decade and centralization of pancreatic surgery is thought to have contributed to this.[30,31] Despite reduction of mortality, major morbidity following pancreatoduodenectomy remains persistently common with a reported incidence ranging between 25% and 30%.[17,32] High morbidity undoubtedly contributes to poor overall outcomes and increased treatment costs.

Pancreatoenteric anastomosis constitutes the Achilles tendon of pancreatoduodenectomy, and leakage from the pancreatic stump the major cause of morbidity in distal pancreatectomy. Because of its serious consequences, significant efforts have been made to reduce the incidence of pancreatic fistula, and numerous studies, randomized trials, and metaanalyses focused on various aspects of its prevention. However, no single surgical technique has been demonstrated to decrease POPF incidence. So far, there is considerable variation of operative techniques in various centers and among pancreatic surgeons over the world.

Pancreatojejunostomy is the commonly used type of pancreatoenteric anastomosis after pancreatoduodenectomy. Comparison between end-to-side, end-to-end, duct-to-mucosa, and the invagination technique has been attempted in numerous randomized studies. However, since a uniform definition of POPF was not available before 2005, fistula rates are not easy to compare.[25] Metaanalyses of randomized studies comparing duct-to-mucosa to invagination pancreatojejunostomy are also available, showing no significant overall difference of POPF occurrence.[33,34] A recent randomized study comparing duct-to-mucosa to invagination pancreatojejunostomy similarly showed no difference in the overall incidence, but demonstrated superiority of the invagination technique with significantly lower rates of POPF in patients with a soft pancreas (10% vs. 42%, p = .010).[35]

Pancreatogastrostomy is an appealing alternative to pancreatojejunostomy, conferring a theoretically smaller risk of POPF through deactivation of the pancreatic enzymes, and absence of trypsin activating enterokinase inside the acidic gastric environment. A multicentre randomized study confirmed a lower incidence of POPF after pancreatogastrostomy, but the overall postoperative complications and mortality were not significantly different among studied groups.[36] In the largest multicentre randomized trial comparing pancreatogastrostomy to pancreatojejunostomy during pancreatoduodenectomy, no significant difference in the rate of POPF could be demonstrated (20% vs. 22%, p = .617). Interestingly, higher rates of significant postoperative hemorrhage, perioperative cerebrovascular accidents, avoidance of long-term pancreatic enzyme supplementation, and some improvement in quality of life parameters were observed in patients with pancreatogastrostomy.[37] A recent metaanalysis of eight randomized studies comparing pancreatogastrostomy with pancreatojejunostomy in 1200 pancreatoduodenectomies recognized a significant reduction of POPF rates and severity with the pancreatogastrostomy technique.[38] However, in a retrospective study of 58 patients undergoing central pancreatectomy, pancreatogastrostomy was associated with a significantly higher incidence and severity of POPF. The authors recommended performing pancreatojejunostomy in older patients, to improve central pancreatectomy outcomes.[39]

Stapled closure of the pancreatic stump and avoidance of a pancreatoenteric anastomosis after PD with a clinically significant POPF rate of only 13.6% was reported in a small retrospective study of patients undergoing pancreatoduodenectomy. The authors concluded that a fistula from the occluded pancreatic remnant is less dangerous than one related to anastomotic dehiscence due to absence of enterokinase-mediated activation of pancreatic enzymes and proposed closure of the pancreatic stump for "high-risk" elderly patients (>65 years), to reduce morbidity related to conventional pancreatic anastomosis.[40] This old idea was supported by some[41] but did not prove to be of benefit in a subsequent randomized study.[42] Similarly, application of fibrin sealants and acrylic glues to lower the incidence of POPF after pancreatoduodenectomy or localized pancreatic resection conferred no apparent clinical benefits. A recent metaanalysis observed a trend toward less postoperative hemorrhage and intraabdominal collections but no difference in terms of mortality, wound infections, reinterventions, or hospital stay.[43]

Kausch-Whipple procedure, the operation first performed by Kausch and consequently improved and reported by Whipple, served as standard pancreatoduodenectomy for 4 decades. Its modification with preservation of the pylorus aimed to avoid unnecessary stomach resection without scarifying oncologic adequacy and long-term results. Several randomized studies and metaanalyses, including the latest update of a Cochrane metaanalysis verified similar mortality, morbidity, and survival comparing them. Still, pylorus-preserving pancreatoduodenectomy was significantly associated with delayed gastric emptying, while operating time, intraoperative blood loss, and need for transfusions were significantly higher in the standard pancreatoduodenectomy group.[11] Delayed gastric emptying is defined as the prolonged aspiration of >500 mL/day from a nasogastric tube (in place for ≥10 days), need for reinsertion of nasogastric tube, or failure of unlimited oral intake by the 14th postoperative day. Regardless of type of reconstruction, delayed gastric emptying is reported in 9%−37% of patients after pancreatoduodenectomy.[44] Antecolic duodenojejunostomy after pylorus-preserving pancreatoduodenectomy has been recommended as the reconstruction technique with lower incidence of delayed gastric emptying.[45] However, a recent metaanalysis comparing duodenal with gastric stump reconstruction techniques after pancreatoduodenectomy could not demonstrate a difference in outcomes including delayed gastric emptying.[46]

Biliary drainage in jaundiced patients before surgery for cancer of the pancreatic head is associated with increased complications. It was initially performed via a percutaneous, transhepatic approach. Despite early enthusiasm, later metaanalyses demonstrated poor overall results.[47] Following advances in endoscopic approach and technology, short-term polyurethane stents could be introduced on an outpatient basis. A multicentre, randomized study that assigned patients to early surgery or surgery following 4−6 weeks of biliary drainage with endoscopically introduced plastic stents demonstrated a significantly higher rate of serious complications in the drainage group, but no difference in postoperative mortality, length of stay, or long-term survival.[48] In a subsequent metaanalysis of biliary drainage first versus major surgery in jaundiced patients suffering mainly with malignant disease (520 patients from six randomized studies, cancer rate 60%−100% per study), similar results were obtained and the safety of routine preoperative biliary drainage was not established.[49] Outside the confines of research trials, preoperative drainage should only be considered for patients with hepatic and/or renal failure and associated coagulopathy. Metal stents are safer to use and less prone to complications. Their use should be considered in the setting of neoadjuvant treatment.[50]

The extend of lymphadenectomy aimed to increase radicality of pancreatic cancer surgery and prolong patient survival has been subject to considerable debate over the years. While standard dissection is removal of the peripancreatic lymph node groups,[51] radical lymphadenectomy involves clearance of paraaortic and celiac axis nodes and occasionally those of the hepatoduodenal ligament and peripancreatic soft tissue. Despite encouraging results from some smaller studies, many randomized studies found no survival advantage following extended lymphadenectomy. A recent metaanalysis of two prospective, randomized studies demonstrated that extended lymphadenectomy in pancreatoduodenectomy prolonged operative time, increasing the need for blood transfusions and the incidence of overall complications. There was no benefit in long-term survival.[52]

Cancers arising in the pancreatic head and uncinate process frequently extend to the retroperitoneal tissues and surround the proximal superior mesenteric artery, on its course behind the superior mesenteric and above the left renal vein. In these circumstances, tumors often invade the periarterial nerve plexus and lymphatics, a sign of local extension and mark of aggressive tumor biology. Extensive infiltration of the arterial wall, especially extending to the intima, constitutes the absolute criterion of unresectability. The accuracy of preoperative staging with multidetector CT to determine resectability is high, approaching 95% under normal circumstances.[53] However, the positive predictive value for unresectability following neoadjuvant treatment drops to 25%.[54] Microscopically infiltrated (R1) medial-posterior transection margins after pancreatoduodenectomy for pancreatic cancer have been associated with worse prognosis.[55] Macroscopically infiltrated margins (R2) confer a worse prognosis than definitive chemoradiotherapy. The anatomic definition of borderline resectable pancreatic cancer describes tumors at high risk for positive resection margins (R1 or R2).[56] Evidence from high-volume centers confirm that with optimal pathology processing approximately, 60%−85% of pancreatectomy specimens originate from R1 resections.[57]

Akimasa Nakao first reported the technique of isolated pancreatectomy in 1993.[58] This was the first description of superior mesenteric artery (SMA) approach prior to transection of the pancreatic neck, the "point of no return" in pancreatoduodenectomy. The superior mesenteric artery and vein were dissected free from the mesentery of the jejunum at the base of the transverse mesocolon and portal circulation was preserved using an antithrombogenic bypass catheter between the portal and femoral veins. This operation facilitated early division of the inferior pancreaticoduodenal artery and meticulous dissection along the superior mesenteric artery, allowing for radical excision and reconstruction of any affected vessels in 80 out of 114 consecutive pancreatoduodenectomies. Perioperative mortality was 9.6%. In 2010, the term "artery first" approach was devised to describe the uncinate first approach to the superior mesenteric artery.[59] It allowed early transection of the mesopancreas and radical soft tissue clearance laterally to the superior mesenteric artery. Excellent hemostasis and shorter portal vein occlusion time could be achieved in patients with locally advanced tumors, frequently requiring venous resection and reconstruction.[60] A recent metaanalysis demonstrated "artery first" pancreatoduodenectomy to be associated with smaller blood loss and requirement for transfusions, POPF, and delayed gastric emptying rates. Despite similar 1- to 3-year overall survival, the "artery first" approach had a lower local and distant recurrence rate.[61]

Training in pancreatic surgery

Training in surgery has traditionally required many years and long hours of apprenticeship in a suitably organized, staffed, and equipped environment, within the confines of a hospital. Resident apprentices were expected to be able to cope with "any emergency that may arise and to perform any operation known to surgery" after successful completion of their training, as William Halsted pointed out over a century ago, during the annual address in medicine delivered in June 1904 at Yale University. He went on to add that this laborious period of training was not suited to "those who so soon weary of the study of their profession."

Since this paradigm was implemented, advances in medical knowledge, technological development, social attitudes, and public expectations dictated some changes in surgical apprenticeship. Surgical practice has been affected by the development of specialties and subspecialties. Training has evolved to produce surgeons in a relatively short period of time and still expect them to deliver the best level of care for patients and their individual needs, communities, and academic establishments. It has become clear that superior care is offered to patients with complex surgical disease when they are cared for by surgeons with high numbers and experience, in hospitals having the necessary infrastructure.[62] Pancreatic surgery subspecialisation is commonly combined with training in hepatobiliary (HPB) surgery and offered to successful candidates as a fellowship program after their certification in general surgery. Other pathways including training in pancreatic surgery are subspecialisation in surgical oncology or transplant surgery. Still, training curricula are variable, and time duration ranges from 1 to 3 years in different programs. In a consensus conference hosted by the Society of Surgical Oncology, the American Hepato-Pancreatico-Biliary Association, and the American Society of Transplant Surgeons, the minimum operation numbers and metrics for quality assessment were defined. Formatted monitoring of both opertive and nonoperative skills was proposed. The necessary number of major pancreatic procedures with trainees as first surgeons ranged from 15 to 25 across programs.[63] Another study recorded substantial variability evaluating HPB fellowship training globally. Significant deviation from structured and standardized recommendations was detected in many participating centers. Most operations undertaken by fellows as primary surgeons involved non-HPB cases, while the ratio between procedures in which fellows assisted versus performed ranged to 80% among centers around the world.[64]

In the United States, more than three-quarters of surgeons who wish to specialize in pancreatic surgery complete a subspecialization fellowship.[65] General surgeons pursue HPB fellowship training to increase their inadequate operative experience in complex pancreatic and HPB surgery. Most surgical residents perform less than twelve major pancreas operations during training in general surgery, while HPB subspecialization is commonly achieved by training with expert teams and leaders in high-volume hospitals.[66] Despite superior outcomes, 2 decades ago only 10% of the hospitals caring for 11% of patients who had a pancreatectomy were high-volume centers.[67] Improvements in healthcare since resulted in a considerable increase in high-volume centers and the annual number of pancreatic resections performed in each. The total number of patients with pancreatic cancer operated in high-volume centers has also multiplied, with over 50% currently receiving care in very high, and 20% in intermediate- and high-volume centers in certain parts of the United States.[68]

Apart from increased operative experience, better outcomes and low mortality reported in high-volume centers after major pancreatic surgery are likely to result from improved ability of medical and nursing personnel to detect complications early and treat them successfully. Interestingly, while complication rates after major pancreatic surgery are reported to be similar, mortality after major complications is almost double in hospitals with high overall mortality.[69] A possible explanation could be the commonly practiced in high-volume centers management of complications with minimally invasive interventional radiology and endoscopy techniques. This results in fewer reoperations and subsequent complications provoking mortality. The availability of an interventional radiology service has been associated with lower perioperative mortality after major pancreatic surgery in any hospital environment.[70] Furthermore, improved results after major pancreatic resections in patients with cancer are likely to be related to neoadjuvant and adjuvant treatments offered to them. Availability of multimodality treatments contributes to improved long-term outcomes.[71]

In the face of increasing worldwide application of minimally invasive pancreatic surgery, there are no global standardized recommendations or formal training programs yet. Minimally invasive distal pancreatectomy has been reported to result in better outcomes for patients with cancer.[72] However, there is lack of results from randomized studies. Aside from decreased postoperative hospitalization, propensity score-matched studies failed to confirm any other benefits of laparoscopy.[73] The value of robotic pancreatic surgery over laparoscopic resections is heavily disputed. Minimally invasive pancreatic resections are favored by experienced surgeons in high-volume centers where reported rates range between 60%−80%.[74] Implementation of minimally invasive techniques on a national level varies between 15% and 30%.[75] Globally, less than 20% of distal pancreatectomies are performed using a minimally invasive approach. The value is even smaller for pancreatoduodenectomies with most surgeons performing less than 40 procedures annually, recommended to achieve favorable results over open resections.[76] Lack of training in minimally invasive pancreatic surgery is the primary explanation for its low utilization. Up to 85% of pancreatic surgeons worldwide are keen to train in minimally invasive pancreatic surgery techniques. A national training program for minimally invasive pancreatic surgery was implemented in the Netherlands from 2014 to 2015 and resulted in a 7-fold increase in minimally invasive distal pancreatectomy rates (from 9% to 47%). Conversion to open, blood transfusions and length of hospitalization decreased. More patients with higher anesthetic risk, pancreatic cancer, and larger tumors were operated with minimally invasive techniques, with no apparent increase in postoperative morbidity that was comparable to expert centers.[77] Participating surgeons were experienced in open pancreatic and laparoscopic surgery. A standardized and reproducible minimally invasive technique was taught using detailed description, video training, and supervision from expert surgeons.

Progress in simulation technology is expected to impact training in pancreatic surgery, through the development of training devices aimed to improve hand-eye coordination and the performance of a variety of simple to intricate surgical tasks. Such systems offer increased safety because trainees acquire basic and complex surgical skills inside the training laboratory, before operating on patients. The training environment is friendly and controlled, allowing trainees to practice without restraints on time or the anxiety of failure in their early experience. Evaluation of the learning progress is objective and measurable. Numerous studies confirmed a significant improvement in operating efficiency, swiftness, and reduction of technical errors in individuals trained with simulators compared to ones taught exclusively in conventional, patient models.[78,79] Training in cadaveric models has similarly been documented to promote surgical skills improvement but requires significant infrastructure and is subject to close regulations.[80]

Accelerated growth of information technology and wide accessibility of Internet resources resulted in the establishment of interactive programs that enable education on patient management. Trainees can navigate through interactive case management scenarios, in which they can order investigations and decide treatment for individual virtual patients. Immediate feedback and identification of areas of weak knowledge can be obtained, allowing for a rich educational experience in the comfort of their chosen place and time.

Pancreatic surgery beyond conventional imaging

Pancreatic disease is complex and when surgical treatment is indicated, optimal results are depended on detailed and accurate preoperative imaging studies. Particularly in the case of pancreatic cancer, surgery offers the only hope for cure but is problematic due to its technically challenging and elaborate nature. CT is the most useful imaging modality for preoperative evaluation of pancreatic cancer. It provides comprehensive details for diagnosis and primary staging, including assessment of invasion of surrounding structures and involvement of vessels. However, it is less sensitive in diagnosing early nodal and metastatic spread. Improvements in technology have brought forward the evolution of multidetector helical CT (MDCT) scanners. They can acquire very thin sliced cuts faster and provide high-resolution images from the area of the pancreas. Pancreatic protocol dual-phase CT typically involves acquisition of images during the arterial and venous phases of contrast injection. Advanced image processing with special software can provide high-quality, volume rendered, 3D reconstructed images as well as curved and standard multiplanar images. Endoscopic ultrasound is more sensitive for the detection of early pancreatic cancer and can detect vascular involvement better than CT.[81] The ability to perform guided fine needle aspiration biopsies assists preoperative diagnosis and helps further management, when considering neoadjuvant or palliative therapy in patients with borderline resectable and advanced disease. Endoscopic ultrasound and MRI are particularly useful in the evaluation of cystic lesions of the pancreas. MRI is highly sensitive and able to highlight fluid-filled cavities, providing high-resolution images of the ductal anatomy, ductal communications, and important details on the structure of small (<3 cm) cystic pancreatic neoplasms.

Poor outcomes in pancreatic cancer can be attributed to several factors including aggressive tumor biology and presentation at an advanced stage. At presentation, 30%−40% of tumors are locally advanced, while 50%−60% are metastatic.[82] In the absence of metastatic disease, radical extirpation of pancreatic cancer offers the best chance for long-term survival. Postoperatively, patients with clear resection margins (R0) have the best prognosis.[83] Median survival after R0 resections varies from 17 to 27 months, while following R1 surgery survival drops to 10.3 months.[84] Since the presence of residual tumor at the resection margin is detrimental to patient survival, redefining the surgical approach to achieve clear margins could be an important step toward improving surgical results. Unfortunately, incomplete resection of pancreatic cancers is still unacceptably high. Depending on the method of specimen interpretation, it occurs in 35%–85% of cases.[57,85] Neoadjuvant chemotherapy or chemoradiotherapy treatment in patients with borderline resectable pancreatic cancer has been linked to improved overall survival, decreased lymph node metastasis, and local recurrence rates, comparable to patients receiving upfront surgery. However, it carries the cost of decreased resectability, particularly for patients who received neoadjuvant chemoradiotherapy. Still, the impact of neoadjuvant treatment in overall survival could be related to systemic control of microscopic metastatic disease. However, local control is also achieved as demonstrated by the decreased local recurrence and lymph node metastasis rates.[86]

Added to advances in the medical treatment of pancreatic disease, image-guided enhancement of surgical accuracy using intraoperative margin assessment and innovative visualization techniques could aid the pancreatic surgeon in his quest for curative resections.

Intraoperative ultrasound (IOUS) can provide real-time guidance for assessment of resectability, decreasing the number of incomplete resections.[87] Its sensitivity and specificity in the detection of vascular involvement are 92% and 95% in patients who have not received neoadjuvant therapy.[88] Laparoscopic ultrasound shares the same high diagnostic value. In patients with locally advanced pancreatic cancer receiving neoadjuvant therapy, CT examination cannot accurately determine the extent of vascular involvement. Compared to CT, IOUS changed the resectability status in one-third of patients at surgical exploration after neoadjuvant therapy.[89]

Near-infrared (NIR) fluorescence is a novel imaging technique that can contribute to the radicality of pancreatic resections by real-time intraoperative visualization of pancreatic cancer deposits and amplification of vital structures. It does not utilize ionizing radiation and can penetrate the superficial layers, revealing targets below. NIR light is invisible and does not change perception of the surgical field, reducing the learning curve and permitting its use in minimally invasive surgery. In a recent study, intraoperative use of a fluorescent labeled anti-CEA antibody was safe and feasible for the detection of primary and metastatic tumor deposits in patients with pancreatic cancer.[90]

Augmented reality (AR) is a real-time, intraoperative imaging technique revealing otherwise invisible anatomic details using composite computer-generated images (3D virtual model) from the synthesis of preoperative imaging and operative field views. It allows for improved accuracy and safety of surgical dissection, ensuring clear margins and avoidance of morbidity from intraoperative iatrogenic injuries. Creation of the composite images represents the main difficulty in AR because operative views are highly variable and change with tissue manipulation or movement due to heartbeat, ventilation and creation of pneumoperitoneum.

A report of AR-assisted pancreatoduodenectomy for periampullary cancer was published in 2013. The 3D virtual model was obtained from preoperative thoracoabdominal CT using special software. The virtual model was superimposed onto the operative field with an endoscope using different visible landmarks. A computer scientist manually registered in real time the virtual and real images using a video mixer. Dissection by the superior mesenteric artery first approach was performed under AR. Operation time was 360 min. Postoperative recovery was uneventful and resection margins were clear at final pathology.[91]

Surgical navigation systems (SNS) utilize preoperative and intraoperative imaging combined with intraoperative tracking of the position and orientation of surgical instruments inside the operative field. This can be particularly useful for minimally invasive surgery because of the otherwise diminished visual and tactile perception. SNS enhance 3D appreciation of the operative anatomy and important anatomic landmarks, promoting accurate localization and complete removal of the lesion. The basic components of an SNS consist of a computer using appropriate navigation software and a suitable display, a preoperative image data source, and an instrument tracking system. The utilization of "CustusX" navigation system during distal pancreatectomy for a cystic pancreatic neoplasm has been recently reported.[92] However, there are no other published accounts of its use in pancreatic surgery.

3D models in pancreatic surgery

Interpretation of high-quality, volume rendered, 3D reconstructed images obtained by processing of standard preoperative radiologic studies can be a useful tool in achieving safe and effective radical pancreatic surgery. 3D reconstructed images cannot surpass the diagnostic accuracy offered by the original preoperative images. However, they can be used to enhance understanding of the complex anatomic interrelations between the disease-bearing pancreas and its ducts, blood vessels, extrahepatic biliary tree, and surrounding organs. Their study could help the surgical team to preoperatively plan an R0 resection and design the dissection line used in surgery, determining if blood vessels can be dissected free or if they need to be excised together with the diseased organ.

Utilization of reconstructed 3D images from MDCT datasets of candidate living donors evaluated for right lobe liver transplantation was originally reported from Japan at the beginning of the century.[93] However, 3D models from MDCT alone could not provide essential for pancreatic surgery comprehensive details about the extrahepatic biliary tree and pancreatic duct configuration. To overcome this problem, a methodology integrating preoperative MDCT and magnetic resonance cholangiopancreatography images evolved, originating also from Japan. It delivered accurate anatomic 3D images used in pancreatic surgical planning.[94,95] Difficulties relating to the acquisition of 3D images with the above methodology were a considerable amount of processing time (originally 3−5 h) and difficulty in 3D image composition because of movement of the abdominal organs caused by respiration.

To overcome it, anatomic landmarks such as the junction between the portal and splenic veins and the bifurcation of the gastroduodenal and hepatic arteries were successfully employed.[94]

Consistency between 15 surgical residents' anatomic drawings from MDCT images and simulated 3D images was assessed using 61 preoperative 3D surgical simulations at the Department of Surgery, University of Tsukuba, Japan. Residents were divided into two groups: junior and senior. The 3D surgical simulation was shown to be useful for preoperative assessment before pancreatic surgery, especially for junior residents.[96] In a different study from the same institution, perioperative outcomes were compared for 117 patients who underwent pancreatoduodenectomy. The patients were divided into two groups: with and without preoperative 3D reconstruction. Factors evaluated were presence of an accessory bile duct, origin of the hepatic artery, confluence patterns of the coronary gastric vein and the inferior mesenteric vein, and intraoperative blood loss. Intraoperative blood loss was significantly reduced in the group with preoperative 3D reconstruction. Based on the results, authors proposed 3D imaging as a useful tool for preoperative assessment before pancreatoduodenectomy.[97] A third study from the same team sought to determine whether 3D measured pancreatic remnant volume is predictive of POPF after pancreatoduodenectomy. Pancreatic remnant volume was measured in 91 patients using 3D reconstructed images, which simulated actual intraoperative pancreatic parenchymal remnant volume. At multivariate analysis, pancreatic remnant volume and other well-known POPF risk factors were studied. Results showed that preoperative 3D measured pancreatic remnant volume is independently predictive of POPF after pancreatoduodenectomy.[98]

Despite originating from a single institution and including a relatively small number of patients, all the above studies highlight the potential value of 3D modeling in pancreatic surgery. 3D images can be used preoperatively to clarify the exact anatomic relationships of the bile duct, major vascular branches (including the hepatic artery and portal vein), pancreas, and liver. Surgeons and the rest of the surgical team can study the individualized, anatomic 3D images in a stress-free environment away from the operating table, being able to design the optimal approach to the pancreas. Ongoing technological progress is expected to improve the quality of preoperative 3D imaging and allow for further applications, improving outcomes in pancreatic surgery. A potential application of 3D images could be the construction of exact anatomic 3D printed models that can be used to practice the operation on an individual patient basis, before entering the operating theater.

3D printing as means of surgical training

The fabrication of physical models from 3D computer-aided designs was originally called rapid prototyping (RP), a term later replaced by 3D printing. The term was introduced during the 1980s to describe the new technologies which made it possible. Computer numeric controlled milling was gradually replaced by additive layer processes. Additive manufacturing is the term commonly used presently. In medicine, additive manufacturing brought about construction of anatomically accurate physical models using datasets derived from medical imaging.[99] RP technology followed the advances in 3D image reconstruction from MDCT datasets. Naturally, the study of physical models offered many benefits and was particularly well received by the surgical community for its advantages over plain radiologic visualization.[100] Physical models allowed for improved comprehension of complex anatomy over both axial and 3D rendered images and ameliorated the localization of lesions and patient outcomes.[101]

Today, 3D printing is possible with a wide variety of materials, including plastics, powders, ceramics, metals, polyether ether ketone (a colorless organic thermoplastic polymer with excellent overall properties), and silicone. Advanced 3D printers can use multiple materials and accurately construct complex models.[102] Limiting factor in the resolution of 3D printing is image acquisition, with many printers capable of delivering detail level superior to what medical scanners are currently able to provide. Some models produced from MRI data have similar accuracy to ones constructed from CT.[103]

In surgical practice, applications of 3D printing include the construction of anatomic models, surgical instruments, and implants or prostheses. It is primarily used in maxillofacial and orthopedic surgery. In a recent extensive metaanalysis, advantages from its implementation included the ability of precise operative planning, high accuracy of the modeling process, and a decreased operating time. However, accuracy was not found to be satisfactory in all studies included in the metaanalysis. The time-consuming process to prepare a model and additional applied cost were further limitations to routine implementation of 3D printing.[104]

In surgical training, simulations using 3D printed models offer a tactile understanding of the operative field anatomy, guidance, and bench practice on the exact operative approach to be performed during actual surgery, as well as planning and tailoring of implants and prostheses.[101,105] Surgical simulations enable surgeons to acquire new skills and prepare for specific operations without the need for practice on living patients, cadaveric, or animal models. By reconstruction of 3D printed models of patients' organs, realistic surgical procedures can be simulated. Recent technological advantages allow the fabrication of exact anatomic models using both preoperative MRI and MDCT datasets. Apart from helping experienced surgeons prepare for difficult operations on a patient-specific basis, surgical simulations with 3D printed models can also facilitate training of new surgeons, overcoming the limitation of donated human tissues and organs available for this.

3D printing technology for pancreatic surgery

The retroperitoneal location of the pancreas and its intimate relationship with the surrounding vital structures contribute to the complex and difficult nature of its surgical manipulation. Pancreatic surgery is rightly considered to be among the most demanding and technically challenging surgical subspecialties. A complete and thorough understanding of each patient's anatomy and unique disease characteristics is essential to ensure safe and successful surgical treatment. However, preoperative planning is often difficult and especially challenging for trainees and less experienced surgeons. Despite its inherent difficulty, perioperative planning is taught to only one-third of general surgical residents.[106]

Pancreatic surgery planning typically involves study of preoperative MDCT or MRI images, evaluation of the pancreas and surrounding vascular structures, and assessment of their potential involvement in the disease process. Experienced surgeons can review two-dimensional images and create a mental 3D impression of the operative anatomy to guide their surgical approach. This is particularly difficult for inexperienced surgeons. 3D printing is an innovative technology in surgical simulation training. 3D printed pancreatic models provide the opportunity to train surgeons handle and manipulate the pancreas and feel its relationships with surrounding anatomical structures, all before entering the operating theater. Study of the printed models gives trainees the opportunity to coordinate their visual and tactile assessment of a patient's operative anatomy. This is superior to plain visual inspection and mimics the interactions taking place during the actual surgical procedure. The trainee is also able to appreciate the presence of individual variations of complex anatomic elements. As the texture of 3D printed models can be accustomed to suit specific training needs, they can provide patient-specific models in any surgical simulation scenario. Furthermore, 3D printing with multiple materials can reproduce the different tissues encountered during surgery with high fidelity, enhancing comprehension of operative anatomy and encouraging rehearsal of specific, difficult steps of the operation.

The ideal 3D printed model should accurately carry tissue feel and handling characteristics encountered during a pancreatic operation. This would permit the safe practice of simulated pancreatic surgery by trainees, inexperienced and experienced surgeons alike, using different approaches and techniques, suited to the individual patient. It could even drive the improvement of pancreatic surgical techniques, tools, and approaches and contribute toward more effective treatment of pancreatic disease.

Studies and experience

Published studies of 3D printed models in pancreatic surgery are few but are expected to increase with evolution and growing utilization of the technique. In a study from China, 10 patients with pancreatic or periampullary neoplasms were preoperatively studied with MDCT. CT images were exported into a Medical Imaging 3D Visualization System for 3D visualization. Standard Template Library (STL) files were exported for 3D printing. Surgical planning and real-time guided operations were performed with 3D printed models. Operating time, intraoperative blood loss and blood transfusions, postoperative hospital stay, and follow-up were recorded in all patients. The resection margins were negative in all cases. There were no significant postoperative complications, and tumor recurrence was not observed in the first 6 months of follow-up. The authors concluded that in patients undergoing surgery for pancreatic and periampullary neoplasms, 3D printing could facilitate preoperative evaluation of the surgical risk, ascertain critical anatomical structures, navigate the surgical procedure in real time, and improve the prognosis of patients.[107]

A study from Canada examined three patients with pancreatic cancer requiring different operative approaches based on their preoperative CT. 3D volume rendered images and 3D printed models were obtained in all. A total of 30 first-year surgical residents were randomized to study the CT and 3D rendered images or 3D printed models and were later subjected to an examination designed to assess and mark their preoperative planning. Trainees who studied the 3D printed models scored significantly higher in preoperative planning. All participants reported a high level of satisfaction with the exercise. Authors concluded that 3D printed models improve the quality of trainee provided operative planning for complex pancreatic surgery.[108]

A report from Chicago described the case of a middle-aged woman with a borderline resectable carcinoma of the pancreatic head. The tumor was shown to involve the gastroduodenal artery on a preoperative CT. Its relationship with the hepatic artery was not clear in the same examination. After appropriate software manipulation of the MDCT datasets, a 3D printed model of the tumor and surrounding structures was constructed and became apparent that the tumor was unresectable. The model was also used for teaching and patient information purposes. The authors concluded that reconstructing traditional imaging to 3D allows observation of previously obscure anatomical details and that high-quality 3D printed models are increasingly useful not only in the clinical setting but also for personalized patient education.[109]

Future directions

3D printing as a tool for surgical planning, training, and treatment has evolved significantly in recent years. However, despite important progress, application of 3D printing technologies in the surgical treatment of pancreatic disease is limited and currently available in only a few centers worldwide. This is partly related to the difficulty in fabrication of pancreatic models combining mechanical characteristics of soft tissue with high resolution anatomic fidelity. In the case of pancreatic surgery, a combination of elastic, harder, and softer materials should be used to precisely simulate the pancreas and its topographic surroundings. An equally desired quality of 3D printed models would be to allow surgical manipulation like real pancreatic tissue, permitting surgeons to safely and reliably practice pancreatic division and anastomosis in surgical simulations. Techniques of additive manufacturing of hydrogels with control over mechanical properties have long been reported and evolved for usage in tissue engineering applications.[110] However, they are yet to be applied in manufacturing of anatomical models for surgical simulation.[111]

In 2016, Celprogen Inc., a United States-based biotechnology company, announced the production of a pancreatic model using additive manufacturing techniques. The 3D printed organ was supported by a scaffold from flexible polylactide, coated with extracellular matrix protein, and then seeded with pancreatic stem cells. This construction allowed seeded cells to potentially differentiate into a functional adult pancreas. Earlier this year, scientists from the Foundation for Research and Science Development in Poland 3D printed the first ever "bionic pancreas." Dr Wszoła and his team collected animal pancreatic cells and mixed them with bioink, a substance that helps the α- and β-cells survive. A 3D printer arranged them in a bioreactor rendering a computer-designed pattern. Blood vessels were printed simultaneously, using a different material. Parts of the 3D printed pancreas were implanted into mice in April 2019. By October 2019, larger parts of the pancreas together with blood vessels will be implanted in pigs. If successful, this could pave the way for 3D pancreas transplantation in humans with type one diabetes.

A plethora of commercial companies are currently offering 3D printing services over the Internet. Patient imaging data can be uploaded and processed and the 3D printed model shipped to the customer. However, the level of interaction between surgeons and such companies is limited by geographic and communication issues, and vital details on what is exactly required is sometimes lost in transit. Furthermore, considerable costs and delays apply. The ideal would be to generate 3D models or even STL files in the place of use. In 2018, a 3D printing company called Materialise NV headquartered in Belgium received FDA approval for 3D printed anatomical model software, used for diagnostic procedures. This could further support adoption of 3D planning and printing and creation of point-of-care 3D printing facilities in United States hospitals. Similarly, university departments and teaching hospitals across the globe motivated by the increasing applications of additive manufacturing technology organize in-house 3D printing services to optimize convenience, interaction, and results.

Future developments in biomaterials and 3D printing techniques will hopefully provide the next generation of pancreatic surgical simulations with natural realism. This would undoubtedly improve training and preoperative planning and increase success rates in pancreatic surgery.

References

1. Rahib L, Smith BD, Aizenberg R, et al. Projecting cancer incidence and deaths to2030: the unexpected burden of thyroid, liver, and pancreas cancers in the United States. *Cancer Res.* 2014;74(11):2913–2921.
2. McDowell BD, Chapman CG, Smith BJ, Button AM, Chrischilles EA, Mezhir JJ. Pancreatectomy predicts improved survival for pancreatic adenocarcinoma: results of an instrumental variable analysis. *Ann Surg.* 2015;261(4):740–745.
3. Ferrone CR, Pieretti-Vanmarcke R, Bloom JP, Zheng H, Szymonifka J, Wargo JA, et al. Pancreatic ductal adenocarcinoma: long-term survival does not equal cure. *Surgery.* 2012;152:S43–S49.

4. Meguid RA, Ahuja N, Chang DC. What constitutes a "high-volume" hospital for pancreatic resection? *J Am Coll Surg*. 2008;206(4):622.e1−622.e9.
5. Schnelldorfer T, Adams DB, Warshaw AL, Lillemoe KD, Sarr MG. Forgotten pioneers of pancreatic surgery: beyond the favorite few. *Ann Surg*. 2008;247:191−202.
6. Halsted WS. Contributions to the surgery of the bile passages, especially of the common bile-duct. *Boston Med Surg J*. 1899;141:645−654.
7. Kausch W. Das Carcinom der Papilla duodeni und seine radikale Entfernung. *Beitrage zur Klinische Chirurgie*. 1912;78:439−486.
8. Whipple AO, Parsons WB, Mullins CR. Treatment of carcinoma of the ampulla of Vater. *Ann Surg*. 1935;102:763−779.
9. Whipple AO. A reminiscence: pancreaticoduodenectomy. *Rev Surg*. 1963;20:221−225.
10. Traverso LW, Longmire WP. Preservation of the pylorus in pancreaticoduodenectomy. *Surg Gynecol Obstet*. 1978;146:959−962.
11. Hüttner FJ, Fitzmaurice C, Schwarzer G, Seiler CM, Antes G, Büchler MW, Diener MK. Pyloruspreserving pancreaticoduodenectomy (pp Whipple) versus pancreaticoduodenectomy (classic Whipple) for surgical treatment of periampullary and pancreatic carcinoma. *Cochrane Database Syst Rev*. 2016;2:CD006053.
12. Gagner M, Pomp A. Laparoscopic pylorus-preserving pancreatoduodenectomy. *Surg Endosc*. 1994;8:408−410.
13. Chen K, Liu XL, Pan Y, Maher H, Wang XF. Expanding laparoscopic pancreaticoduodenectomy to pancreatichead and periampullary malignancy: major findings based on systematic review and meta-analysis. *BMC Gastroenterol*. 2018;18(1):102.
14. Giulianotti PC, Coratti A, Angelini M, et al. Robotics in general surgery: personal experience in a large community hospital. *Arch Surg*. 2003;138(7):777−784.
15. Zureikat AH, Moser AJ, Boone BA, et al. 250 robotic pancreatic resections: safety and feasibility. *Ann Surg*. 2013;258:554−559. discussion 559-62.
16. Daouadi M, Zureikat AH, Zenati MS, et al. Robot-assisted minimally invasive distal pancreatectomy is superior to the laparoscopic technique. *Ann Surg*. 2013;257:128−132.
17. van Rijssen LB, Koerkamp BG, Zwart MJ, et al. Nationwide prospective audit of pancreatic surgery: design, accuracy, and outcomes of the Dutch Pancreatic Cancer Audit. *HPB (Oxford)*. 2017;19(10):919−926.
18. Parikh P, Shiloach M, Cohen ME, Bilimoria KY, Ko CY, Hall BL, et al. Pancreatectomy risk calculator: an ACSNSQIP resource. *HPB (Oxford)*. 2010;12(7):488−497.
19. Yoshioka R, Yasunaga H, Hasegawa K, Horiguchi H, Fushimi K, Aoki T, et al. Impact of hospital volume on hospital mortality, length of stay and total costs after pancreaticoduodenectomy. *Br J Surg*. 2014;101(5):523−529.
20. Pratt WB, Callery MP, Vollmer CM. Risk prediction for development of Pancreatic fistula using the ISGPF classification scheme. *World J Surg*. 2008;32:419−428.
21. Callery MP, Pratt WB, Kent TS, Chaikof EL, Vollmer Jr CM. A prospectively validated clinical risk score accurately predicts pancreatic fistula after pancreatoduodenectomy. *J Am Coll Surg*. 2013;216(1):1−14.
22. Han IW, Kim H, Heo J, et al. Excess intraoperative fluid volume administration is associated with pancreatic fistula after pancreaticoduodenectomy: a retrospective multicenter study. *Medicine*. 2017;96(22):e6893.
23. Kanda M, Fujii T, Suenaga M, et al. Estimated pancreatic parenchymal remnant volume accurately predicts clinically relevant pancreatic fistula after pancreatoduodenectomy. *Surgery*. 2014;156(3):601−610.

24. Iacono C, Verlato G, Ruzzenente A, et al. Systematic review of central pancreatectomy and metaanalysis of central versus distal pancreatectomy. *Br J Surg.* 2013;100(7): 873–885.

25. Bassi C, Dervenis C, Butturini G, et al. Postoperative pancreatic fistula: an international study group (ISGPF) definition. *Surgery.* 2005;138(1):8–13.

26. Bassi C, Marchegiani G, Dervenis C, et al. The 2016 update of the International Study Group (ISGPS) definition and grading of postoperative pancreatic fistula: 11 years after. *Surgery.* 2017;161(3):584–591.

27. Daskalaki D, Butturini G, Molinari E, Crippa S, Pederzoli P, Bassi C. A grading system can predict clinical and economic outcomes of pancreatic fistula after pancreaticoduodenectomy: results in 755 consecutive patients. *Langenbeck's Arch Surg.* 2011;396(1): 91–98.

28. Kim CG, Jo S, Kim JS. Impact of surgical volume on nationwide hospital mortality after pancreaticoduodenectomy. *World J Gastroenterol.* 2012;18:4175–4181.

29. Nimptsch U, Krautz C, Weber GF, Mansky T, Grützmann R. Nationwide In-hospital Mortality Following Pancreatic Surgery in Germany is Higher than Anticipated. *Ann Surg.* 2016;264(6):10821090.

30. Topal B, Van de Sande S, Fieuws S, Penninckx F. Effect of centralization of pancreaticoduodenectomy on nationwide hospital mortality and length of stay. *Br J Surg.* 2007; 94(11):13771381.

31. Pal N, Axisa B, Yusof S, et al. Volume and outcome for major upper GI surgery in England. *J Gastrointest Surg.* 2008;12(2):353–357.

32. Hallet J, Mahar AL, Tsang ME, Lin Y, Callum J, et al. The impact of peri-operative blood transfusions on post-pancreatectomy short-term outcomes: an analysis from the American College of Surgeons National Surgical Quality Improvement Program. *HPB.* 2015;17(11):975–982.

33. Sun X, Zhang Q, Zhang J, et al. Meta-analysis of invagination and duct-to-mucosa pancreaticojejunostomy after pancreaticoduodenectomy: an update. *Int J Surg.* 2016;36(Pt A):240–247.

34. Zhang S, Lan Z, Zhang J, et al. Duct-to-mucosa versus invagination pancreaticojejunostomy after pancreaticoduodenectomy: a meta-analysis. *Oncotarget.* 2017;8(28): 46449–46460.

35. Singh AN, Pal S, Mangla V, et al. Pancreaticojejunostomy: does the technique matter? A randomized trial. *J Surg Oncol.* 2018;117(3):389–396.

36. Topal B, Fieuws S, Aerts R, et al. Pancreaticojejunostomy versus pancreaticogastrostomy reconstruction after pancreaticoduodenectomy for pancreatic or periampullary tumours: a multicentre randomised trial. *Lancet Oncol.* 2013;14:655–662.

37. Keck T, Wellner UF, Bahra M, et al. Pancreatogastrostomy versus pancreatojejunostomy for RECOnstruction after PANCreatoduodenectomy (RECOPANC, DRKS 00000767): perioperative and longterm results of a multicenter randomized controlled trial. *Ann Surg.* 2016;263(3):440–449.

38. Que W, Fang H, Yan B, et al. Pancreaticogastrostomy versus pancreaticojejunostomy after pancreaticoduodenectomy: a meta-analysis of randomized controlled trials. *Am J Surg.* 2015;209(6):1074–1082.

39. Borel F, Ouaissi M, Merdrignac A, et al. Pancreatico-jejunostomy decreases postoperative pancreatic fistula incidence and severity after central pancreatectomy. *ANZ J Surg.* 2018;88(1-2):77–81.

40. Mauriello C, Polistena A, Gambardella C, et al. Pancreatic stump closure after pancreatoduodenectomy in elderly patients: a retrospective clinical study. *Aging Clin Exp Res.* 2017;29(Suppl 1):35−40.

41. Reissman P, Perry Y, Cuenca A, et al. Pancreaticojejunostomy versus controlled pancreaticocutaneous fistula in pancreaticoduodenectomy for perianipullary carcinoma. *Am J Surg.* 1995;169(6):585588.

42. Tran K, Van Eijck C, Di Carlo V, et al. Occlusion of the pancreatic duct versus pancreaticojejunostomy: a prospective randomized trial. *Ann Surg.* 2002;36(4):422−428.

43. Orci LA, Oldani G, Berney T, et al. Systematic review and meta-analysis of fibrin sealants for patients undergoing pancreatic resection. *HPB (Oxford).* 2014;16(1):3−11.

44. Zebri A, Balzano G, Patuzzo R, et al. Comparison between pylorus-preserving and Whipple pancreatoduodenectomy. *Br J Surg.* 1995;82:975−979.

45. Tani M, Terasawa H, Kawai M, et al. Improvement of delayed gastric emptying in pylorus-preserving pancreaticoduodenectomy: results of a prospective, randomized, controlled trial. *Ann Surg.* 2006;243(3):316−320.

46. Hüttner FJ, Klotz R, Ulrich A, Büchler MW, Diener MK. Antecolic versus retrocolic reconstruction after partial pancreaticoduodenectomy. *Cochrane Database Syst Rev.* 2016;9(9):CD011862.

47. Sewnath ME, Karsten TM, Prins MH, et al. A meta-analysis on the efficacy of preoperative biliary drainage for tumors causing obstructive jaundice. *Ann Surg.* 2002;236:17−27.

48. van der Gaag NA, Rauws EA, van Eijck CH, et al. Preoperative biliary drainage for cancer of the head of the pancreas. *N Engl J Med.* 2010;362:129−137.

49. Fang Y, Gurusamy KS, Wang Q, et al. Pre-operative biliary drainage for obstructive jaundice. *Cochrane Database Syst Rev.* 2012;9:CD005444.

50. Mullen JT, Lee JH, Gomez HF, et al. Pancreaticoduodenectomy after placement of endobiliary metal stents. *J Gastrointest Surg.* 2005;9:1094−1104.

51. Tol JAMG, Gouma DJ, Bassi C, et al. Definition of a standard lymphadenectomy in surgery for pancreatic ductal adenocarcinoma: A consensus statement by the International Study Group on Pancreatic Surgery (ISGPS). *Surgery.* 2014;156(3):591−600.

52. Orci Lorenzo A, Meyer Jeremy, et al. A meta-analysis of extended versus standard lymphadenectomy in patients undergoing pancreatoduodenectomy for pancreatic adenocarcinoma. *HPB.* 2015;17(7):565−572.

53. Lu DS, Reber HA, Krasny RM, Kadell BM, Sayre J. Local staging of pancreatic cancer: criteria for unresectability of major vessels as revealedby pancreatic-phase thin-section helical CT. *Am J Roentgenol.* 1997;168:1439−1443.

54. Valls C, Andía E, Sanchez A, et al. Dual-phase helical CT of pancreatic adenocarcinoma: assessment of resectability before surgery. *Am J Roentgenol.* 2002;178:821−826.

55. Jamieson NB, Foulis AK, Oien KA, et al. Positive mobilization margins alone do not influence survival following pancreaticoduodenectomy for pancreatic ductal adenocarcinoma. *Ann Surg.* 2010;251:1003−1010.

56. Isaji S, Mizuno S, Windsor JA, et al. International consensus on definition and criteria of borderline resectable pancreatic ductal adenocarcinoma 2017. *Pancreatology.* 2018;18(1):2−11.

57. Delpero JR, Bachellier P, Regenet N, et al. Pancreaticoduodenectomy for pancreatic ductal adenocarcinoma: a French multicentre prospective evaluation of resection margins in 150 evaluable specimens. *HPB.* 2014;16:20−33.

58. Nakao A, Takagi H. Isolated pancreatectomy for pancreatic head carcinoma using catheter bypass of the portal vein. *Hepato-Gastroenterology*. 1993;40:426−429.
59. Weitz J, Rahbari N, Koch M, Buchler MW. The artery first approach for resection of pancreatic head cancer. *J Am Coll Surg*. 2010;210:e1−e4.
60. Rose JB, Rocha F, Alseidi A, Helton S. Posterior 'superior mesenteric artery first' approach for resection of locally advanced pancreatic cancer. *Ann Surg Oncol*. 2014; 21:1927−1928.
61. Negoi I, Hostiuc S, Runcanu A, et al. Superior mesenteric artery first approach versus standard pancreaticoduodenectomy: a systematic review and meta-analysis. *Hepatobiliary Pancreat Dis Int*. 2017;16:127−138.
62. Goodney PP, Stukel TA, Lucas FL, Finlayson EV, Birkmeyer JD. Hospital volume, length of stay, and readmission rates in high-risk surgery. *Ann Surg*. 2003;238:161−167.
63. Jeyarajah DR, Berman RS, Doyle M, et al. Consensus conference on North American training in hepatopancreaticobiliary surgery: a review of the conference and presentation of consensus statements. *Am J Transplant*. 2016;16:1086−1093.
64. Raptis DA, Clavien PA, International Hepato-Pancreato-Biliary Association (IHPBA) Education and Training Committee. Evaluation of Hepato-Pancreato-Biliary (HPB) fellowships: an international survey of programme directors. *HPB (Oxford)*. 2011;13(4): 279−285.
65. Borman KR, Vick LR, Biester TW, et al. Changing demographics of residents choosing fellowships: longterm data from the American Board of Surgery. *J Am Coll Surg*. 2008; 206:782−788.
66. Sachs TE, Ejaz A, Weiss M, Spolverato G, Ahuja N, Makary MA, et al. Assessing the experience in complex hepatopancreatobiliary surgery among graduating chief residents: is the operative experience enough? *Surgery*. 2014;156:385−393.
67. Fong Y, Gonen M, Rubin D, Radzyner M, Brennan MF. Long-term survival is superior after resection for cancer in high-volume centers. *Ann Surg*. 2005;242:540−547.
68. Stitzenberg KB, Sigurdson ER, Egleston BL, et al. Centralization of cancer surgery: implications for patient access to optimal care. *J Clin Oncol*. 2009;27(28):4671−4678.
69. Ghaferi AA, Birkmeyer JD, Dimick JB. Variation in hospital mortality associated with inpatient surgery. *N Engl J Med*. 2009;361:1368−1375.
70. Joseph B, Morton JM, Hernandez-Boussard T, Rubinfeld I, Faraj C, Velanovich V. Relationship between hospital volume, system clinical resources, and mortality in pancreatic resection. *J Am Coll Surg*. 2009;208:520−527.
71. Yang R, Cheung MC, Byrne MM, et al. Survival Effects of Adjuvant Chemoradiotherapy After Resection for Pancreatic Carcinoma. *Arch Surg*. 2010;145(1):49−56.
72. Mehrabi A, Hafezi M, Arvin J, et al. A systematic review and meta-analysis of laparoscopic versus open distal pancreatectomy for benign and malignant lesions of the pancreas: it's time to randomize. *Surgery*. 2015;157:45−55.
73. De Rooij T, Jilesen AP, Boerma D, Bonsing BA, Bosscha K, van Dam RM, et al. A nationwide comparison of laparoscopic and open distal pancreatectomy for benign and malignant disease. *J Am Coll Surg*. 2015;220(3):263−270.e1.
74. Rutz DR, Squires MH, Maithel SK, Sarmiento JM, Etra JW, Perez SD, et al. Cost comparison analysis of open versus laparoscopic distal pancreatectomy. *HPB*. 2014;16(10): 907−914.
75. de Rooij T, Besselink MG, Shamali A, et al. Pan-European survey on the implementation of minimally invasive pancreatic surgery with emphasis on cancer. *HPB (Oxford)*. 2016;18(2):170−176.

76. van der Geest LG, van Rijssen LB, Molenaar IQ, de Hingh IH, Groot Koerkamp B, Busch OR, et al. Volume-outcome relationships in pancreatoduodenectomy for cancer. *HPB*. 2016;18(4):317—324.

77. de Rooij T, van Hilst J, Boerma D, Bonsing BA, Daams F, van Dam RM, et al. Impact of a nationwide training program in minimally invasive distal pancreatectomy (LAELAPS). *Ann Surg*. 2016;264:754—762.

78. Vergis A, Steigerwald S. Skill Acquisition, Assessment, and Simulation in Minimal Access Surgery: An Evolution of Technical Training in Surgery. *Cureus*. 2018;10(7): e2969.

79. Chang L, Satava RM, Pellegrini CA, Sinanan MN. Robotic surgery: identifying the learning curve through objective measurements of skill. *Surg Endosc*. 2003;17: 1744—1748.

80. Anastakis DJ, Regehr G, Reznick RK, Cusimano M, Murnaghan J, Brown M, Hutchison C. Assessment of technical skills transfer from the bench training model to the human model. *Am J Surg*. 1999;177:167—170.

81. Kala Z, Valek V, Hlavsa J, Hana K, Vanova A. The role of CT and endoscopic ultrasound in pre-operative staging of pancreatic cancer. *Eur J Radiol*. 2007;62:166—169.

82. Gillen S, Schuster T, Zum Büschenfelde CM, Friess H, Kleeff J. Preoperative/neoadjuvant therapy in pancreatic cancer: a systematic review and meta-analysis of response and resection percentages. *PLoS Med*. 2010;7(4):e1000267.

83. Neoptolemos JP, Stocken DD, Dunn JA, Almond J, Beger HG, Pederzoli P, et al. Influence of resection margins on survival for patients with pancreatic cancer treated by adjuvant chemoradiation and/or chemotherapy in the ESPAC-1 randomized controlled trial. *Ann Surg*. 2001;234(6):758—768.

84. Garcea G, Dennison AR, Pattenden CJ, Neal CP, Sutton CD, Berry DP. Survival following curative resection for pancreatic ductal adenocarcinoma. A systematic review of the literature. *JOP*. 2008;9:99—132.

85. Kato K, Yamada S, Sugimoto H, Kanazumi N, Nomoto S, Takeda S, et al. Prognostic factors for survival after extended pancreatectomy for pancreatic head cancer: influence of resection margin status on survival. *Pancreas*. 2009;38(6):605—612.

86. Nagakawa Y, Sahara Y, Hosokawa Y, et al. Clinical Impact of Neoadjuvant Chemotherapy and Chemoradiotherapy in Borderline Resectable Pancreatic Cancer: Analysis of 884 Patients at Facilities Specializing in Pancreatic Surgery. *Ann Surg Oncol*. 2019; 26:1629—1636.

87. Piccolboni D, Ciccone F, Settembre a, Corcione F. Laparoscopic intra-operative ultrasound in liver and pancreas resection: Analysis of 93 cases. *J Ultrasound*. 2010;13(1): 3—8.

88. Shin LK, Brant-Zawadzki G, Kamaya A, Jeffrey RB. Intraoperative ultrasound of the pancreas. *Ultrasound Q*. 2009;25:39—48 [quiz].

89. van Veldhuisen E, Walma MS, van Rijssen LB, et al. Added value of intra-operative ultrasound to determine the resectability of locally advanced pancreatic cancer following FOLFIRINOX chemotherapy (IMAGE): a prospective multicenter study. *HPB*. 2019; 21(10).

90. Hoogstins CES, Boogerd LSF, Sibinga Mulder BG, et al. Image-Guided Surgery in Patients with Pancreatic Cancer: First Results of a Clinical Trial Using SGM-101, a Novel Carcinoembryonic Antigen-Targeting, Near-Infrared Fluorescent Agent. *Ann Surg Oncol*. 2018;25:3350.

91. Marzano E, Piardi T, Soler L, et al. Augmented reality-guided artery-first pancreatico-duodenectomy. *J Gastrointest Surg*. 2013;17(11):1980–1983.

92. Sánchez-Margallo JA, Langø T, Hofstad EF, Mårvik R, Sánchez-Margallo FM. *Laparoscopic Pancreas Surgery: Image Guidance Solutions, Laparoscopic Surgery*. 2017. Arshad M. Malik, IntechOpen.

93. Kamel IR, Kruskal JB, Pomfret EA, Keogan MT, Warmbrand G, Raptopoulos V. Impact of Multidetector CT on Donor Selection and Surgical Planning Before Living Adult Right Lobe Liver Transplantation. *Am J Roentgenol*. 2001;176(1):193–200.

94. Oshiro Y, Sasaki R, Nasu K, Ohkohchi N. A novel preoperative fusion analysis using three-dimensional MDCT combined with three-dimensional MRI for patients with hilar holangiocarcinoma. *Clin Imag*. 2013;37(4):772–774.

95. Miyamoto R, Oshiro Y, Nakayama K, et al. Three-dimensional simulation of pancreatic surgery showing the size and location of the main pancreatic duct. *Surg Today*. 2017;47: 357.

96. Miyamoto R, Oshiro Y, Nakayama K, Ohkohchi N. Impact of Three-Dimensional Surgical Simulation on Pancreatic Surgery. *Gastrointest Tumors*. 2017;4:84–89.

97. Miyamoto R, Oshiro Y, Sano N, Inagawa S, Ohkohchi N. Three-dimensional surgical simulation of the bile duct and vascular arrangement in pancreatoduodenectomy: A retrospective cohort study. *Ann Med Surg*. 2018;36:17–22.

98. Miyamoto R, Oshiro Y, Sano N, Inagawa S, Ohkohchi N. Three-Dimensional Remnant Pancreatic Volumetry Predicts Postoperative Pancreatic Fistula in Pancreatic Cancer Patients after Pancreaticoduodenectomy. *Gastrointest Tumors*. 2018;5:90–99.

99. Winder J, Bibb R. Medical rapid prototyping technologies: state of the art and current limitations for application in oral and maxillofacial surgery. *J Oral Maxillofac Surg*. 2005;63(7):1006–1015.

100. Shiraishi I, Yamagishi M, Hamaoka K, Fukuzawa M, Yagihara T. Simulative operation on congenital heart disease using rubber-like urethane stereolithographic biomodels based on 3D datasets of multislice computed tomography. *Eur J Cardio Thorac Surg*. 2010;37(2):302–306.

101. Müller A, Krishnan KG, Uhl E, Mast G. The application of rapid prototyping techniques in cranial reconstruction and preoperative planning in neurosurgery. *J Craniofac Surg*. 2003;14(6):899–914.

102. Salmi M, Paloheimo KS, Tuomi J, Wolff J, Mäkitie A. Accuracy of medical models made by additive manufacturing (rapid manufacturing). *J Cranio-Maxillofacial Surg*. 2013;41(7):603–609.

103. Eley KA, Watt-Smith SR, Golding SJ. Three-dimensional reconstruction of the craniofacial skeleton with gradient echo magnetic resonance imaging ("Black Bone"): What is currently possible? *J Craniofac Surg*. 2017;28(2):463–467.

104. Martelli N, Serrano C, van den Brink H, Pineau J, Prognon P, Borget I, El Batti S. Advantages and disadvantages of 3-dimensional printing in surgery: A systematic review. *Surgery*. 2016;159(6):1485–1500.

105. Kalejs M, von Segesser LK. Rapid prototyping of compliant human aortic roots for assessment of valved stents. *Interact Cardiovasc Thorac Surg*. 2009;8:182–186.

106. Snyder RA, Tarpley MJ, Tarpley JL, Davidson M, Brophy C, Dattilo JB. Teaching in the operating room: results of a national survey. *J Surg Educ*. 2012;69(5):643–649.

107. Fang C-H. Application of 3D printing technique in the diagnosis and treatment for pancreatic and periampullary neoplasms. *HPB*. 2016;18:e357.

108. Zheng YX, Yu DF, Zhao JG, Wu YL, Zheng B. 3D Printout Models vs. 3D-Rendered Images: Which Is Better for Preoperative Planning? *J Surg Educ*. 2016;73(3):518−523.
109. Andolfi C, Plana A, Kania P, Banerjee P, Stephen S. Usefulness of Three-Dimensional Modeling in Surgical Planning, Resident Training, and Patient Education. *J Laparoendosc Adv Surg Tech*. 2016:1−4.
110. Bajaj P, Marchwiany D, Duarte C, Bashir R. Patterned three-dimensional encapsulation of embryonic stem cells using dielectrophoresis and stereolithography. *Adv Healthc Mater*. 2013;2(3):450−458.
111. Moroni L, Burdick JA, Highley C, Lee SJ, Morimoto Y, Takeuchi S, Yoo JJ. Bio-fabrication strategies for 3D in vitro models and regenerative medicine. *Nature Rev Mater*. 2018;3(5):21−37.

Three-dimensional printing and hepatobiliary surgery

Andreas I. Tooulias, MD, MSc [1], Maria V. Alexiou, BSc, MSc [2], Georgios Tsoulfas[3]

[1]*General Surgeon, HPB Fellow, Surgical Department, School of Medicine, Faculty of Health Sciences, Aristotle University of Thessaloniki, Thessaloniki, Greece;* [2]*Molecular Biologist and Geneticist, Surgical Department, School of Medicine, Faculty of Health Sciences, Aristotle University of Thessaloniki, Thessaloniki, Greece;* [3]*Associate Professor of Transplantation Surgery, Chief of the Department of Transplantation Surgery, School of Medicine, Faculty of Health Sciences, Aristotle University of Thessaloniki, Thessaloniki, Greece*

Introduction: the introduction of three-dimensional printing in liver surgery

During the last decade, the evolution of advanced imaging methods and computer-based technologies has led to the increased use of three-dimensional (3D) printing in the medical field and especially in general surgery and all the different surgical specialties and subspecialties as well.[1,2] 3D printing is a process of successive adding of a material in a layer-by-layer way, resembling the conventional inkjet printing. Since 2013, when the first-attempted 3D printing application in liver surgery was described,[3] there have been several important and remarkable efforts in order for 3D printing technology to constitute a valuable tool in liver surgery. Education and training on human organ models, profound study of disease models, education and training of students and residents, preoperative planning, intraoperative assessment of complex surgical operations that demand accuracy, postoperative evaluation, and patient counseling are fields where 3D printing is involved.[4] It appears to be a valuable tool for the surgeon in order to plan complex surgical operations carefully, with great accuracy and with fewer complications.

Despite the significant digital revolution, thanks to which radiology provides the extraction (or acquisition) of highly detailed and informative medical images,[5] the clear understanding of anatomical structures remains puzzling in some cases.[6] However, the comprehension of an organ's anatomy is of outmost importance for the surgeon in order to plan and conduct an operation. That means that the surgeon's team should have at their disposal detailed information, so as to interpret the extracted medical images. The conventional analysis of two-dimensional (2D) images obtained from radiology and the analysis of 3D virtual reconstructions[5,7] facilitate the anatomical understanding, which still needs to be optimized. Hence, the development of an imaging method that represents the real anatomy of interest in a precise

3D Printing: Applications in Medical Surgery. https://doi.org/10.1016/B978-0-323-66193-5.00006-X

manner is necessary. In this way, the surgeon would be focused on the preoperative planning and the surgical operation itself. 3D printing technology has been targeting the shortcomings of the above methods.[8–10] Since 1983, when Chuck Hull[11] invented 3D printing, until nowadays, this technology has been used in multiple fields including medicine, where it has led to continuous progress.[12] The inherent accuracy of the 3D printing method, its low cost, and the fact that the images acquired from multidetector computed tomography or magnetic resonance (MRI) could be quickly translated into a physical object of the anatomy of interest justify the broadened range of 3D printing applications in surgery.

The majority of intrahepatic masses requiring resection, in adults, includes hepatocellular carcinoma (HCC) and isolated or few intrahepatic metastases (e.g., colorectal metastasis).[13] According to the World Cancer Report 2014 released by WHO in 2014,[14] HCC ranks first place among all categories of carcinomas based on its prevalence and second place based on its mortality across the world, whereas it is second in prevalence and third in mortality in the Chinese mainland, where it is also first regarding total number of new cases.

HCC is known to be a very serious and complex pathological situation concerning its clinical management, due to its tendency to spread to surrounding intrahepatic structures.[15] There is limited data evaluating the clinical value and feasibility of 3D-printed liver models in HCC and in diagnostic reporting for HCC. Thus, further exploration is needed and warranted especially in cases where a surgical operation is considered as a viable intervention for treatment and reporting of imaging characteristics is crucial.[15–18] Reviewing the international bibliography, there are no large-scale studies suggesting qualitative and/or quantitative methods so as to meet the need for holistic evaluation of the clinical applications of 3D-printed liver structures apart from small-scale pilot study and/or case studies.[19]

In addition to HCC, the most frequently seen malignant mass in the liver is metastatic liver disease. Liver metastases are tumors that have spread to the liver from other malignant sites.[20] The secondary hepatic tumors are reported to be 18–40 times more common than primary hepatic malignancies in Western populations.[21] The statistics indicate that half of the patients suffering from liver malignancies have primary colorectal cancer (CRC), which constitutes a leading cause of cancer-associated death in Western countries and the third most frequent cause of cancer-related death in the world.[22] Approximately, 25%–30% of patients affected with CRC develop liver metastases during the course of their disease.[23,24] Apart from CRC, there are also additional primary tumors of the gastrointestinal tract that give rise to secondary liver disease, including esophageal ($\sim$1%–2%) and gastric carcinomas ($\sim$5%–9%), pancreatic and intestinal neuroendocrine tumors ($\sim$1%), biliary tract cancers ($\sim$5%–10%), as well as pancreatic ductal adenocarcinomas ($\sim$14%) and gastrointestinal stromal tumors (<1%). Other malignant sites outside the gastrointestinal tract that lead to liver malignancies include the breast (<1%–2%), lung (12%–20%), kidney (1%–2%) cancers and melanoma (<1%) and are rare.[25,26] Until nowadays, the estimated 5-year overall survival for all patients with stage IV colorectal cancer is 13%.[27] Treatment approaches for patients with metastatic CRC can be classified as (1) curative or potentially curative (this identifies a group of patients where liver metastases may be resectable), (2) noncurative with active treatment intent (most patients fall into this group), or (3) palliative intent.[20,27] Unfortunately, despite the progress in oncological medication and surgical techniques, only about 25% of patients affected are amenable to resection, which is regarded as the only way to achieve cure.[26]

The implementation of 3D printing in the field of liver transplantation[3] is extremely interesting. It has been reported that 3D-printed liver models have been used in order to have a tactile structure both of the donor's and the recipient's livers. These models have been used so that the surgeon is able to better identify anatomical landmarks, optimize preoperative planning, and avoid the large-for-size or small-for-size syndrome.[28] Furthermore, it is mentioned that the mean errors of the measurements are <4 mm for the whole liver and <1.3 mm for the diameter of the vessels.[3]

Liver diseases, especially those requiring surgical treatment, have implemented this state-of-the-art technique for many applications in liver surgery. Until nowadays, liver resection constitutes the first-line procedure available for liver cancer that guarantees successful treatment. Regardless of the latest technological progress, liver resection remains a challenging procedure especially for residents and/or young surgeons. The excellent knowledge of liver anatomy is extremely crucial for the different types of intricate liver resections, whether they are anatomical or not. However, each patient is different, meaning that there are always anatomical variations present. Furthermore, the knowledge of the anatomical relationships among the branches of Glisson's sheath, the hepatic veins, and the tumor is essential for safe and accurate liver interventions as well.[29]

The progress made in 3D visualization technology and more updated 3D printing technology has offered more accessible approaches to HCC and/or a variety of liver lesions. Despite the fact that 3D printing method cannot replace the technique, the ability, and the experience of a surgeon, it remains a beneficial technology providing accurate, personalized, graspable, and tactile 3D liver models with the lesion in question. Specifically, 3D-printed liver models may be helpful in the resection of hepatic tumors through demonstrating the relationship of the tumor and its location within hepatic segments with surrounding structures, thus helping with issues such as invasion or proximity to major hepatic or portal veins, arteries, and bile ducts.[30]

The clinical use of the 3D-printed liver models in hepatic surgeries

The liver is an organ with complex anatomy and physiology, rendering the hepatectomy one of the most difficult surgical operations. Thus, 3D models are beneficial to comprehend the liver's complex and highly variable anatomical characteristics.[3,31–34] There is a variety of studies in the literature examining the feasibility of the 3D printing liver model's application in the clinical use. The quantitative analysis of these studies have demonstrated the accurate replication of complex liver anatomical structures and tumors with the differences between printed models and original source images or reference images ranging from 0.20% to 20.8%.[35]

There are three stages during a liver resection, when the surgical team can evaluate the clinical use of the 3D liver model and adjust it to the needs of each patient individually. These stages are preoperative, intraoperative, and postoperative. There are plenty of case studies that support that 3D liver models are extremely useful clinical tools during all the stages needed for a liver lesion resection and for living donor liver transplant procedures.[3,17,34,36–38] The majority of available data describe the role of 3D printing in the preoperative stage.[4,7,39–41] Reviewing the bibliography, there are plenty of studies reporting the use of 3D-printed liver models in order to develop a better understanding of the organ's anatomy, the lesion's location, and surrounding structures' interactions during the preoperative planning.[17,28,31,32,34,37,38,42–46]

Preoperatively, the precise anatomical characterization of vascular and biliary network and the volumetric accuracy are necessary in order to plan the surgery with more accuracy and safety. 3D printing technology contributes to that, as it provides detailed imaging of the target anatomy, the geometry, and the volume of the liver. In other words, it provides a mean for getting deeply familiarized with the patient's anatomy prior to surgery. Furthermore, it could help the surgeon evaluate patients with challenging anatomy so as to decrease possible intraoperative complications.[3] Interestingly, it was reported[47] that a minor hepatectomy was avoided as the presence of the 3D model revealed that the tumor was unresectable. There are a lot of reports in the international bibliography that underline the effectiveness of the 3D-printed model when referring to a variety of surgical operations including hepatic surgeries.[3,4,39,41] More specifically, the 3D-printed model can help the surgeon localize the targeted part of the liver, delineate the tumor, and specify the resection lines or the dissection planes. Furthermore, the printed models have the advantage of tactile sense, thus allowing the surgeons (students and residents, as well) to practice and plan the resection achieving in this way the goal of personalized and precision medicine.[48]

Admittedly, the majority of the studies report satisfying results regarding the effectiveness of the 3D-printed liver models during the preoperative design. Nevertheless, the absence of randomized controlled trials (RCTs) does not allow a thorough evaluation of all the clinical outcomes.[49]

During the surgical procedure, the presence of the 3D model in the operating room is very helpful for localizing quickly and with advanced accuracy the hepatic tumor(s). The fact that the 3D model is portable is one of the major advantages of 3D printing especially in cases of difficult orientation, where the model serves for intraoperative reassessment[7,39,40] and guidance of intraoperative procedures.[35] In conclusion, the preoperative organization of the hepatic resection with the aid of a 3D model comes with advantages such as the decrease of the surgical time, the reduction of possible intraoperative complications, and the avoidance of blood product transfusions. All the above act cumulatively for minimizing the postoperative complications and the hospitalization period as well.

It is very interesting that the surgeon can not only design the surgical plan but also personalize the postoperative treatment of each patient based on the 3D-printed model.

3D-printed liver models as educational and training tools in surgery

Apart from their usefulness in the preoperative planning and intraoperative assessment, the 3D-printed liver models have served as important tools for the education and training of medical students and residents in liver surgical techniques. This revolutionary technique has been applied in surgical and medical education as it can address the requirement for high-quality visualization of the interior architecture, tactile feedback, and highly reproducible structures. There are plenty of studies supporting that the 3D imaging technology contributes to the better understanding of the liver's anatomy and the tumor's location.

For example, according to such a study, it was demonstrated that the 3D visualization and 3D-printed models contributed to improved understanding of the hepatic anatomy and pathology, when compared with the traditional anatomical atlases as a learning method ($P < .05$).[50] This makes the interaction of technology and modern surgery essential. The new generations of doctors and especially surgeons should be aware of the advances in technology, while at the same time showing a level of comfort in using them that will allow to benefit their patients. 3D-printed liver models come from individualized patient-specific imaging data allowing the elaborate recognition of anatomical landmarks and/or pathological characteristics.

A few RCTs have been conducted in recent years, and the results highlight the effectiveness of the 3D model among a variety of participants including medical students and junior—senior surgeons and residents. It is interesting that during the evaluation of the given anatomy on 3D-printed model and computed tomography (CT) scan, 3D reconstruction, and cadavers, 3D-printed models contributed more to identifying key anatomical elements.[40,50,51] It is important to realize that the advancement of technology has led to the reproduction of hollow structures with such properties that mimic the native human tissue and/or organ.[6,52] Such structures represent a new age for surgical simulation. This means that the surgeons of any expertise, and especially trainees, can train themselves in as many tasks as the 3D-printed models can reproduce, whatever the purpose of simulation might be: improving a certain skill through multiple repetitions of the same exercise, testing novel surgical devices outside the operating room, or getting ready for a real intervention before it takes place on the patient.[53]

Training is not only for novice surgeons but also for those surgeons who are going to perform a liver resection and is extremely important in order to develop and continuously improve their surgical skills. Until recently, cadaver models constituted the gold standard for medical practice.[54] However, there are limitations that have led to cadaver laboratories being an inefficient method due to cost, procurement, and reproducibility.[55] A 3D-printed model can overcome some of the limitations of the cadaver's use and help the specialists to optimize the conditions of their practice so as to organize the surgical plan in a more efficient manner, which will ultimately benefit the patient the most.

A hepatic resection is a team effort. The surgical team consists of the surgeons, the operating room nurses, and the anesthesiologists. 3D models can achieve the goal of bringing everyone together and training all of them as a team. Furthermore, the surgeons have the time to explain the surgical steps and the anatomy of the patient's liver to the surgical team. They can describe possible difficulties that may arise during the surgery, so that the team will be prepared to avoid them. Everyone will have the time to get ready. It is well known that a steady, trained team has better outcomes and is more efficient, more accurate, and consequently ready to avoid major complications. Eventually, the surgical team will be more specialized throughout the time, and they will be equipped with "tools" for the next step if needed during the operation, foe example, the anesthesiologists would be ready for providing additional drugs, the operating room nurses would be ready for giving surgical tools, the surgeons would be knowledgeable of alternate plans (plan B).

3D-printed models as useful tools for patient and family counseling before the surgical operation

The fact that the 3D-printed model is portable facilitates its demonstration to the patient from the surgeon's team before the operation aiming to provide more convincing information concerning the patient's overall health situation and the possible complications.[7,40] It is worthy to mention that the patients develop a better understanding of their liver damage, the reasons for which the surgery is needed, and the most important is that the feeling of safety and confidence between physician and patient is increased. It is very important for the patient and the family that they see their own anatomical model with the lesion in question. The presence of the model stimulates various questions concerning the surgery, the kind of the damage and the technical details of the operation and what kind of outcome should be expected.[7]

This detailed briefing is summarized in the consent form that will mention the type of the surgical operation and the possible complications. The result is a detailed and "as good as can be" consent form and process.

Limitations of 3D printing technology in hepatic surgeries

Regardless of the increasing application of 3D printing technology, mostly in the planning of a surgical procedure, the cost and the time required are limitations that need to be overcome. Concerning the cost of the process, it is variable and depended on the consumables used and/or the preferable size of the printed model (full-size or scaled-down). The data resulting from different studies suggest a variable cost ranging from the lowest USD13 to as high as USD2000 with a high-quality, full-sized liver model printed with photopolymer resin, which can cost up to USD2000.[35] The software and hardware of the technique used, the kind of the printer, the selected materials, the desired model's size could contribute to the cost's increase. The reduction of the cost is vital for the improvement of the feasibility and the clinical value. It is even more important if we consider that one of the side benefits of this new technology is that it can be used to promote global surgery. Specifically, technology such as 3D printing can be used to help print instruments or help demonstrate parts of the surgery, and thus prove to be of immense help in parts of the world with limited resources.

As for the time required, it is divided in the time needed for the processing of the image, segmentation, editing of data for 3D printing, and the time spent for the printing process.[35] The processing of the image, segmentation, and editing of data for 3D printing are depended on the software used and the user's familiarity. However, the duration of the printing according to the data published so far ranges from 11 to 100 h.[3,37,38,42,43,56] It is important to mention the fact that the time is much lesser than when the creation of the liver models is based on patient-specific imaging data.[57] The duration of the whole process is described in a study, where the authors report that they needed 160 h in order to print the liver model from the image's segmentation until the final 3D structure.[31]

In addition, the time needed for the production of a model restricts the application of 3D-printed models in emergency cases that demand immediate treatment.

Conclusion: 3D printing applications in surgery is a revolution in the medical field

In 2018, the Radiological Society of North America Special Interest Group on 3D Printing published initial guidelines for medical 3D printing appropriateness, which included a number of organ- or system-based appropriateness criteria.[58] However, those guidelines did not include indications for abdominal, hepatobiliary, and gastrointestinal 3D printing.

In this chapter, the data advocate for the systematic use of 3D printing in the clinical evaluation of liver lesions. It is concluded that 3D-printed liver models have been used to enhance the surgeon's comprehension of the highly variable and complex liver anatomy.[3,31,32,34,50] As mentioned above, the liver resection is a complicated task requiring full understanding of each patient's specific anatomical and pathological characteristics in order to ensure optimal surgical outcomes.[15–17,36,59,60] The inherent 3D-printed model accuracy is crucial when evaluating the feasibility as it ensures precision and safety during the designation of effective surgical planning.[19] Although it is apparent that 3D liver models can be very useful tools in intraoperative navigation and orientation, they are not yet able to replace the intraoperative visualization methods (e.g., Doppler ultrasound and cholangiography).[3,17,34,37] Furthermore, a specialist should take into account that there is the risk of inconsistencies in the orientation and location of measurements for the individual anatomical landmarks.[35]

Overall, 3D printing technology represents a new age in liver surgery. Apart from the benefits of this new technology, there are also some limitations. Unquestionably continued technological improvements and developments would overcome any obstacles. The cost of time and money could be decreased by optimizing the perspectives of the available software and hardware.

It is worth mentioning that 3DP technology is not intended to entirely replace the conventional imaging methods such as CT and MRI. The purpose is the evaluation of all the available imaging methods and the translation of the 3D-printed model in such way that the surgeon could perform a hands-on simulation before the liver resection and design a detailed and sufficient operative plan in the absence of a time-pressured surgical environment.

Despite the fact that the use of 3D-printed applications in hepatobiliary surgery is in its infancy, the inherent anatomical and geometrical accuracy of these constructs paves the way for the goal of printing whole organs that can change medicine and surgery as we know it.

Co-financed by the European Union and Greek national funds through the Operational Program Competitiveness, Entrepreneurship and Innovation, under the call RESEARCH? CREATE - INNOVATE (project code:T1EDK-03599).

References

1. Giannopoulos AA, Steigner ML, George E, et al. Cardiothoracic applications of 3-dimensional printing. *J Thorac Imag*. 2016;31:253–272.
2. Chae MP, Rozen WM, McMenamin PG, et al. Emerging applications of bedside 3D printing in plastic surgery. *Front Surg*. 2015;2:25.
3. Zein N, Hanouneh I, Bishop P, Samaan M, Eghtesad B, Quintini C, et al. Three-dimensional print of a liver for preoperative planning in living donor liver transplantation. *Liver Transplant*. 2013;19(12):1304–1310.
4. Malik HH, Darwood ARJ, Shaunak S, Kulatilake P, El-Hilly AA, Mulki O, Baskaradas A. Three-dimensional printing in surgery: a review of current surgical applications. *J Surg Res*. 2015;199:512–522.
5. Doi K. Diagnostic imaging over the last 50 years: research and development in medical imaging science and technology. *Phys Med Biol*. 2006;51:R5–R27.
6. Rengier F, Mehndiratta A, von Tengg-Kobligk H, Giesel FL. 3D printing based on imaging data: review of medical applications. *Int J Comput Assist Radiol Surg*. 2010;(5):335–341.

7. Pietrabissa A, Marconi S, Peri A, Pugliese L, Auricchio F. From CT scanning to 3-D printing technology for the pre-operative planning in laparoscopic splenectomy. *Surg Endosc*. 2015;30(1):366−371.

8. Tack P, Victor J, Annemans L. 3D-printing techniques in a medical setting: a systematic literature review. *Biomed Eng Online*. 2016;15:115.

9. Kim GB, Lee S, Kim H, Yang DH, Kim Y, Kyung YS, et al. Three-dimensional printing: basic principles and applications in medicine and radiology. *Korean J Radiol*. 2016; 17(2):182−197.

10. Ventola CL. Medical applications for 3D printing: current and projected uses. *Pharmacol Ther*. 2014;39:704−711.

11. Hull CW. *Apparatus for Production of Three-Dimensional Objects by Stereolithography*. United States Patent US 4,575,330. 1986:1−16.

12. Gross BC, Erkal JL, Lockwood SY, Chen C, Spence DM. Evaluation of 3D printing and its potential impact on biotechnology and the chemical sciences. *Anal Chem*. 2014;86: 3240−3253.

13. Gani F, Thompson VM, Bentrem DJ, Hall BL, Pitt HA, Pawlik TM. Patterns of hepatic resections in North America: use of concurrent partial resections and ablations. *HPB*. 2016;18(10):813−820.

14. Cancer IAFR. *World Cancer Report 2014*. Geneva: WHO; 2014.

15. Ertel AE, Shah SA. Surgical approaches to hepatocellular carcinoma. *Semin Roentgenol*. 2016;51:88−94.

16. Memeo R, De'Angelis N, De Blasi V, Cherkaoul Z, Brunetti O, Longo V, Piardi T, Sommacale D, Marescaux J, Mutter D, Pessaux P. Innovative surgical approaches for hepatocellular carcinoma. *World J Hepatol*. 2016;8:591−596.

17. Souzaki R, Kinoshita Y, Ieiri S, Hayashida M, Koga Y, Shirabe K, Hara T, Maehara Y, Hashizume M, Taguchi T. Three-dimensional liver model based on preoperative CT images as a tool to assist in surgical planning for hepatoblastoma in a child. *Pediatr Surg Int*. 2015;31:593−596.

18. Choi JY, Lee JM, Sirlin CB. CT and MR imaging diagnosis and staging of hepatocellular carcinoma: part II. Extracellular agents, hepatobiliary agents, and ancillary imaging features. *Radiology*. 2014;273:30−50.

19. Witowski JS, Coles-Black J, Zuzak TZ, Pedziwiatr M, Chuen J, Major P, Budzynki A. 3D printing in liver surgery: a systematic review. *Telemed J E Health*. 2017;23:1−5.

20. Milette S, Sicklick JK, Lowy AM, Brodt P. Molecular pathways: targeting the microenvironment of liver metastases. *Clin Cancer Res*. 2017;23(21):6390−6399.

21. Namasivayam S, Martin DR, Saini S. Imaging of liver metastases: MRI. *Cancer Imag*. 2007;7:2−9.

22. Adam R, De Gramont A, Figueras J, Guthrie A, Kokudo N, Kunstlinger F, Loyer E, Poston G, Rougier P, Rubbia-Brandt L, et al. The oncosurgery approach to managing liver metastases from colorectal cancer: a multidisciplinary international consensus. *Oncologist*. 2012;17(10):1225−1239.

23. Manfredi S, Lepage C, Hatem C, Coatmeur O, Faivre J, Bouvier AM. Epidemiology and management of liver metastases from colorectal cancer. *Ann Surg*. 2006;244(2): 254−259.

24. Hackl C, Neumann P, Gerken M, Loss M, Klinkhammer-Schalke M, Schlitt HJ. Treatment of colorectal liver metastases in Germany: a ten-year population based analysis of 5772 cases of primary colorectal adenocarcinoma. *BMC Cancer*. 2014;14:810.

25. Hoyer M, Erichsen R, Gandrup P, Norgaard M, Jacobsen JB. Survival in patients with synchronous liver metastases in central and northern Denmark, 1998 to 2009. *Clin Epidemiol*. 2011;3(Suppl 1):11−17.

26. Turdean S, Gurzu S, Turcu M, Voidăzan S, Sin A. Liver metastases: incidence and clinicopathological data. *Acta Med Marisiensis*. 2012;58(4):254−258.

27. Sag AA, Selcukbiricik F, Mandel NM. Evidence-based medical oncology and interventional radiology paradigms for liver-dominant colorectal cancer metastases. *World J Gastroenterol*. 2016;22(11):3127−3149.

28. Leng S, Chen B, Vrieze T, Kuhlmann J, Yu L, Alexander A, Matsumoto J, Morris J, McCollough CH. Construction of realistic phantoms from patient images and a commercial three-dimensional printer. *J Med Imaging*. 2016;3:033501.

29. Kuroda S, Kobayashi T, Ohdan H. 3D printing model of the intrahepatic vessels for navigation during anatomical resection of hepatocellular carcinoma. *Int J Surg Case Rep*. 2017;41:219−222.

30. Ballard D, Wake N, Witowski J, Rybicki FJ, Sheikh A. Radiological Society of North America (RSNA) 3D printing special interest group (SIG) clinical situations for which 3D printing is considered an appropriate representation or extension of data contained in a medical imaging examination: abdominal, hepatobiliary, and gastrointestinal conditions. *3D Print Med*. 2020;6(1):13.

31. Witowski JS, Pedziwiatr M, Major P, Budzynski A. Cost-effective personalized, 3D-printed liver model for preoperative planning before laparoscopic liver hemihepatectomy for colorectal cancer metastases. *Int J Comput Assist Radiol Surg*. 2017;12:2047−2054.

32. Madurska MJ, Poyade M, Eason D, Rea P, Watson AJM. Development of a patient-specific 3D-printed liver model for preoperative planning. *Surg Innovat*. 2017;24:145−150.

33. Watson RA. A low-cost surgical application of additive fabrication. *J Surg Educ*. 2014;71:14−17.

34. Xiang N, Fang C, Fan Y, Yang J, Zeng N, Liu J, Zhu W. Application of liver three-dimensional printing in hepatectomy for complex massive hepatocarcinoma with rare variations of portal vein: preliminary experience. *Int J Clin Exp Med*. 2015;8:18873−18887.

35. Perica ER, Sun Z. A systematic review of three-dimensional printing in liver disease. *J Digit Imag*. 2018;31:692−701.

36. Alkhouri N, Zein NN. Three-dimensional printing and pediatric liver disease. *Curr Opin Pediatr*. 2016;28:626−630.

37. Igami T, Nakamura Y, Hirose T, Ebata T, Yokoyama Y, Sugawara G, Mizuno T, Mori K, Nagino M. Application of a three-dimensional print of a liver in hepatectomy for small tumors invisible by intraoperative ultrasonography: Preliminary experience. *World J Surg*. 2014;38:3163−3166.

38. Oshiro Y, Mitani J, Okada T, Ohkohchi N. A novel three-dimensional print of liver vessels and tumors in hepatectomy. *Surg Today*. 2017;47:521−524.

39. Martelli N, Serrano C, van den Brink H, Pineau J, Prognon P, Borget I, El Batti S. Advantages and disadvantages of 3-dimensional printing in surgery: a systematic review. *Surgery*. 2016;159(6):1485−1500.

40. Marconi S, Pugliese L, Botti M, Peri A, Cavazzi E, Latteri S, et al. Value of 3D-printing for the comprehension of surgical anatomy. *Surg Endosc*. 2017;31(10):4102−4110.

41. Li C, Cheung F, Fan VC, Ka Kit Leung G. Application of three-dimensional printing in surgery. *Surg Innovat*. 2017;24(1):82−88.

42. Perica E, Sun Z. Patient-specific three-dimensional printing for pre-surgical planning in hepatocellular carcinoma treatment. *Quant Imag Med Surg*. 2017;7(6):668−677.

43. Soejima Y, Taguchi T, Sugimoto M, Hayashida M, Yoshizumi T, Ikegami T, Uchiyama H, Shirabe K, Maehara Y. Three-dimensional printing and biotexture modeling for preoperative simulation in living donor liver transplantation for small infants. *Liver Transplant*. 2016;22:1610−1614.

44. Wang JZ, Xiong NY, Zhao LZ, Hu JT, Kong DC, Yuan JY. Review fantastic medical implications of 3D printing in liver surgeries, liver regeneration, liver transplantation and drug hepatotoxicity testing: a review. *Int J Surg*. 2018;56:1−6.

45. Takagi K, Nanashima A, Abo T, Arai J, Matsuo N, Fukuda T, Nagayasu T. Three-dimensional printing model of liver for operative simulation in perihilar cholangiocarcinoma. *Hepatogastroenterology*. 2014;61:2315−2316.

46. Baimakhanov Z, Soyama A, Takatsuki M, Hidaka M, Hirayama T, Kinoshita A, Natsuda K, Kuroki T, Eguchi S. Preoperative simulation with a 3-dimensional printed solid model for one-step reconstruction of multiple hepatic veins during living donor liver transplantation. *Liver Transplant*. 2015;21:266−268.

47. Igami T, Nakamura Y, Oda M, Tanaka H, Nojiri M, Ebata T, Yokoyama Y, Sugawara G, Mizuno T, Yamaguchi J, Mori K, Nagino M. Application of three-dimensional print in minor hepatectomy following liver partition between anterior and posterior sectors. *ANZ J Surg*. 2018;88:882−885.

48. Matsumoto JS, Morris JM, Foley TA, Kuhlamann JL, Nesberg LE, Vrtiska TJ. Three-dimensional physical modeling: applications and experience at Mayo clinic. *Radiographics*. 2015;35:1989−2006.

49. Bangeas P, Tsioukas V, Papadopoulos V, Tsoulfas G. Role of innovative 3D printed models in the management of hepatobiliary malignancies. *World J Hepatol*. 2019;11(7):574−585.

50. Kong X, Nie L, Zhang H, Wang Z, Ye Q, Tang L, Li J, Huang W. Do three-dimensional visualization and three-dimensional printing improve hepatic segment anatomy teaching? A randomized controlled study. *J Surg Educ*. 2016;73:264−269.

51. Fasel JH, Aguiar D, Kiss-Bodolay D, Montet X, Kalangos A, Stimec BV, Ratib O. Adapting anatomy teaching to surgical trends: a combination of classical dissection, medical imaging, and 3D-printing technologies. *Surg Radiol Anat*. 2016;38:361−367.

52. Rasheed K, Mix D, Chandra A. Numerous applications of 3D printing in vascular surgery. *Ann Vasc Surg*. 2015;29(4):643−644.

53. Pugliese L, Marconi S, Negrello E, Mauri V, Peri A, Gallo V, Auricchio F, Pietrabissa A. The clinical use of 3D printing in surgery. *Updates Surg*. 2018;70(3):381−388.

54. Blaschko SD, Brooks HM, Dhuy SM, Charest-Shell C, Clayman RV, McDougall EM. Coordinated multiple cadaver use for minimally invasive surgical training. *J Soc Laparoendosc Surg*. 2007;11:403−407.

55. Waran V, Narayanan V, Karuppiah R, Pancharatnam D, Chandran H, Raman R, et al. Injecting realism in surgical training-initial simulation experience with custom 3D models. *J Surg Educ*. 2014;71:193−197.

56. Bucking TM, Hill E, Robertson JL, Maneas E, Plumb AA, Nikitichev DI. From medical imaging to data to 3D printed anatomical models. *PloS One*. 2017;12:e0178540.

57. Javan R, Herrin D, Tangestanipoor A. Understanding spatially complex segmental and branch anatomy using 3D printing: liver, lung, prostate, coronary arteries, and circle of willis. *Acad Radiol*. 2016;23:1183−1189.

58. Chepelev L, Wake N, Ryan J, Althobaity W, Gupta A, Arribas E, et al. Radiological Society of North America (RSNA) 3D printing special interest group (SIG): guidelines for medical 3D printing and appropriateness for clinical scenarios. *3D Print Med.* 2018;4(1): 11.
59. Yao R, Xu G, Mao SS, Yang HY, Sang XT, Sun W, Mao YL. Three-dimensional printing: review of application in medicine and hepatic surgery. *Cancer Biol Med.* 2016;13: 443−451.
60. Soon DS, Chae MP, Pilgrim CH, Rozen WM, Spychal RT, Hunter-Smith DJ. 3D haptic modelling for preoperative planning of hepatic resection: a systematic review. *Ann Med Surg.* 2016;10:1−7.

3D printing in gynecology and obstetrics

Angelos Daniilidis, MD, PhD, MSc, BSCCP, DFFP, MIGS [1],
Theodoros D. Theodoridis, MD, PhD [2], **Grigoris F. Grimbizis, MD, PhD** [2]

[1]*2nd Department of Obstetrics and Gynaecology, Hippokratio General Hospital, Aristotle University of Thessaloniki, Thessaloniki, Greece;* [2]*1st Department of Obstetrics and Gynaecology, Aristotle University of Thessaloniki, Thessaloniki, Greece*

Introduction

The three-dimensional (3D) illustration technology developed throughout the 1980s, but it has made a huge progress over the last 10 years. While most of the printers have a commercial use, the 3D imaging and printing is a developing application, which helps doctors in diagnosis, therapeutic planning, and possibly the cure of patients with complicated diseases. The evolution has been significant especially during the last decade, walking toward thrilling evolution. The 3D printing, known as additives production, is a process of 3D total data use for the production of tactile natural objects from digitized models. This is accomplished through the setting of material consecutive levels like plastic, ceramic, or glass, which corresponds to a string of cross sections for the vulnerable 3D objects printing. The 3D printing was not only successfully used for the creation of additional limps, hearing aid, and dental devices but also for the development of regenerated tissues. Certain medical specialties focused on the technology use for the creation of customized implants through the illustration printing with magnetic resonance imaging (MRI) or computerized tomography (CT), as well for the guidance of surgical approach with assessment of the patient's anatomy model.

3D printer types

There are numerous 3D printers, each one with its advantages and disadvantages. It is important to take the institutional targets into consideration, as well as the anticipated model use, depending on the medical specialty. The printers can be divided into two main groups. The first group consists of the printers that perform additional processes and the second one of the printers that execute reductive processes. The basic idea behind the 3D printing is that of the inkjet printer, which adds isolated ink dots to give an illustration, and a 3D printer adds material that is required by following orders of a digital file.

The technology of additive construction is performed on printers of different shapes and sizes regardless of the 3D printer type or the material used, whereas the 3D printing process follows the same basic steps. It starts with the creation of a 3D drawing from the object desired by the specialist, by using CAD (computer-aided design). The digital model could also emerge through the use of some 3D scanner or by downloading a file through the Internet.

The modeling printers with the fusion deposition method (FDM), widely known as material extrusion printers, belong to the common types of additional 3D illustration. A lot of FDM devices are able to print on different kinds of material like ABS, PLA, TPE/TPU, nylon fiber, soluble material, and polypropylene. The advantages of this kind of printer are its low cost, the low cost of the material, the available cords, and the spare parts, as well as the easy installation and use. Due to the quality of these devices, the really high analysis prints can be difficult, the printing time for complicated anatomic structures can be extremely high, and the options of the material and color are limited. To continue with, it is worth mentioning the selective laser sintering, the selective laser melting printers, and the melting printers with electron beams. These devices are similar to the printers SLA/DLP, by using resin. The sintering warms the material while maintaining the porosity. The melting warms the material further by making it a homogenous part. While the printers can produce models on materials that are available in the devices mentioned above, like the ceramics and other metals and alloys, their size and cost can be prohibitive for many healthcare institutions.

Simple printers are also available, including laminating object construction devices (LOM). With this technology, the thin material layers (paper, plastic, metal) are collided to each other and then cut with a thin blade or laser. More layers can be added later and the process is repeated until the model is fulfilled. The potential benefit of this technology is the variety of the materials that can be used. Some of these materials are very cheap and easily recycled, like paper. The LOM printers tend to be so big and expensive that they could limit the institutional use at the moment.

Clinical application of 3D printing in gynecology

Although the last 20 years were characterized by the total domination of the two-dimensional (2D) ultrasonography as the basic tool of gynecology and obstetrics, the future belongs to the 3D illustration, and even 3D printing. The 3D ultrasonography is already applied as diagnostic tool in gynecology and obstetrics, despite the debated opinions on its essential contribution. Even though the illustration of the embryo's face inside the uterus is unique, this approach has not been widely accepted by the specialists. However, the 3D ultrasonography has been directly accepted due to its really useful diagnostic applications.

The accomplishment of the 3D illustration was first fulfilled by Kossoff et al.,[1] who succeeded in replacing the normal linear core with the cylindrical 3D, in order to illustrate the size of the tissue examined. This core was not likely to be applied in obstetrics since the vaginal access was not possible. Another research team, however, of Baba,[2] succeeded in creating 3D pictures by receiving sequential sections of the examined tissue with the transducer movement. These pictures come into the computer memory as a mass, while the saved data can be edited with the section reconstruction, the surface rendering, and the volume rendering.[2]

The potential for the practical application in the field of gynecology and obstetrics will possibly include three basic development fields:

- Use of 3D standardized models for simulation and preoperative surgical planning of complex processes: The introduction of this technology in pelvic surgery has shown an improving diagnosis due to the better 3D assessment of pathology. In a principle where a successful surgery depends on the evaluation of the soft tissues levels and their anatomy, the preoperative interdisciplinary conversation and simulation contribute to the prediction of potential complications, allowing us to design the best surgical strategy. This can lead to decreased operation time and the effective use of the device.[3−5]
- Education of scientists and informing the patients having had complications: For the apprentices, the extended anatomy knowledge is completed by the 2D illustration and can be further enhanced with more intensive education by using 3D models. Furthermore, patients who have suffered complications, like accidental urethral injury, can be informed by using tactile models of their real injuries so that their injury can be explained and interventions can be discussed.
- Research in the tissue planning and bioprinting: The research could increase the use possibility of tissue planning and biological printing in order to help the ovary regeneration or the restoration of the embryo's face on a pelvic level.[4,5]

Several bibliographical data prove that the 3D illustration offers multiple advantages in contrast to the 2D illustration as well as the other diagnostic approaches. A benefit of the 3D ultrasonography contrary to the 2D one, and to expand the case, the benefit of 3D printing, is the fact that a reproduction of every selected mass can be fulfilled. One characteristic case is the uterus illustration in a coronary section. Moreover, the 3D mass illustration and printing can be realized in three rectangle shots by offering a complete examination at the same time.[6,7]

In addition, another benefit of the 3D printing is the case of the pelvis organ mass assessment regardless of their shape. The mass competency constitutes the nowadays popular application of 3D ultrasonography in obstetrics, since its consequence is the embryo's face illustration. We have to mention up to this point that the 3D real-time illustration in obstetrics has a disadvantage due to the possibility of artifacts, which are usually caused from the intense movement of the embryo or from the fact that anatomic structures (i.e., hands, the placenta or the umbilical cord) intervene giving a fallible picture. This possibly constitutes the most significant cause of the nontotal acceptance of the 3D real-time ultrasonography in obstetrics. On the other hand, in gynecology, the pelvis organs do not move, and with the intravaginal strategy, the approach of the examined organs takes place without the intervention of anatomic clues, by preventing the appearance of artifacts, which results in the unreliability of the uterus illustration. This also constitutes the main cause of the 3D ultrasonography and printing wide acceptance in gynecology.[8]

The uterus can easily be observed through the intervaginal ultrasonography due to its small size, as well as its small distance from the core. Thus, the ultrasonography illustration and the 3D printing is feasible, regarding the diagnosis of pathological findings. The 2D ultrasonography does not offer a satisfying illustration in coronary section, and as a result, other diagnostic approaches are used, like hysterosalpingography, diagnostic hysteroscopy, and laparoscopy, so that birth defects can be diagnosed. The uterus printing and imagine in coronary section is possible through the 3D illustration during the intercellular phase of the cycle, when the endometrium is particularly thick and the endometrial cavity is distinctly separated from the myometrium.

Jurcovic et al.,[9] in order to study the diagnostic reliability of the 2D and 3D ultrasonography, by using hysterosalpingography, included 61 women in their work, having a series of miscarriages or subfertility, and they observed that there was total agreement between the 3D ultrasonography and the hysterosalpingography, regarding the uterus characterization as normal or not, whereas the 2D ultrasonography showed really fallible positive results. Similar results are published by Raga et al.,[10] comparing the 3D ultrasonography data to those of hysterosalpingography and diagnostic laparoscopy. The value of the 3D ultrasonography for the diagnosis of birth defects is emphasized by Merz's team.[11] Thus, it is perceivable that the 3D ultrasonography is able to be used in diagnosing a routine, regarding the uterus birth defects contrary to the normally used methods. Taking the next step, using the obtained 3D images, we can produce 3D models, which will be easily used for better visualization.

Another important parameter that regards the 3D ultrasonography and printing use in the daily diagnosis is the possibility of regenerating and processing the picture after the examination has finished. The uterus 2D ultrasonography could be used as a first-level screening test, in case there is suspicion of uterus birth defects while a detailed examination with a 3D imaging and printing could significantly help.

One of the most important dilemmas of the ultrasonography examination of women with irregular vaginal bleeding is the differential diagnosis of focal or generalized pathology of the endometrium. Women with pervasive malfunction usually undergo an endometrial biopsy, so that a malignancy is excluded. On the contrary, women with focal malfunctions, like polyps or submucous fibroids, undergo a surgical hysteroscopy. Although there are several references that prove that the 2D transvaginal ultrasonography is a reliable method for the diagnosis of focal endometrium pathological findings, there are other references as well, which claim that the diagnostic accuracy can be improved with physiological saline injection into the endometrial cavity. These opinions have expanded nowadays in the field of 3D ultrasonography.[12] Bonilla-Musoles et al.[13] studied 36 women with postmenopausal bleeding by using 2D intervaginal ultrasonography, hysterosalpingography hysteroscopy, and 3D ultrasonography. In four women with focal malfunctions, the 3D ultrasonography totally achieved the right diagnosis, whereas the 2D one lost two from four polyps. In another study of 23 women with endometrial polyps, La Torre[14] proved that the specificity of the 2D ultrasonography was only 69%. This result increased to 88% with the use of 3D ultrasonography combined with 3D printing, and up to 100% with the 3D sonohysterography combined with 3D printing.

Versellini et al.[12] studied the level of agreement between ultrasonography and hysteroscopy diagnosis of submucous fibroids preoperatively and observed that both strategies were equally reliable with the ultrasonography having a lower sensitivity of the submucous fibroids screening level. Pretorius et al.[15] have recently compared the position of the submucous fibroids that were diagnosed with the strategy of the 3D sonohysterography by the process of their hysteroscopy removal. The removal took place in 47% of the women with diagnosed fibroids through the 3D sonohysterography, yet only 5% of the women showed serious ultrasonography findings. Although the study is retroactive, the diagnostic value of the 3D ultrasonography is fully proven in the preoperative assessment of the uterus fibroids.

The 2D ultrasonography is frequently used for the assessment of the endometrium oval-shaped size. However, with the help of the 3D ultrasonography, its evaluation achieves a more accurate determination of its limits and a size evaluation with sections of 1−2 mm through a computer. In another interesting study, Lee et al.[6] observed that the endometrial size is changing according to the menstrual cycle within 0.2−5.5 mL, and there are high differences among individuals. The value of the endometrial thickness measurement on incidental postmenopausal women has been indicated by Gruboeck et al.[16] as an accurate diagnostic tool. This group studied women whose endometrium cancer diagnosis was conducted with sensitivity 100% and specialty 98%, taking into consideration 13 mL as tumor limit. This result was compared to endometrium thickness measurement, which indicated sensitivity 83% and specialty 88%, taking the limit of 15 ml into consideration.[16] In all of the above studies, we realize that 3D printed models would help even more the accurate diagnosis of these conditions. A study by Aluwe et al.[17] has mentioned the use of 3D printing of five ovaries with endometrial cancer preoperatively. The soft tissues levels (STL) were created through MRI pictures with 3D models printed later. The CT pictures of produced models were compared with the patient's MRI. Specialists have realized that the lightly countable mistakes were accepted and that the models are useful for the preoperative planning. On the doctors' side as well on the patients', the 3D models were proven as an effective tool for the patients' education. Throughout the same year, Ajao et al.[18] were led to the construction of a deeply endometrium filtering caruncle, which included the uterus back side and a patient's voltage. A 3-Tesla magnet was used to take a picture of the pelvis MRI, including the 3D pictures which depict illustration sections of 1 mm. The DICOM saved data were converted into STL ones. A 3D representative model was later created. The patient underwent total laparoscopic hysterectomy, left oophorectomy, right tubal excision, and endometriosis excision. The patient's uterus had a normal size, but the left ovary was collided into the pelvis side. In the laboratory, a colorectal caruncle between 2 and 3 cm was observed, which corresponds to the malfunction that was seen in the 3D printed model. Because of the software connected with the MRI to available model, this model was not available before the surgery and was later compared to intraoperative findings. This model agreed to the intraoperative finding in comparison with the caruncles position and their topographic connection to the environment.

The contribution of ultrasonography to cervical cancer diagnosis is limited. However, two projects are mentioned regarding the diagnostic ability of the 3D ultrasonography in the research of this pathological entity. Chou et al.[19] support that the conclusions of the 3D ultrasonography examination of cervical cancer are better connected to the tumor of the pathological histological sample. Suren et al.[20] have observed that the vessel architecture of benign and malignant malfunctions, which was studied with 3D power Doppler, shows some differences. This is why it is anticipated that the 3D illustration role will be substantiated for the cervical cancer research, and 3D printing is enhancing it.

Throughout the last two decades, great efforts have been made so that there is an improvement in the diagnostic reliability of the ultrasound in the preoperative assessment of the adnexal masses. Although there are numerous positive results, regarding the ultrasonography diagnosis of ovarian cancer, there are still some questions. The great difficulty in the evaluation of ovarian tumor is the fact of the wide spectrum of the histological types and the multiplicity of their morphological features. The adnexal mass evaluation becomes more difficult because of the consecutive morphological changes that take place to the ovary throughout the menstrual cycle and due to the fact that similar pictures can be depicted of benign and malignant situations.

Two studies have been conducted regarding the role of the 3D ultrasound in the research of the ovary tumor morphological analysis. The number of infiltrating epithelial tumors was small, but a borderline tumor was mentioned, whereas there was none of epithelial type. Both studies draw the conclusion that the 3D ultrasonography has definitely more advantages than the 2D one, regarding the adnexal tumor research. The work of Hata et al.[21] is referred to the transabdominal 3D illustration, whereas this of Bonilla-Musoles et al.[22] to the transvaginal 3D. The 3D illustration for the adnexal mass research offers a detailed illustration of hyperechogenic sites of dermoid cysts while giving the opportunity of the illustration of papillary protrusions of cystic sites through the Vocal strategy (3D volume calculation), with which we can revolve an angle on predefined degrees, having as a result the finding global illustration. Still the 3D ultrasonography is not able to replace the clinical examination, the 2D ultrasonography, the pulsing Doppler, and the oncogene markers at the diagnostic approach of ovary cancer. There is no doubt that the surface rendering mode and the 3D power Doppler provide new and thrilling possibilities of ovary cysts research.

Furthermore, the evaluation of the fallopian tubes situation constitutes a regular diagnostic approach, particularly of people with subfertility. The hysterosalpingography and the diagnostic laparoscopy constituted the reliable test regarding the pathology of fallopian tubes. Randolph et al.[23] were the first to be involved with the diagnostic value of the ultrasound in the research of this topic. Throughout the last decade, an ultrasound salpingography has been described as a newly accepted alternative method. Nevertheless, problems do exist in this strategy, like the illustration weakness of the whole fallopian tube in one picture, difficulty in depicting the fringe and the pelvic limp, and the diffusion of the contrast into the minor pelvis.

Sladkevicius et al.[24] have studied the contrast flow through the fallopian tubes with power Doppler and concluded that the 3D power Doppler, as well as the hysterosalpingography and the diagnostic laparoscopy, contribute to the research of the subfertility. Kiyokawa et al.[25] have announced that recent work, through which ultrasound salpingography is compared to 3D ultrasound, can be entirely depicted along the fallopian tube and that the whole process becomes faster and better. Yet, the high percentage of false positive results, regarding the fallopian tubes obstruction, decreases the strategy sensitivity to 83%.[25] Rempen[26] has recently announced that the endometrial cavity shape, as depicted with the 3D ultrasound, is asymmetric to women with endometrial pregnancy and symmetric to those with ectopic pregnancy. Yet, with the use of contemporary 2D transvaginal core ultrasounds, the ectopic pregnancy diagnosis is based on the direct overview of its sac, outside the endometrial cavity, despite the evaluation of the uterus alterations. The uterus examination in coronary section with the 3D ultrasound achieves the evaluation of the embryo sac position in conjunction with the endometrial cavity, particularly when it is not easily recognizable.

Researchers claim that the 3D printing on an incident of deep filtering endometriosis can be proven as a beneficial addition to the standard preoperative illustration forms.[1] In addition for patients who undergo an assisted regenerating program, the follicles size is better illustrated with the 3D compared to the 2D. However, this fact does not define success since the follicles increased size, as well as the increase of their layers, constitute typical ultrasonography criteria of polycystic ovaries, and are connected to the increase of androstenedione in blood. The 3D ultrasonography can offer a better and more objective evaluation of the ovary layer, and as a result, it can contribute to the further understanding of pathophysiology of the polycystic ovaries syndrome. For specific occasions of deep infiltrating endometriosis that affect the multiple organ systems (pelvis, urinary tract, bowels), specialists can decide if the 3D models are particularly useful in the preoperative planning in advance regarding the operative excision size and the need for additional operative processes.

Other possible applications of 3D printing in operative gynecology include muscle excision and surgery for specific Müllerian malformations. Under the spectrum of the limitation of laparoscopy and robotics muscle excision, smaller fibroids can remain accidently throughout these processes. The uterus 3D models with a different color can contribute to a more solid ground process. Moreover, a tangible model in complicated occasions of multiple muscle excision can define the best position for hysterectomies, limiting in this way the unnecessary and ineffective sections. Women with Müllerian malfunctions in which a hysterectomy is indicated often undergo a preoperative MRI as part of the evaluation of the reproduction and urinary system. The 3D rendering of malfunctions of the uterus lowest part or the cervix could describe more accurately the vessels and ureter connection to the uterus.[27]

Tudela et al.[28] used ultrasound prenatal measurements for the length and the radius of the cervix to construct adapted 3D printed vaginal pessaries. Hakim et al.[29] have constructed vaginal stents and dilators of adapted shapes and sizes by computer data, which come from the tomographic material. In the Radiotherapeutic Oncology, the 3D printing has been used to a limited number of patients for the construction of vaginal cylinders for vaginal brachytherapy.[30]. Sethi et al.[31] have mentioned 3D adapted vaginal applicators that were used in brachytherapy on patients with postoperative vaginal anatomy.

Finally, the creation of bioadditive ovaries on mice has been made easier through the use of 3D printing. Laronda et al.[32] have created structural discs type 3D porous gelatin with inflexibility in order to mime the ovary tissues in a size of a duct. After substantiating their detection in vitro, the 3D implants were implanted, which resembled with ovaries in mice with ovariectomy. This scaffolding had numerous folliculars on different maturity levels. In the course of time, the development of these ovaries showed the folliculogenesis and also the development of the blood vessels in the whole scaffolding. Furthermore, three of the seven mice with 3D printed ovaries were proven as fertile and gave descendants.

Clinical application of 3D printing in obstetrics

The medical illustration systems, which are designed to give 3D information from human organs through nonoperative methods (like the ultrasounds), are considered even more developed and play a significant role, leading to the confirmation of the medical illustration strategies. The 3D ultrasonography constitutes the development of regular ultrasounds and was directly applied on the prenatal control that in conjunction with the 3D printing enables the future parents to "feel" the embryo before its birth.

Throughout the first 3 months of pregnancy the embryo is depicted during the ultrasound carrying out of the nuchal translucency, where we can see an accurate illustration of arms, legs, the face, and of course the nasal bone. Moreover, we can recognize the connections among the embryo, the developing placenta, and the cavity of amniotic fluid. In women with fibroids, the connections among the placenta development, the circulation, and the fibroids can be better assessed and the danger for potential miscarriage can be calculated more accurately.

Economides et al.,[33] in a research that they conducted in order to determine the embryo's sex, studied 200 women throughout the first 3 months of pregnancy. The data used from the 3D ultrasonography were gathered, saved, and analyzed, and they stated their opinion regarding the sex of each embryo and the measurement of the angle between the genetic caruncle and the skin that covers the sacrum. The results of this study were that both examiners achieved correct diagnosis of the embryo's sex in 150 women (81.5%), whereas in the rest 18.5%, either both or one of the two could not accurately determine it. In total, a correct diagnosis of the embryo sex was achieved in 85.3% of cases. The measurement of the angle that was achieved was particularly satisfying, whereas the gestational age did not affect the embryo's sex diagnosis.[33]

At the end of the second trimester, the detailed ultrasound is conducted. This examination is the most important one for the prenatal control. Throughout it, all the embryo's anatomical systems are thoroughly investigated. Regarding the central nervous system, a detailed check is conducted for the brain anatomy, and pathological situations like hydrocephalus, brain birth defects, and agenesis of different brain parts can be excluded. In addition, spinal column defects are assessed, like spina bifida and skeletal and limp defects, just as polydactylism and deficits. A particularly impressive 3D illustration use is that of cavity evaluation of the embryo's brain during the seventh to the eighth week of gestation. By this age, the hemispheres as well as the brain with its connections to the third ventricle can be visible. The study of the premature fetal brain development opens a new door for science in neuroanatomy development. Malfunctions of the neural tube can be determined more easily with the 3D use, while there is an ability to analyze the data and better assess the anatomy. Through the 3D ultrasonography and after the printing, the potential malfunctions of the nervous system can be visible, like in the occasion of cyst hygroma in a very premature level.

Moreover, the 3D and four-dimensional (4D) ultrasonography gives the ability of an impressive illustration of the embryo's face. Diagnostically, the presence of spina bifida can be assessed, while in comparison with the 2D ultrasonography, the section level can be noticed more accurately. It is worth mentioning that the 4D illustration can be particularly beneficial in the neurological assessment of the limp movement, while it is able to predict the clinical seriousness of an open spina bifida because the neurological symptoms are directly connected to malfunction level. The spina bifida morbidity includes clinical features like paraplegia, esthetical deficits, intestine dysfunction, and urinary incontinence. The prenatal diagnosis of spina bifida recognizes ossification centers and deficits on skin, whereas the cranial suture and the brain sources are successfully assessed. When a sufficient face picture is obtained, the study can be enhanced more with the revolving of the 3D picture, by using "cine loop." Between the 20th and 22nd week, the outline of the eyes, the nose, and the lips can be easily recognized, the ears construction is sufficiently determined, and malfunctions can be assessed, as well as their connections to the surrounding parts like the chicks, the mouth, the nose, and the chin.[34]

The sufficient prenatal fetal diagnosis can significantly help the genetic consultation, the miscarriage possibility, a surgery preparation, and general prognosis. Particularly for the cleft lip, the prenatal diagnosis is difficult because of the soft tissues acoustics that surround the constructions. Therefore, the 3D ultrasonography is really beneficial with the suitable revolving of the structures saved data.

Moreover, with an average sight of the face, a more accurate diagnosis of a potential micrognathia is possible. Micrognathia is a face malfunction characterized from a small chin. The embryos that have micrognathia have an increased risk of a karyotype malfunction. An underdeveloped chin in the embryo can be enough to cause polyhydramnio or respiratory problems after birth. Furthermore, its presence can be connected to the infant's nutrition problems and more than one surgery may be necessary. The main advantage of the 3D ultrasound for the definition of micrognathia is located in its ability to represent the real median plane structure of the embryo's facial profile.

The heart constitutes the most difficult embryo's system for examination. It is a mobile organ that consists of many anatomic structures and vessels. With the modern strategies of the 4D ultrasonography, we can check these structures, demonstrate properly the vessels, and exclude many birth defects. It is believed that it can of much use for better detection of the heart and valve malfunctions. The 3D ultrasonography has a great strength to show the evolution of the cardiovascular system. It is also considered that the fetal sound cardiography will be the main helping strategy in 3D illustration, mostly when regarding to small defects that appear in many and different sights, and there is no possibility of a consecutive illustration of this interaction.[35]

There is a clear improvement in the diagnosis of urogenital malfunctions. We can better assess the fetal urinary bladder size, as well as the cyst presence in kidneys. Moreover, the fetal sex can be assessed by the 3D ultrasounds, as well as the malfunctions diagnosis.

With the use of the above described 3D ultrasonography strategies, the osseous structures like bones and limbs can be clearly depicted. The developing malfunctions can be defined with really great reliability. The vertebrae, the ribs, and the collarbone can be well depicted, as well as the general appearance of the fetal body, and as an example, it is mentioned that the 3D ultrasonography particularly contributes to the detection of spina bifida in a 10-week embryo in conjunction with the last menstruation. Regarding the limbs, the 3D ultrasound is almost the ideal tool for the assessment of the arms and legs completeness. The 3D ultrasonography appears to be superior than the 2D one in the assessment and the counting of the fetal fingers (74% vs. to 53%). However, the mass revolving was the strategy that made the difference. It is anticipated that the real-time 3D or 4D ultrasonography will be able to assess the arm function, and more specifically the hand function. The publications of Plocekinger et al and Budorick et al were really convincing studies regarding the assessment of both fetal limbs. A problem that was expressed from both studies was the inability to study arms and legs because of their quick movement. The 4D ultrasound can be the answer to this problem.[36]

Lee et al have recorded an incident where the phocomelia syndrome was diagnosed with the 3D ultrasound use. The skeletal dysplasia has also been an object of various reports regarding the 3D ultrasonography use. According to the study of Ruano et al.,[37] it was published that the 3D ultrasonography use can be of benefit for the perinatal diagnosis of skeletal dysplasia. Thus, they used the 3D helical computerized tomography (3D-HCT) as well as the ultrasound of two dimensions (2D) in six situations of embryos with skeletal dysplasia, and the results of these examinations were compared to the radiological findings after birth. Three of these cases were achondroplasia, two for incomplete osteogenesis type II and one for chondrodysplasia. The diagnosis in all these situations took place between the 27th and 36th pregnancy week. The study results were that with the 3D and the 3D-HCT use, all six situations of skeletal dysplasia were diagnosed in comparison with the 2D ultrasonography, where only four of the six situations were diagnosed.

Merz et al.[35] published a step forward in the diagnosis of urogenital abnormalities by using 3D ultrasound, for example, the diagnosis of the bloating of the urinary bladder has been helped enough by the technique of 3D. According to the authors, it is feasible to evaluate the volume of the fetal bladder as well as the presence of cysts in the fetal kidneys. In addition, the fetal sex can be determined with 3D ultrasound, so the diagnosis of genital abnormalities could be a real possibility.

According to Nicolaides et al.,[38] nasal bone was examined in 120 stored data from single pregnancies between 11 and 14 weeks of fetal age collected by interventricular 3D ultrasound. The data collection followed the conventional 2D ultrasound that had demonstrated the presence of nasal bone. The data were assembled with original 2D images in transverse, coronal, mesoevelian, paraboviral, and lateral longitudinal incision of the fetal skull. The conclusions that appeared from this research showed that using 3D, the degree in which the presence of nasal bone in a given prefabricated area can be demonstrated depends mainly on the quality of the original 2D image.

The natural models have an impact on the planning of medical interventions.[39] It can also be used in fetal medicine for educational purposes.[40,41] The combination of images obtained by different methods, such as ultrasonography and MRI, can lead to a better understanding in the evaluation of complex diseases.[42] Previous studies have used ultrasound and 3D models. The team of Blaas and colleagues calculated the embryo's tumors in the first trimester of pregnancy by transforming the fetal area into a virtual model. Nelson et al.[8] 3D-US data were converted into a set of polygons representing a surface that could be transferred to various types of rapid prototype equipment in order to create a solid 3D object. This was considered the first attempt to convert 3D data into physical models.

The possible fetal syndromes are recognized with specific anomalies and abnormalities models. Some of these defects might be of minor importance, like those of ears or of fingers. We should keep in mind, however, that with 3D ultrasonography and 3D printing, the doctor is provided with new available imaging tools, which will help him identify the anomalies better and associate them with a possible syndrome. Therefore, both techniques have been reported to aid in prenatal diagnosis of ichthyosis, short ribs with polydactyly, the Klippel-Trenaunay-Weber syndrome, and the Apert or Pfeiffer syndromes.

Down's syndrome is often diagnosed by the bone structure anomalies, like the broadened iliac angles. Hence, measuring these angles is not possible with 2D ultrasonography, due to the complex pelvic anatomy, which prevents the ideal measurements of the area. The iliac angles are in correlation with the fetal age. We must emphasize that a perfectly median sagittal view of the fetal face must be obtained, like the one that can be obtained with the 3D ultrasound, in order to have the perfect measurements. 3D printing is then used to provide more accurate models.

Until now, no comparative study is available, to support the superiority of 3D printing or 3D sonography, over the 2D sonography. But it is clear that 3D imaging and printing helps accurately and easily to specify various fetal brain anomalies. One of the most important diagnoses that is more accurately identified with 3D imaging is the complete absence of the mesolobium. With 3D imaging and printing, we can reconstruct the median level of the brain. Without the latter, the diagnosis is extremely difficult to be made.

Color Doppler use in Obstetrics is mainly focusing in the placenta, uterine arteries, and, in a smaller degree, in the fetal circulation. The advantage of being able to take a closer and direct look at the vessels, either with 3D ultrasound or even better with 3D printed models, is that you can examine these vessels in situ, in their normal position in the fetal body. Despite this fact though, the estimation of the tissue infusion is appearing to be problematic with the 3D Doppler, and new techniques are being examined for this purpose, like vascular flow index.

To sum up, 3D imaging and 3D printing technologies are the newest addition to fetal imaging, due to the technological inventions and findings. It is expected to change the way of fetal imaging in the most revolutionary way.

The use of 3D printing for doctor's education

The 3D imaging and printing use or the quick production of prototypes in medical simulation (MS) education seems to have a great progress. A specific approach has been studied in neurosurgery, plastic surgery, and cardiovascular surgery. However, limited data support the use of this technology in gynecologic practice.

The MS constitutes a significant technical approach of the educational gap by providing the ability of the accurate learning and practice of rich knowledgeable and practical skills in a safe environment, as well as the global evaluation, and also the constructive learning from the instructor and the apprentice or intern.

Specifically, some of the main advantages and reasons of using the MS are given below:

1. Revision practice: It enables practice on a repetitive basis in the same or different scenario with different levels of difficulty.
2. They are easily incorporated in university projects and courses of medical specialty.
3. Customized education: The apprentice can develop an interaction type with the simulator.
4. Adaptation to different learning strategies.
5. Quantitative evaluation: The apprentice's performance is quantified and compared. The ability of objective and quantitative evaluation of the confrontation kind of a clinical scenario constitutes one of the most crucial goals in education.
6. A possibility of interfeedback exists during learning for the future improvement and adaptation of the scenario itself and the student's performance (debriefing).
7. Educational effectiveness: A realistic simulation of clinical incidents and scenarios takes place with the aid of patterns and/or simulators that allow learning of complex skills and knowledge.
8. Multifunctionality—team training): The simulation provides the education ability of medical personnel from different specialties and different education levels.

9. Practice in complicated and rare incidents: This may be the most important advantage of MS since it provides the learning and practice ability in extra complicated incidents with a variable difficulty level.

10. The models arisen are of high accuracy and provide the practice ability of operational skills in a realistic way.[43–45]

Thus, it becomes perceivable that a 3D illustration can be regarded as a valuable tool of education and practice. It is considered as a new educational way that replaces the processes of a real incident confrontation with artificial models.[46] Anatomic structures are regenerated, as well as entire or partial clinical incidents in a reliable way under realistic conditions, leading the apprentice or intern to effectiveness. Therefore, the learning is encouraged through the experimentation and the methodology of trial-and-error, having in this way the opportunity of revising the incident as well as "pausing" it and returning to a previous moment, during the confrontation of a clinical incident for leading and advice reasons without negative results.

We need to emphasize yet that the 3D illustration is advisable for supplementary reasons and not for replacement of the traditional educational way, given the importance of the previously mentioned educational advantages, so that the trainee (student/apprentice/junior doctor) is equipped with the suitable self-confidence, before being asked to handle an incident.

In comparison with the surgery field, a relatively limited number of simulators have been developed, which are used for the learning and practice of specific actions, like the clinical examination of the internal genitals, as well as birth simulations, which are equipped with suitable mechanical parts for the realistic execution of natural birth. However, some of the virtual reality laparoscopy simulators consist of gynecological operations in their software, like the confrontation of ectopic pregnancy.

The application of MS in the field of gynaecology obstetrics for the practice of diagnostic as well as therapeutic routines aims to the improvement of the engaged anatomic clues, the increase of the doctor's self-confidence, and the cooperation among the doctors. The amniocentesis learning with the aid of ultrasounds, the assessment of the embryo's position, the birth problems confrontation, and the urgent gynecologic incidents confrontation are educational points of great importance for the trainee in gynecology and obstetrics.

Conclusion

3D printing produces virtual models. It has gained a lot of dynamic in recent years, due to the high performance of software applied in the fields of engineering, architecture, and design. It is easy for using, making it easier to visualize 3D images, making it especially useful in gynecology and obstetrics.

The use of 3D printed models might be the future for medical education, as well as the way to explain health conditions, complications, or surgical procedures. The production of specifically designed tools or devices might help in certain diseases, malignancies, or deformities. The future of 3D printing, as we mentioned previously, might even help infertility treatments.

The segmentation and reconstruction techniques that have been developed in fetal modeling could be applied for the construction of virtual and natural models derived from ultrasound, MRI, and CT imaging, individually or in combination. 3D printing and physical models in the near future will facilitate the tactile and interactive study of complex anomalies in obstetrics. These techniques can also be very useful for the future for the couples interested in having the opportunity to recreate a 3D model with the physical characteristics of their fetus, allowing a more direct emotional connection with the unborn child.

References

[1] Kossoff G, Griffiths KA, Kadi AP, Warren. Principles of three-dimensional volume imaging insonography. In: Baba K, Jurkovic D, eds. *Three-dimensional Ultrasound in Obstetrics and Gynecology*. Carnforth: Parthenon Publishing; 1997:21–28.

[2] Baba K. Basis and principles of three-dimensional ultrasound. In: Baba K, Jurkovic D, eds. *Three-dimensional Ultrasound in Obstetrics and Gynecology*. Carnforth: Parthenon Publishing; 1997:1–20.

[3] D'Urso P, Earwaker W, Barker T, Redmond M, Thompson R, Effeney D, Tomlinson F. Custom cranioplasty using stereolithography and acrylic. *Br J Plast Surg*. 2000;53: 200–204.

[4] Guarino J, Tennyson S, McCain G, Bond L, Shea K, King H. Rapid prototyping technology in for surgeries of the pediatric spine and pelvis: benefits analysis. *J Pediatr Orthop*. 2007;27:955–960.

[5] Hurson C, Tansey A, O'Donnchadha B, Nicholson P, Rice J, McElwain J. Rapid prototyping in the assessment, classification and preoperative planning of acetabular fractures. *Injury*. 2007;38:1158–1162.

[6] Lee A, Sator M, Kratochwil A, et al. Endometrial volume change during spontaneus menstrual cycles: volumetry by transvaginal three-dimensional ultrasound. *Fertil Steril*. 1997;68:831–835.

[7] Tulandi T, Watkin K, Tan SL. Reproductive performance and three-dimensional ultrasound volume determination of polycystic ovary: following laparoscopic ovarian drilling. *Int J Fertil Wom Med*. 1997;42:436–440.

[8] Nelson TR, Pretorius DH, Hull A, Riccabona M. Sources and impact of artifacts on clinical three-dimensional ultrasound imaging. *Ultrasound Obstet Gynecol*. 2000;16:374–383.

[9] Jurkovic D, Geipel A, Gruboek K, et al. Three-dimensional ultrasound of the assessment of the uterine anatomyand detection of congenital anomalies: acomparison of hysterosalpingography and two dimension sonography. *Ultrasound Obstet Gynecol*. 1995; 5:233–237.

[10] Raga F, Bonilla-Musoles F, Blans G, Osborn NG. Congenital Mullerian anomalies: diagnostic accuracy of three-dimensional ultrasound. *Fertil Steril*. 1996;65:523–528.

[11] Merz E. Three-dimensional transvaginal ultrasound in gynecologic diagnosis. *Ultrasound Obstet Gynecol*. 1999;14:81–86.

[12] Versellini P, Cortesi I, Oldani S, et al. The role of transvaginal ultrasonography and outpatient diagnostic hysteroscopy in the evaluation of patient with menorrhagia. *Hum Reprod*. 1997;12:1768−1771.

[13] Bonilla - Musoles F, Raga F, Osborn NG, et al. Threedimensional hysterosonography for the study of endometrial tumors: comparison with conventional transvaginal sonography hysterosalpigography and hysteroscopy. *Gynecol Oncol*. 1997;65:245−252.

[14] La Torre R. Transvaginal sonographic evaluation of endometrial polyps: a comparison with tow dimensional and three dimensional contrast sonography. *Clin Exp Obstet Gynecol*. 1999;26:171−173.

[15] Pretorius DH, Becker E, Lev-Toaff AS. Impact of sonohysterography of the management of women with uterine myomas. *Ultrasound Obstet Gynecol*. 2001;18(suppl):2.

[16] Gruboeck K, Jurkovic D, Lawton F, et al. The diagnostic value of endometrial thickness and volume measurements by three-dimensional ultrasound in patients with postmenopausal bleeding. *Ultrasound Obstet Gynecol*. 1996;8:272−276.

[17] Sayed Aluwee SAZB, Zhou X, Kato H, Makino H, Muramatsu C, Hara T, Matsuo M, Fujita H. Evaluation of pre-surgical models for uterine surgery by use of three-dimensional printing and mold casting. *Radiol Phys Technol*. 2017;10(3):279−285. https://doi.org/10.1007/s12194-017-0397-2. Epub 2017 Apr 12.PMID: 28405900.

[18] Ajao MO, Clark NV, Kelil T, Cohen SL, Einarsson JI. Case report: three-dimensional printed model for deep infiltrating endometriosis. *J Minim Invasive Gynecol*. 2017; 24(7):1239−1242.

[19] Chou CY, Hsu KF, Wang ST, Huang SC. Accuracy of three-dimensional ultrasonography in volume estimation of cervical carcinoma. *Gynecol Oncol*. 1997;66:89−93.

[20] Suren A, Osmers R, Kuhn W. 3D color power angio imaging: a new method to assess intracervical vascularization in benign and pathological conditions. *Ultrasound Obstet Gynecol*. 1998;11:133−137.

[21] Hata T, Yanagihara T, Hayashi K, Yamashiro C, Ohnishi Y, Akiyama M, Manabe A, Miyazaki K. Three-dimensional ultrasonographic evaluation of ovarian tumours: a preliminary study. *Hum Reprod*. 1999;14(3):858−861. https://doi.org/10.1093/humrep/14.3.858. PMID: 10221729.

[22] Bonilla-Musoles F, Raga F, Osborne NG. Three-dimensional ultrasound evaluation of ovarian masses. *Gynecol Oncol*. 1995;59(1):129−135. https://doi.org/10.1006/gyno.1995.1279. PMID: 7557598 Clinical Trial.

[23] Randolph GR, Ying YK, Maier DB. Comparison of real-time ultrasonography, hysterosalpigography and laparoscopy/hysteroscopy in the evaluation of uterine anomalies and tubal patency. *Fertil Steril*. 1986;46:828−832.

[24] Sladkevicius P, Campbell S. Advanced ultrasound examination in the management of subfertility. *Curr Opin Obstet Gynecol*. 2000;12(3):221−225. https://doi.org/10.1097/00001703-200006000-00009. PMID: 10873123 Review.

[25] Kiyokawa K, Masuda H, Fuyuki F. Three-dimensional hysterosalpigo-contrast sonography as an outpatient procedure to assess infertile women: a pilot study. *Ultrasound Obstet Gynecol*. 2000;16:648−654.

[26] Rempen A. The shape of the endometrium evaluated with three-dimensional ultrasound: an additional predictor of extrauterine pregnancy. *Hum Reprod*. 1998;13:450−454.

[27] Yoong W, Cresswell K, Moffatt J, Mead R, Laverick B, Szarko M. The application of 3D printing technology in obstetrics and gynaecology. *Obstet Gynaecol*. 2015;17(1):3−4.

[28] Tudela F, Kelley R, Ascher-Walsh C, Stone JL. Low cost 3D printing for the creation of cervical cerclage pessary used to prevent preterm birth. *Obstet Gynecol*. 2016;127:154S.

[29] Hakim J, Oluyemisi A, Buskmiller C, Krishnamurthy R, Cohn W, Dietrich JE. Innovative use of 3D printers in gynecology. *J Pediatr Adolesc Gynecol.* 2015;28(2):e67.

[30] Ricotti R, Vavassori A, Bazani A, Ciardo D, Pansini F, Spoto R, et al. 3D-printed applicators for high dose rate brachytherapy: dosimetric assessment at different infill percentage. *Phys Medica.* 2016;32(12):1698−1706.

[31] Sethi R, Cunha A, Mellis K, Siauw T, Diederich C, Pouliot J, et al. Clinical applications of custom-made vaginal cylinders constructed using three-dimensional printing technology. *J Contemp Brachytherapy.* 2016;8(3):208−214. Termedia Publishing.

[32] Laronda MM, Rutz AL, Xiao S, Whelan KA, Duncan FE, Roth EW, et al. A bioprosthetic ovary created using 3D printed microporous scaffolds restores ovarian function in sterilized mice. *Nat Commun.* 2017;8:15261.

[33] Michailidis GD, Papageorgiou P, Morris RW, Economides DL. The use of three-dimensional ultrasound for fetal gender determination in the first trimester. *Br J Radiol.* 2003;76(907):448−451. https://doi.org/10.1259/bjr/13479830. PMID: 1285770.

[34] Benacerraf BR, Shipp TD, Bromley B. How sonographic tomography will change the face of obstetric sonography: a pilot study. *J Ultrasound Med.* 2005;24(3):371−378.

[35] Merz E. Risk calculation of fetal chromosomal defects in the first trimester. *Ultraschall Med.* 2005;26(5):377−378. PMID: 16312030 English, German. No abstract available.

[36] Cannon JW, Stoll JA, Salgo IS, Knowles HB, Howe RD, Dupont PE, Marx GR, del Nido PJ. Real-time three-dimensional ultrasound for guiding surgical tasks. *Comput Aided Surg.* 2003;8(2):82−90.

[37] Ruano R, Molho M, Roume J, Ville Y. Prenatal diagnosis of fetal skeletal dysplasias by combining two-dimensional and three-dimensional ultrasound and intrauterine three-dimensional helical computer tomography. *Ultrasound Obstet Gynecol.* 2004;24(2): 134−140.

[38] Nicolaides KH, Heath V, Spencer K, Nix AB. Nuchal translucency and gestational age. *Prenat Diagn.* 2004;24(10):833−834.

[39] Armillotta A, Bonhoeffer P, Dubini G, et al. Use of rapid prototyping models in the planning of percutaneous pulmonary valved stent implantation. *Proc Inst Mech Eng H.* 2007;221:407−416.

[40] Werner H, Dos Santos JRL, Fontes R, et al. Virtual bronchoscopy in the fetus. *Ultrasound Obstet Gynecol.* 2011;37:113−115.

[41] Werner H, Lopes dos Santos JR, Fontes R, et al. Virtual bronchoscopy for evaluating cervical tumors of the fetus. *Ultrasound Obstet Gynecol.* 2013;41:90−94.

[42] Robiony M, Salvo I, Costa F, et al. Virtual reality surgical planning for maxillofacial distraction osteogenesis: the role of reverse engineering rapid prototyping and cooperative work. *J Oral Maxillofac Surg.* 2007;65:1198−1208.

[43] Chen S, Pan Z, Wu Y, Gu Z, Li M, Liang Z, Zhu H, Yao Y, Shui W, Shen Z, Zhao J, Pan H. The role of three-dimensional printed models of skull in anatomy education: a randomized controlled trial. *Sci Rep.* 2017;7:575.

[44] Cornwall J. The ethics of 3D printing copies of bodies donated for medical education and research: what is there to worry about? *Australas Med J.* 2016;9:8−11.

[45] Lim KH, Loo ZY, Goldie SJ, Adams JW, McMenamin PG. Use of 3D printed models in medical education: a randomized control trial comparing 3D prints versus cadaveric materials for learning external cardiac anatomy. *Anat Sci Educ.* 2016;9:213−221.

[46] Gaba DM. The future vision of simulation in healthcare. *Qual Saf Health Care.* 2004; 13(S1):i2−i10.

Further reading

[1] Baek MH, Kim DY, Kim N, Rhim CC, Kim JH, Nam JH. Incorporating a 3-dimensional printer into the management of early-stage cervical cancer. *J Surg Oncol*. 2016;114: 150–152.

[2] Bartellas MP. Three-dimensional printing and medical education: a narrative review of the literature. *Univ Ottawa J Med*. 2016;6:38–43. University.

[3] Bartellas M, Ryan S, Doucet G, Murphy D, Turner J. Three-dimensional printing of a hemorrhagic cervical cancer model for postgraduate gynecological training. *Cureus*. 2017;9(1):e950.

[4] Blaas HG, Taipale P, Torp H, et al. Three-dimensional ultrasound volume calculations of human embryos and young fetuses: a study of the volumetry of compound structures and its reproducibility. *Ultrasound Obstet Gynecol*. 2006;27:640–646.

[5] Bonilla F, Raga F, Osborn N. Three-dimensional ultrasound evaluation of ovarian masses. *Gynecol Oncol*. 1995;59:129–135.

[6] Goudie C, Shanahan J, Gill A, Murphy D, Dubrowski A. Investigating the efficacy of anatomical silicone models developed from a 3D printed mold for perineal repair suturing simulation. *Cureus*. 2018;10(8):3181. https://doi.org/10.7759/cureus.3181.

[7] Merz E, Welter C. 2D and 3D Ultrasound in the evaluation of normal and abnormal fetal anatomy in the second and third trimesters in a level III center. *Ultraschall der Med*. 2005;26(1):9–16.

[8] Miller J, Ahn E, Garcia J, Miller G, Satin A, Baschat A. Ultrasound-based three-dimensional printed medical model for multispecialty team surgical rehearsal prior to fetoscopic myelomeningocele repair. *Ultrasound Obstet Gynecol*. 2018;51:836–840.

[9] Nelson TR, Bailey MJ. Solid object visualization of 3D ultrasound data. *J Med Imaging*. 2000;3982:26–34.

[10] Sayeed Aluwee SAZB, Hiroaki I, Xiangrong Z, Hiroki K, Hiroshi M, Takeshi H, et al. Patient-specific model generation by using 3D printing and its application to surgical planning of uterine fibroid removal. *Tech Rep Med Imag*. 2016;116(160):1–4.

[11] Sladkevicius P. Three-dimensional power doppler imaging of the fallopian tube. *Ultrasound Obstet Gynecol*. 1999;13:287.

[12] VanKoevering K, Morrison R, Prabhu S, Ladino Torres M, Mychaliska G, Treadwell M, et al. Antenatal three-dimensional printing of aberrant facial anatomy. *Pediatrics*. 2015; 136(5):e1382–e1385.

[13] Werner Jr H, Santos JL, Belmonte S, Ribeiro G, Daltro P, Gasparetto EL, et al. Applicability of three-dimensional imaging techniques in fetal medicine. *Radiol Bras*. 2016; 49(5):281–287.

[14] Lee W. 3D fetal ultrasonography. *Clin Obstet Gynecol*. 2003;46:850–867.

3D printing in neurosurgery

**Alkinoos Athanasiou[1,2], Torstein R. Meling[3,4], Alexandros Brotis[5],
Alessandro Moiraghi[3], Konstantinos Fountas[5], Panagiotis D. Bamidis[6],
Ioannis Magras[1]**

[1]*Department of Neurosurgery, AHEPA University General Hospital, Aristotle University of
Thessaloniki (AUTH), Thessaloniki, Greece;* [2]*Lab of Medical Physics, School of Medicine, Aristotle
University of Thessaloniki, Thessaloniki, Greece;* [3]*Service de Neurochirurgie, Hôpitaux
Universitaires de Genève (HUG), Geneva, Switzerland;* [4]*Faculty of Medicine, University of
Geneva, Geneva, Switzerland;* [5]*Department of Neurosurgery, Larisa University General Hospital,
University of Thessaly, Volos, Greece;* [6]*Professor of Medical Physics, Medical Informatics and
Medical Education, Lab of Medical Physics and Digital Innovation, Department of Medicine,
School of Health Sciences, Aristotle University of Thessaloniki, Thessaloniki, Greece*

Abbreviations

2D	Two-dimensional
3D	Three-dimensional
3DP	Three-dimensional printing
AVM	Arteriovenous malformation
CAD	Computer-aided design
CNS	Central nervous system
CSF	Cerebrospinal fluid
CT	Computed tomography
CTA	Computed tomographic angiography
DAVF	Dural arteriovenous fistula
DICOM	Digital Imaging and Communications in Medicine
DLGG	Diffuse low-grade glioma
DSA	Digital subtraction angiography
DTI	Diffusion tensor imaging
EANS	European Association of Neurosurgical Societies
EVD	External ventricular drainage
EVT	Endoscopic third ventriculostomy
fMRI	Functional magnetic resonance imaging
LITT	Laser interstitial thermal therapy
MRA	Magnetic resonance angiography
MRI	Magnetic resonance imaging
PLA	Polylactic acid
PMMA	Polymethyl methacrylate

3D Printing: Applications in Medical Surgery. https://doi.org/10.1016/B978-0-323-66193-5.00008-3

R&D	Research and Development
RIM	Radiotherapy immobilization masks
SEBS	Styrene-ethylene-/.butylene-styrene

Introduction

Three-dimensional (3D) printing (3DP) constitutes a rather new technology that is based on computer-aided design (CAD) models and on layer-by-layer additive manufacturing process. 3DP, as a process, permits the rapid manufacturing of high-fidelity 3D models using dedicated printers.[1] This technology emerged in the 1980s and through the 1990s was used mainly for rapid prototyping in industry. Gradual advances during the last decade in precision, printable material range, and reduced production costs, as well as affordability of the technology itself (to the point of commercial home 3D printers), have both increased the viability of industrial production based on 3DP and greatly expanded its range of applications. Numerous innovations and novel approaches started to involve affordable many biomedical applications.[2,3] Medical equipment, implanted materials, and prostheses, as well as cell printing, are nowadays well within the range of this technology, while current 3DP biomedical research includes highly innovative themes such as manufacturing pathological tissue and organ models, personalized implants, targeted therapeutic delivery, bioactive and biodegradable scaffolds, and even living organ fabrication.[4] Neuroscience applications such as peripheral nerve regeneration through 3D microprinted conduits and scaffolds can be considered among the most advanced research themes currently pursued.[4,5]

Concerning the medical practice state of the art, Neurological Surgery is widely considered to be among the most demanding and intricate medical specialties, as it deals with fine and highly critical neural and vascular elements. Even the most standard neurosurgical interventions or the most common pathological conditions involve and affect neural and neurovascular tissues with little to no room for error. Various novel approaches of 3DP technology for Neurosurgery applications have been already tried out and described in the literature, including but not limited to fabrication of educational or training models and prototyping of implant materials. Complicated skull base tumors have been visualized using composite virtual models and 3D printed solid fabrications in order to illustrate critical skull base anatomy, including large vessels, cranial nerves, sinuses, and areas such as the cerebellopontine angle.[6,7] Realistic high-fidelity neuroanatomical models of the dural venous sinuses have greatly facilitated the understanding of cerebral and cerebellar circulation for medical students, trainees, and experts alike.[8]

While 3DP does not yet belong into standard neurosurgical practice, the variety and novelty of possible applications underline the expected impact of this technology to the field. As such, during the past few years, attempts have also been made in order to study, advance, and predict the applications of this novel technology within the specialty of Neurosurgery. The growth of the field has been rapidly accelerating and, while a systematic review in 2016 would include less than 40 relevant studies for a period of 2011–15,[3] numerous papers have been published during the more recent years, coinciding with the progress and maturity of 3DP technology.

We can broadly categorize this progress into four main distinct directions for the use of 3DP technologies within the prism of Neurological Surgery, and we can also envision further progress and future steps for each one of them. While serious overlap exists between directions, we will attempt to categorize the field into the following:

(1) the delineation of vascular physiological anatomy and its associated disorders, such as aneurysms and arteriovenous malformations (AVMs), would allow for better understanding of lesion-specific characteristics on a case-to-case basis and, also, for optimal planning of clipping or endovascular treatment;

(2) the stereotactic visualization of complex central nervous system (CNS) tumors and their associations to normal structures, such as intraventricular or base skull tumors in particular, could significantly improve postoperational morbidity associated with cranial nerve or deep structure compromise;

(3) the study of spine deformities and planning of treatment with regards to biomechanical implications of applied instrumentation could improve overall safety and efficacy of these treatments and also reduce instrumentation failure and sagittal balance disorders;

(4) the study of normal CNS anatomy for educational purposes and of simple case models, such as disc herniation, can improve both theoretical and practical education of young neuroscientists and neurosurgical residents, reduce the need for cadaveric studies, increase availability and exposure to specific approaches and surgical techniques, and "flatten" learning curves for basic neurosurgical operations. Further uses of 3DP technologies have also been described with relation to Neurosurgery, such as the engineering and prototyping of implants, devices, and equipment.

The aforementioned approaches to implementing 3DP technology to the field of Neurosurgery are elaborated below, at the sections of this chapter, where we attempt a comprehensive review of the advances and achievements of this technology mainly in vascular neurosurgery, neurooncology, spine surgery, surgical education, and prototyping. We attempt to identify the key potential of 3DP technology for each approach with regard to anatomical education, preoperative planning, surgical training, and intraoperative applications, while identifying and discussing the limitations still met, as well as envisioning the future milestones to be achieved.

Vascular neurosurgery
A new frontier in preoperative planning and surgical training

Cerebrovascular neurosurgery demands high-quality procedural outcomes in combination with optimal safety levels. Pathologies as aneurysms, AVM, and dural arteriovenous fistulae are often complex structures that require a deep understanding of their 3D configuration and of surrounding anatomical structures in order to treat them properly. However, the interpretation of medical images has historically been limited to two-dimensional (2D) media such as textbooks and computer screens. In contrast, 3D printers allow medical images to be converted into real 3D structures.[9,10] The main advantage of this technology is the noninvasive visualization of anatomical structures for diagnosis, surgical planning, and education for both trainees and patients. The possibility to create customized, high-resolution models is considered one of the most interesting innovations in surgical training, being at the same time a useful rehearsal for experienced surgeon facing very complex cases and a possibility of intensive and immersive training for residents.[11–13] For these reasons, 3DP is considered an effective method of training, offering realistic anatomical reconstruction that may facilitate surgical skills acquisition, particularly in this era of reduced exposure to the operative room, as reported in a recent survey by the European Association of Neurosurgical Societies (EANS) Young Neurosurgeons and EANS Training Committee.[14–16]

Surgical planning

Despite the evolution of radiologic imaging over past decades, with the introduction of 3D computed tomographic angiography (3D-CTA) and digital subtraction angiography (DSA) in daily practice, a great importance is given to the ability of the surgeon to mentally reconstruct very complex vascular anatomy and project it into patient's head. Even in the case of 3D rendering reconstruction, those images are often visualized on flat 2D screens, making the evaluation of depth and anatomical relationships between pathological and normal structures difficult. In this environment, the use of 3DP can provide real patient-specific and high-fidelity physical models (Fig. 8.1), which can be visualized from any angle, representing a potentially more advantageous method of visualization. In addition, due to recent technical developments, this approach has become faster and cheaper, constituting a real amendment to traditional radiological techniques, enabling physical representation of complex vascular networks.[17–19] In a recent systematic literature review by *Randazzo et al.*, 36 articles

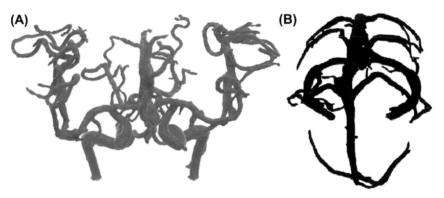

(A) **(B)**

FIGURE 8.1

Three-dimensional (3D) printed models of intracranial arteries (A) and veins (B) reproducing a normal anatomy, useful for educational purposes for residents, students, or patients (these products are part of the Kezlex series manufactured by Ono and Co., Ltd., Tokyo, Japan).

reported research experiences with 3DP in the neurosurgical field, 12 of which were related to cerebrovascular applications. This reflects a larger interest in this technique compared to other fields of neurosurgery like neurooncology, functional neurosurgery, or spine surgery, in which this technique is to date less represented in the literature.[3] Surgical planning can be improved, thanks to 3D printed models also in some cases of pediatric patients needing treatment for AVMs and cranial malformations facilitating the approach and reducing the time of surgery.[20,21]

The use of artificial models for neurosurgical planning was described way before the 3DP technique was available. In 1986, Schultz et al. made use of 3D acrylic and plastic models to foreplan of a craniopagus twins' separation. Consultation with medical artists and prosthetists was important to create exact models of the patients.[22] The use of physical models for planning surgery on craniopagus twins has been reported also in the "3D printing era": A special emphasis is attributed to the importance of these models to understand 3D relationships between vascular structures that are shared by the twins. The possibility to simulate expendable models, bony and skin reconstruction as well the reproduction of venous anatomy that was correlated to cerebral angiography were proven particularly useful for surgical planning. The models were crucial to choose the most effective surgical strategy, after a 360 degrees anatomical evaluation, permitting the design of tailored instruments (surgical table, head holders, stereotactic frame …), allowing to better coordinate multiple teams.[23,24]

D'Urso et al. were the first to replicate the cerebral vasculature morphology of patients in a solid material. Nineteen artificial models were obtained by downloading native images from CTA and MRA onto a dedicated computer workstation. Raw image data were then converted to a format compatible with a stereolithography apparatus for manufacturing the models. Initial 3D reconstructions were performed using a volume rendering technique. The segmentation between vessels and bone was achieved by image thresholding and structures unconnected to the main arterial tree were removed using a 3D connectivity function. The contour data were then used to create the final object file that was sent to the stereolithography device. In the manufacturing process, a laser beam solidified layers of a photosensitive liquid resin monomer according to the cerebral vasculature contours. The resulting object was then rigidified in an ultraviolet oven. The utility of these models was subjectively assessed by the neurosurgeons in charge after the operation. They reported that the 3D models accurately represented the cerebral vasculature and the aneurysm relationships except in one case (in a patient who presented an endosaccular thrombus). Thus, this tactile anatomic overview would help even an inexperienced surgeon to quickly understand the spatial organization of the aneurysm without requiring a complex mental reconstruction from multiple images or replacement of the vascular volume. The authors reported that the models helped to position the patient's head with respect to the most appropriate approach angle and were also helpful for understanding the 3D anatomy, giving the surgeon more confidence during the procedure. It was also possible to try the appropriate aneurysm clip in terms of length, shape, and orientation on the artificial model (Fig. 8.2), thereby developing a new type of direct simulation.[25,26]

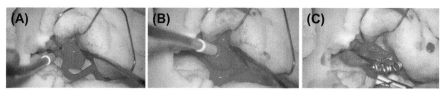

FIGURE 8.2

Middle cerebral artery aneurism three-dimensional (3D) model (A) designed to reproduce an intraoperative aneurismal rupture (B) for training in controlling bleeding and emergency clipping (C) (this product is part of the Kezlex series manufactured by Ono and Co., Ltd., Tokyo, Japan).

Kimura et al. made 3D elastic hollow models of individual cerebral aneurysms for the purpose of preoperative simulation and surgical training (3 retrospective and 7 prospective cases). They also applied a stereolithographic technique and used a prototyping machine to build the model from a rubber-like polymer hardened under ultraviolet light, according to the vessel wall anatomy. The aneurysm model was then fixed with either flexible wires or plastic clay, according to the selected approach, and oriented along the surgical view. Finally, under the operating microscope, various types of aneurysm clips were applied to determine the most appropriate size, shape, and orientation. In one case of a deep-seated vertebrobasilar aneurysm, they designed a solid 3D model that included the aneurysm, vessels, and cranial base bone. They then created a craniotomy and simulated the access to the aneurysm. The goal of developing these models was to represent a real 3D arterial tree in order to simulate preoperatively the surgical repair of intracranial aneurysms (with regard to selection of clip properties and orientation). This technique might also assist young neurosurgeons in developing their own surgical strategy and allow them to confront the potential difficulties of an approach and clip application in a narrow corridor. Unfortunately, these simulation techniques lack any representation of surrounding brain structures, which is one of the main aspects restricting accessibility and maneuverability during aneurysm surgery. Furthermore, when looking at anatomic accuracy, the authors acknowledged difficulties in replicating small arteries and avoiding contamination of the solid 3D models by venous components that could only be distinguished from the arterial component by an experienced vascular neurosurgeon. In two cases using these models, the aneurysm neck was also poorly depicted because of the limited definition of native images combined with suboptimal segmentation of the vasculature, which is operator dependent. Another drawback of these methods is the absence of information concerning the thickness or biomechanical properties of the aneurysm wall and parent vessels, which could be useful in predicting their deformability during clipping. Although these interesting techniques are quite expensive and the preparation of a single model takes usually several days, making such simulations is not applicable to emergency situations like ruptured intracranial aneurysms.[26,27]

Kondo et al. reported their experience with 22 patients where unruptured intracranial aneurysms were reproduced in 3D printed models from 3D-CTA. The authors found that the microsurgical anatomy of skull bones, main arteries, and the vascular lengths was molded with high-level accuracy, concluding that 3D printed models prepared by this procedure are useful for neurosurgical simulation.[28]

Endovascular applications

Numerous groups have reported encouraging results in terms of accuracy in reproducing complex vascular structures using this technology.[13,18,21,28-33] Based on existing publications, significant differences between preoperative imaging and 3D printed models were only observed in a few cases and on specific areas, attesting to the accuracy and fidelity in reproducing intracranial vessels and surrounding anatomical structures. In particular, *Ionita et al.* used a printer able to manufacture 3D phantoms with up to 17 different materials to reproduce endovascular models for clot-retrieving procedures in case of an ischemic stroke. They were able to print ultrafine 16 μm layers, which is ideal for details, complex geometries, and very thin walls (as it is for intracranial vascular structures). For rigid materials, the accuracy in each printed plane was between 20 and 85 μm for features smaller than 50 mm and up to 200 μm for full model size. The net printing area was $255 \times 252 \times 200$ mm. For soft materials, the layer-resolution was about 32 μm and up to 200 μm in-plane accuracy. The phantoms were tested in three steps: X-ray imaging, procedure simulations, and cone beam computerized tomography (CT) for geometry accuracy verification. Each phantom was connected to a peristaltic pump, and planar and rotational angiography was performed on each one. For complex phantoms, vessel patency and qualitative assessment of the flow were obtained. The phantom models are extremely accurate; the geometry differences between the phantom and the patient geometry were of the order of the voxel size, less than 125 μm. This benefit makes this technology very useful for device development testing and medical research.[34] Mechanical behavior of the catheter and the haptic feedback sensed by the interventionist were very similar to that experienced clinically. Clots were easy to deliver at the desired location, and they were not removed by the flow in the system. Sometimes clot fragmentation occurred because of the procedure and resulted in blockage of more distal branches, similarly to situations seen in some clinical cases. To demonstrate the accuracy and the reliability of the 3D printed models, *Namba et al.* tried to determine the shape of the microcatheter inserted for aneurysm coiling and were able to correctly predict it in 10 consecutive patients.[32]

Surgical training

Printed vascular networks have been utilized to replicate hemodynamics within an aneurysm and to practice clipping procedures: through a better understanding of vascular anatomy, this technology seems to lead to an easier surgical

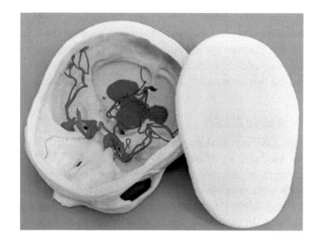

FIGURE 8.3

Three-dimensional (3D) printed model of the skull base with intracranial arteries and a right middle cerebral artery aneurism, useful for simulated surgical approaches (this product is part of the Kezlex series manufactured by Ono and Co., Ltd., Tokyo, Japan).

planning.[29,35] To assess the potential application in neurovascular training, *Mashiko et al.* used three patient-specific models composed of a trimmed skull, an elastic, retractable brain, and a hollow elastic aneurism with its parent artery. The brain models were created using 3D printers via a casting technique, whereas the artery models were made by 3DP and a lost-wax technique. Trainees succeeded in performing the simulation in line with an actual surgery, and their skills tended to improve upon completion of the training.[35] Based on existing experiences, we can imagine that in the future, the use of 3D printed phantoms will play a more important role in surgical training, partially replacing the standard training on cadavers (Fig. 8.3). The principal advantage of 3DP is that it is possible to reproduce a real disease, in order to reproduce and subsequently train on real cases, making it possible to reproduce it every time needed.

Neurooncology

Space-occupying lesions increase the complexity of the cerebral anatomy. Depending on the tumor location, normal tissues are distorted, anatomical planes are difficult to separate, and the associations between the anatomical structures change. As a consequence, sellar tumors frequently encase the carotid artery and compress the optic chiasm; cerebellopontine angle tumors distort the brain stem and facial nerve; and gliomas deform the major association pathways, including the corticospinal tract and the visual pathway. The end result is that traditional landmarks are rendered useless, spatial orientation becomes a difficult task, and the choice of the optimal treatment plan is challenging, with an increased risk of damage of delicate structures, including the neural elements and vessels. Furthermore, the surgical learning curves turn out to be steeper for young neurosurgical trainees to achieve the targeted safety levels, and doctor-to-patient communication is inevitably obstructed. Initially, rapid prototyping models were constructed based on data acquired from CT and CTA, limiting their use in skull base lesions. Of note, the latter are mostly benign in terms of histology, but are associated with significant morbidity and mortality due to their proximity to critical structures. With the broad use of advanced magnetic resonance imaging (MRI) modalities, their use was extended to intraparenchymal glial tumors, as well. Functional MRI was employed to delineate eloquent cortical areas, whereas diffusion tensor imaging (DTI) facilitated the visualization of the major neural tracts, such as the pyramidal tract and the corpus callosum. Nowadays, 3D printed models are regarded as a promising accessory tool in cerebral neurooncology, involving a constantly enlarging field. They assist in surgical planning and their use extends from simple surgical biopsy to open surgery, transnasal endoscopic surgery, and stereotactic laser interstitial thermal therapy (LITT). Meanwhile, the role of 3D models harboring a tumor has been frequently used in neurosurgical training and in communicating with the patients. Finally, the use of 3DP technology has also been described in the construction of radiotherapy immobilization masks (RIM).

Surgical planning

The ultimate objective in oncological neurosurgery is the gross total lesion removal while maintaining the functional integrity of the patient. In turn, precision microneurosurgery demands excellent understanding of the personalized neuroanatomy, in addition to the basic anatomical knowledge. It is really important for the treating surgeon to understand the spatial relation of the tumor with adjacent eloquent areas and tracts, particularly for intraaxial tumors (Table 8.1).

The significant contribution of 3D printed models in the surgical planning of **extra-axial lesions** was initially recognized by the late 1990s, when Abe et al. evaluated the use of 3DP models in the management of seven patients with skull base tumors.[36] The models were constructed based on skull bone CT data, while handmade models of the lesion and the adjacent nerves and vessels were added to the model. The authors concluded that the skull base was accurately fabricated, including its foramina and mastoid air cells, and the models were useful in the successful management of all seven patients. However, they recognized that the sellar and upper clival regions were not well reproduced due to artifacts in the CT scan. Muellman et al. studied the usefulness of 3DP models in the surgical planning of three patients with petroclival tumors.[41] The models were constructed using the stereolithography methods, while the tumor was highlighted with acrylic paint. The authors reported significant variability in terms of exposure among different approaches that was useful in the choice of the optimal approach. Kondo et al. reported on the utility of 3DP models using various density meshes for tumor replication.[39] The models were based on CTA, MRI, and DSA data to replicate the skull,

Table 8.1 Summary table of studies focusing on the role of 3D printed models in surgical planning in neurooncology.

Author	Objective	Study design	Primary lesion	Dataset	Replicated structures	Results
Abe (1998, Japan)[36]	Qualitative evaluation of 3DP models for surgical planning and simulation.	Retrospective cohort; N = 7 patients	Skull base lesions	Bone CT of the skull base	Fabricated skull model using stereolithography, and handmade models of the tumor, major vessels, and cranial nerves.	The skull base was accurately fabricated, including the cranial base foramens and mastoid air cells. However, sellar and upper clival regions were not well reproduced due to artifacts in the CT scan. Surgery in all seven patients was uneventful.
Oishi (2013, Japan)[37]	Qualitative evaluation of interactive presurgical simulation applying advanced 3DP imaging and modeling techniques.	Retrospective cohort; N = 12 patients	Skull base or deep intracranial tumors	CT, CTA, Gd 3D SPGR MRI, TOF-MRA, DSA	Fabricated models of the skull, intracranial vessels and nerves, and space-occupying lesion using the selective laser sintering method.	Microscopic observation of color-printed plaster models provided substantial utility in confirming realistic surgical anatomies.
Spottiswoode (2013, Germany)[38]	Qualitative and quantitative evaluation of 3DP models using functional MRI in surgical planning of deep-seated cerebral tumors.	Retrospective cohort; N = 2	Lesions in the proximity of the motor cortex	T1-WI 3D MPRAGE MRI and fMRI of the hand and foot motor tasks	Patient 1: the entire cerebrum and cerebellum; Patient 2: a Smaller brain region. The lesion and fMRI regions were manually painted.	The models were shown to have acceptable accuracy, with a mean dimensional error of less than 0.5 mm.

Study						
Kondo (2016, Japan)[39]	Qualitative evaluation of 3DP models with a skull base tumor by 12 neurosurgeons. Various density meshes replicated the tumor.	Retrospective cohort; N = 4	Skull base lesions at the petroclival region	CTA, Gd 3D MRI, and DSA	Fabricated models of the skull, blood vessels, tumor, and brain stem.	The internal carotid artery, basilar artery, and brain stem and the positional relationships of these structures with the tumor were significantly more visible in the 3DP models with mesh tumors than in the 3DP models with solid or no tumors.
Lan (2016, China)[40]	Qualitative evaluation of 3DP models for surgical planning and simulation.	Retrospective cohort; N = 3	NA	CT, CTA, and MRI (including DTI and fMRI)	Skull intracranial vessels and nerves, brain tumors, eloquent areas, and conduction bundles.	The model accurately showed the spatial relation between tumor and intracranial vasculatures, tractus pyramidalis, and functional areas, which was helpful in selecting the optimal surgical approach and to avoid damage to brain function.
Muelleman (2016, USA)[41]	Qualitative evaluation of 3DP models in skull base surgical planning by measuring the fidelity of printed anatomical structures and comparing tumor exposure afforded by different approaches.	Retrospective cohort; N = 3	Petroclival tumors	Skull base or temporal bone CT and brain MRI	Tumor and bone using stereolithography. The tumor was highlighted using acrylic paint.	The 3DP models were useful for preoperative planning. Significant variability in exposure was noted between the models for similar or identical approaches. A notable drawback is that the printing process did not replicate mastoid air cells.

Continued

Table 8.1 Summary table of studies focusing on the role of 3D printed models in surgical planning in neurooncology.—*cont'd*

Author	Objective	Study design	Primary lesion	Dataset	Replicated structures	Results
Lau (2017, Australia)[42]	Quantitative evaluation of a 3DP model of a brain tumor in a pediatric patient to delineate the tumor and its surrounding anatomical structures.	Case presentation	Pilocytic astrocytoma	Gd MRI	Cerebellum and brain tumor.	3DP model was found to provide realistic visualization of brain anatomical structures and tumor and enhance understanding of pathology in relation to the surrounding structures. The mean difference in diameter measurements of the brain tumor was 0.53 mm (0.98%) between the 3DP model and computerized model.
Thawani (2017, USA)[43]	Quantitative evaluation of 3DP modeling with intraparenchymal lesions and the associated white matter tract anatomy by faculty and residents using a five-grade Likert scale.	Cross-sectional; N = 3 patients	Diffuse low-grade gliomas	T2 and FLAIR MRI	Tumor, corticospinal tract, arcuate fasciculus, and corpus callosum using the stereolithography method.	We found that faculty scores ranged from 4.25 to 5.0 (mean 4.75) and resident (postgraduate years 3 −6) scores ranged from 4.6 to 5.0 (mean 4.77).
Cingoz (2019, Turkey)[44]	Quantitative evaluation of 3 DP models for transnasal endoscopic pituitary surgery in terms of length of surgery and length of hospitalization.	Prospective control trial; 12 patients	Pituitary adenoma	Paranasal sinus CT images	Nasal cavity, sphenoid sinus opening, nasolacrimal channel, internal carotid artery, optic channel, nasal conchae, and sphenopalatine foramen.	The average operation duration of surgery in patients with and without 3DP modeling was 106 and 152 min, respectively. Similarly, the average hospital stay of patients with and without 3DP modeling was 3 and 6 days, respectively. All differences were statistically significant ($p < .01$).

tumor mass, intracranial vessels, and brain stem. The authors concluded that mesh tumors enhanced the understanding of the anatomical relations between the tumor lesion and the neighboring structures when compared to the solid models. Lately, Cingoz et al. evaluated the utility of 3DP models for transnasal endoscopic pituitary surgery in terms of the duration of surgery and the length of hospitalization.[44] The average operation duration of surgery in patients with and without 3DP modeling was 106 and 152 min, respectively. Similarly, the average hospital stay of patients with and without 3DP modeling was 3 and 6 days, respectively. All differences were statistically significant (p < .01).

The use of 3DP in the surgical planning extends to the management of **intraaxial tumors**. Oishi et al. performed a qualitative evaluation of the addition of a 3DP model to the presurgical simulation in the management of 12 patients with skull base or deep intracranial tumors.[37] The models were constructed using the selective laser sintering method from CT and MRI data, and replicated multiple structures, including the skull, intracranial vessels and nerves, and the space-occupying lesion. The authors reported that the microscopic observation of the printed models provided realistic representation of the surgical anatomies. In another accuracy study, Spottiswoode et al. quantified the accuracy of the 3D models of two patients with lesions in the proximity to the motor cortex. The accuracy of the technique was estimated both theoretically and by printing a geometrical phantom, with mean dimensional errors of less than 0.5 mm observed.[38] The models were constructed based solely on data from the MRI, including functional MRI for the hand and foot motor tasks. In a step further, Lan et al. constructed craniocerebral models for brain tumor resection, depicting the pyramidal tract, the optic tract and optic radiation, and a number of functional areas that are obvious during surgery, in addition to the tumor.[40] This is facilitated using actual size 3D models printed based on functional MRI and DTI. Similarly, experts and residents qualitatively evaluated the accuracy of 3DP models with diffuse low-grade gliomas (DLGGs) and the associated white matter tract anatomy in a cross-sectional study using a 5-point Likert scale.[43] T2 weighted images and fluid attenuated inverse recovery images were used to replicate the DLGG and along with the corticospinal tract, arcuate fasciculus, and corpus callosum. The authors reported high satisfaction scores from both the experts (4.75) and the residents (mean 4.77).

The experience with lesions within the **posterior cranial fossa** is limited. Lau et al. studied the accuracy of a 3DP model depicting the cerebellum with a pilocytic astrocytoma of a 6-year-old child to delineate the tumor and its surrounding structures.[42] The authors reported that the model provided a realistic visualization of the regional anatomical structures, with a mean difference in the tumor's diameter as high as 0.53 mm in comparison to the computerized model.

Neurosurgical training

The role of 3DP models in neurosurgical training has been studied mainly through cross-sectional studies. They are realistic, enhance learning, and are well accepted by both experts and trainees (Table. 8.2). Warran et al. created four exact replicas that differentiated various tissue structures into skin, bone, dura, tumor, and

Table 8.2 Summary table of studies focusing of neurosurgical training in cases with intracranial tumors.

Author	Objective	Study design	Dataset	Structures	Measured parameters	Results
Waran (2014, Malaysia)[45]	Quantitative evaluation of 3DP modeling in training surgeons to perform a frameless biopsy.	Cross-sectional; 8 trainees and 2 experts	CT and MRI from a patient with a thalamic deep-seated lesion	Skin, bone, dura, tumor, and surrounding brain	Number of attempts at registration and performing a brain biopsy, and the time to successful biopsy.	An average of 2.5 attempts and 8 –9 min were required for a successful registration of the navigation. The number of attempts to successful biopsy was from 2 to 5, for 22 min.
Waran (2013[46] Malaysia)	Qualitative evaluation of 3DP models to simulate common neurosurgical procedures using navigation systems.	Cross-sectional	CT from 3 patients with hydrocephalus, right frontal lesion, and a midline clival meningioma	Two skull models, and 1 model with a skin layer over the skull	The ability in registration, planning, and navigation on two navigation systems.	All models were accurately assessed using both navigation system and perform the necessary simulations as planned.
Waran (2014, Malaysia)[47]	Qualitative evaluation of multimaterial 3DP models to enhance training in surgical simulations.	Cross-sectional; 3 trainees and 1 expert	CT of a patient with a frontal cortically located brain tumor	Skin, bone, dura, tumor, and brain	Pliability, handling, and texture of replicated tissues using a 4-point scale.	The use of the 3DP yields the creation of more realistic models with multiple tissues, which allow for an improved training experience.
Waran (2015, Malaysia)[48]	Qualitative evaluation of 3DP models with intraventricular fluid to train surgeons on EVT and intraventricular biopsy.	Cross-sectional; 12 trainees and 3 experts	CT and MRI from a patient with hydrocephalus and pineal tumor	Skin, bone, dura, CSF, interventricular septum, fornices, choroid plexus, tumor, vessels, and blood	The surgeons assessed the models on a number of areas based on a 5-point Likert scale.	Surgical procedure: 4.6; surgical anatomy score: 3.2; the ventriculostomy procedure score: 3; biopsy procedure score: 4.

Study	Purpose	Study design	Imaging modality	Structures	Outcome measure	Results
Lin (2018, China)[6]	Qualitative evaluation of 3DP cranial nerve models for skull base tumor surgery training.	Cross-sectional; 16 experts	3D T1-WI TFE and DTI of two sellar tumor and one acoustic neuroma cases	Skull, brain, tumor, blood vessels, optic chiasm, and facial nerve	Accuracy, practicability and an overall satisfaction using a 5-point scale.	Accuracy score: 3.94; practicability score: 4.14; and overall evaluation: 3.8.
Lin (2018, China)[49]	Qualitative evaluation off 3DP models in enhancing the learning curve of surgery of tuberculum sellae meningioma.	Prospective cohort; 3DP group: 22; atlas group: 20	CTA and MRI from 4 patients with tuberculum sellae meningioma	Skull, tumor, vessels, and optic chiasm	Pretest and postexamination on 14 items. Each correct answer was awarded 1 point.	Posttest scores and score differences were significantly higher in the 3DP model group. The study group did not affect the mean operating time.
Kondo (2019, Japan)[50]	Evaluation of 3DP model of the petrous bone with an epidermoid petroclival tumor case for surgical training in combined transpetrosal surgery.	Cross-sectional; 13 experts	CT, MRI, and DSA	Skull, petrous bone, auditory ossicles, fallopian canal, cochlea, semicircular canal, brain stem, CN V, VII, and VIII, intracranial vessels	Anatomic reproducibility using a 4-point Likert scale and the distance estimation between a set of landmarks.	Anatomic reproducibility was consistent between the 3D images and the 3DP models. The error between estimated and measured distances between 3 out of 11 anatomic sites was smaller for the 3DP model than the 3D image. The error in the 3D printed model was smaller than in the 3D image for all 11 sites.

surrounding the brain, from a patient with a deep-sited thalamic pathology ([45] After a thorough theoretical seminar on surgery of intracranial pathologies, four trainees and two experts performed frameless biopsies. The total time required for biopsy acquisition and the procedural successes were recorded. Trainees required 22 min and 2 to 5 attempts to plan and successfully perform a frameless biopsy. On the other hand, the two experts succeeded in their first attempt and the whole process lasted for about 16 min. In addition, 3DP models were useful and accurate to simulate common neurosurgical procedures.[46] The same authors assessed the utility of multimaterial of 3D printed models to enhance training through basic neurosurgical steps, from navigation and planning to craniotomy and simple tumor excision.[47] The models clearly delineated the skin, subcutaneous tissues, bone, dura, normal brain, and a tumor with satisfactory results. In particular, the tissue characteristics of the surgical models were good, despite the stiff feeling of the skin and the absence of vessels in the dura. The bone behaved like the natural bone as the perforator stopped at the dural interface and the footplate of the cutter was able to separate the dural layer from the bone. But above all, the models showed excellent compatibility with the navigation devices, allowing for accurate registration and surgical planning. In a study by Kondo et al., 13 experts focused the role of 3DP models of the petrous bone with an epidermoid petroclival tumor case for surgical training and combined transpetrosal surgery.[50] The models were constructed based on CT, MRI, and DSA and replicated the petrous bone in great detail, including structures such as the auditory ossicles, fallopian canal, cochlea, semicircular canals, and major cranial nerves. The anatomic reproducibility was consistent between the 3D images and the 3DP models. The error between estimated and measured distances between 3 out of 11 anatomic sites was smaller for the 3DP model than the 3D image. The error in the 3D printed model was smaller than in the 3D image for all 11 sites.

Printed 3D prototypic models are useful in enhancing learning. More specifically, Lin et al. studied the utility of 3D printed models in enhancing the learning curve of surgery of tuberculum sellae meningioma.[49] A cohort of 20 trainees studied using a color atlas and a second group of 22 trainees studied using 3DP models. The pretest and posttest scores on 14 items were recorded. The posttest scores and score differences were significantly higher in the 3DP model group. The study group did not affect the mean operating time. Both expert neurosurgeons and trainees welcome the 3DP models in neurosurgical training with great satisfaction. Twelve trainees and three experts evaluated 3DP models with pineal tumor and intraventricular fluid during a workshop on endoscopic third ventriculostomy (ETV) and intraventricular biopsy using a 5-point Likert scale.[48] The models were constructed based on CT and MRI data to replicate multiple structures, including the interventricular septum, fornices, choroid plexus, and intracranial vessels. The authors reported moderate to high satisfaction scores with regard to the surgical anatomy (3.2/5), surgical procedure (4.6/5), ETV (3/5), and intraventricular biopsy (4/5). Similarly, 16 experts evaluated the accuracy, practicability, and overall satisfaction of 3DP models with major cranial nerves in skull base tumor surgery training, using a 5-point Likert scale.[6] The accuracy score was as high as 3.94/5, while the predictability and overall satisfaction scores were 4.14/5 and 4/5, respectively.

Application in radiotherapy

3DP technology has been adopted in the construction of RIM. The latter are built based on CT data of the head and neck (Table 8.3). Fisher et al. employed the Hausdorff distance to analyze CT slices obtained by rescanning a phantom with a printed mask in position. The authors reported that with a median "worse" tolerance of approximately 4 mm for more than 80% of the slices, printed masks could achieve similar levels of immobilization to those of systems common in clinical use.[51] Moreover, Laycock et al., performed a preclinical evaluation on the dosimetric properties of 3 material used for 3DP RIM.[52] The study concluded that the majority of the possible candidate 3DP materials under study resulted in very similar attenuation of the therapeutic radiotherapy beam. Finally, Pham et al. performed a quantitative evaluation of 3DP RIM using the Dice similarity coefficient, Hausdorff distance, differences in centroid positions and angular deviations and recorded dosimetric differences.[53] According to their findings, the mean Dice similarity coefficients and mean Hausdorff distance were 0.985 and 0.9 mm, respectively, the mean centroid vector displacement was equal to 0.5 mm, and the mean angular deviation of the 3D printout from the original volume for the Pitch, Yaw, and Roll were 1.1, 0.59, and 0.79, respectively.

In a step forward, Brandmeir et al. used custom 3DP technology to construct customized stereotactic frames for LITT in five patients with brain lesions.[54] Patient CT and MRI with three to four skull fiducials were used to determine the appropriate trajectory to the lesion. At the planning completion, the authors constructed a 3D frame with the patient approval. A week after, the patient returned to the hospital for the LITT using the customized frame. In two cases, the surgeons performed an equal number of lesion biopsies. The placement of the catheters was accurate in all cases without perioperative complications. Finally, radiotherapy thermoplastic immobilization masks, molded onto customized 3D models, have been tested for potential dosimetric differences secondary to inaccuracies in the rotational positioning in 11 patients with excellent results.[53]

Limitations

The use of 3D prototypic models has long been associated with a lengthy printing process (24–48 h) and high cost, and both parameters increase proportionally to the complexity of the model.[36] At the same time, a number of limitations in the use of 3DP in neurooncology have been recognized. To start with, there are important differences in the physical properties of 3DP models from the equivalent cranial components.[50] Current models are often made of heat-deformable materials, whereas the binder is water-soluble preventing irrigation. A large amount of plaster dust is generated during the drilling process. Fine structures are frequently missed, including the small vessels and nerves, and the arachnoidal system of intracranial cisterns.[48] At the same time, blood and cerebrospinal fluid (CSF) hemodynamics are difficult to replicate. Thus, 3DP models are characterized by the absence of bleeding risk to allow for the training on the use of electrocoagulation, and there is no brain shift due to CSF loss.[40,48,49] The quality of the models is further limited by artifacts that are attributed to the quality of the 3D imaging, resolution of the

Table 8.3 Summary table of studies focusing on the use of 3DP technology in the construction of radiotherapy immobilization masks, 3DP stereotactic frames for laser thermal therapy, and in neurooncologic patient education.

Author	Study design	Objective	Dataset	Evaluation	Results
3DP radiotherapy immobilization masks (RIMs)					
Fisher (2014, UK)[51]	Laboratory experimental study	Preclinical evaluation of a 3DP RIM	CT data	Hausdorff distance was used to analyze CT slices obtained by rescanning a phantom with a printed mask in position.	With a median "worse-case" tolerance of approximately 4 mm for more than 80% of the slices, printed masks can achieve similar levels of immobilization to those of systems currently in clinical use.
Laycock (2015, UK)[52]	Laboratory experimental study	Preclinical evaluation on the dosimetric properties of three materials used for 3DP RIM	CT and MRI data	Measurement of the therapeutic radiotherapy beam attenuation produced by three materials suitable for 3DP.	The majority of the possible candidate 3D printing materials tested, resulted in very similar attenuation of the therapeutic radiotherapy beam.
Pham (2018, Canada)[53]	Retrospective cohort; N = 11	Quantitative evaluation of 3DP RIM	CT data	Accuracy (dice similarity coefficient, Hausdorff distance, differences in centroid positions, and angular deviations) and dosimetric differences.	Mean dice similarity coefficients: 0.985; mean Hausdorff distance: 0.9 mm; mean centroid vector displacement: 0.5 mm; mean angular deviation of the 3D printout from the original volume for the pitch, yaw, and roll were 1.1, 0.59, and 0.79, respectively.

3DP stereotactic frames for laser interstitial thermal therapy (LITT)

Brandmeir (2016, USA)[54]	Retrospective cohort; N = 5	Qualitative and quantitative evaluation	CT and MRI data	Intraoperative MRI	Intraoperative and postoperative imaging studies confirmed the accurate placement of the LITT catheter and the lesion created. Mean operating room time for all patients was 45 min but only 26 min when excluding the cases in which a biopsy was performed.

Patient education

van de Belt (2018, The Netherlands)[55]	Survey; 11 patients	Qualitative evaluation of 3DP models of tumors including surrounding functional areas in terms of health literacy, decision-making, and satisfaction by the patients.	CT and MRI data	Semistructured interviews	The model improved patients' understanding about their situation; patients reported that it was easier to ask their neurosurgeon questions based on their model and that it supported their decision about preferred treatment. A perceived barrier for using the 3D model was that it could be emotionally confronting, particularly in an early phase of the disease. Positive effects were related to psychological domains, including coping, learning effects, and communication.

rapid prototyping systems, the printing method, and the quality of the materials used.[38] Finally, the choice of the optimal training method among cadaveric courses, workshops on 3DP models, and textbook atlases should take into consideration existing differences in spatial imagination and learning efficiency among the trainees.[6]

Spine
From simple spine models to surgical planning

Rapid prototyping of spinal elements and models, especially of bony structures, is a rather simple procedure and the use of such models for teaching, planning, and training could be considered a logical next step.[56,57] Not only bone appears to be easily reproduced by 3DP technology in shape and even in texture or weight 56 but also the accuracy of the method regarding complex bones (Fig. 8.4), such as those of the spine, has been already demonstrated.[57,58] To this effect, a wide variety of imaging data are routinely available during the examination of spinal anatomy and spinal pathologies, including functional X-rays, CT and MRI scans, and bone density scans, among others, offering a lot of data to be used in 3DP of spine models and other implementations. As with cerebral tumors, complex pathologies of the spine can be fabricated using 3DP for preoperative planning and visualization. This was demonstrated in the case of complex paraspinal schwannomas in the cervical, thoracic, and sacral regions by Stone et al.[59] who used 3DP to preoperatively assess the complexity of those pathologies, namely their size, location, degree of bony erosion, and vascular or neural compression.[59]

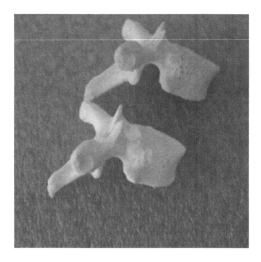

FIGURE 8.4

A three-dimensional (3D) printed human thoracic vertebra, compared to the human tissue used for its design as described by Baskaran et al.[57]

Prototyping for spinal operations

Beyond teaching, visualization, and haptic familiarization with the particularities of the spine and its pathologies, the aforementioned abundance of information and the relative simplicity of the application with regard to the spine have led to an increasing use of 3DP for prototyping templates and aides for spine surgery, attempting to make surgical planning and execution safer and easier. While this utility has been uncommon in other neurosurgical subspecialties, such as vascular neurosurgery or neurooncology, in spine surgery, a number of studies can be identified to use this approach. Sugawara et al were among the first to demonstrate a multistep procedure and technique for the rapid prototyping and intraoperative use of patient-specific laminar templates (guides) for the insertion of pedicle screws at the thoracic spine.[60] The research team used CT data and 3D imaging software to calculate and preoperatively plan screw trajectories. Using 3DP technology, they manufactured patient-specific guide templates that incorporated those trajectories. These templates were used during the operation to assist in achieving the preplanned screw trajectories, while the success of the method was evaluated using postoperative CT scans that showed minimal deviation from the planned trajectory of 0.87 ± 0.34 mm at coronal pedicle midpoint.[60] A prospective multicenter evaluation of the above-described procedure over 103 patients and a total of 813 screws at the cervical and thoracic level demonstrated a remarkable 98.5% accurate screw placement without cortical violation and no neural or vascular injury.[61] The same research team also adapted their procedures and techniques in order to expand the possible applications, investigating the use of 3D printed guides for the treatment of atlantoaxial instability.[62] In a study on canines, they demonstrated 3D modeling of C1 and C2 vertebrae, plate and screw planning, and 3D fabricated acrylic screw guide templates (Fig. 8.5), performing operations with an equally high degree of success and accuracy, as well as high clinical benefit to the canine atlantoaxial instability.[62] As such, the importance of such a procedure in many spinal instrumentation operations, where instrumentation misplacement and subsequent neural and vascular injury are considered not-so-uncommon but possibly devastating complications, becomes apparent and deserves further investigation and

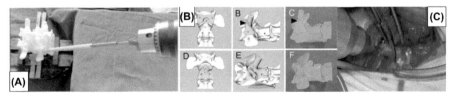

FIGURE 8.5

Improving the trajectory spine instrumentation has been facilitated computer-assisted three-dimensional (3D) printed custom drill guides. In (A), Shao et al.[63] describe transpedicular transdiscal lumbar screw fixation. Kamishina et al.[62] demonstrated atlantoaxial fixation with 3D printed drill guide: in (B) the computer-aided design (CAD)-assisted design, while in (C), intraoperative placement of guide and drill positioning.

benchmarking against imaging guidance system assisted operations. What can be also considered of great importance and greatly in favor of this proposed procedure is that it appears to feature good reproducibility, as a number of other research teams have published similar investigations and variations. Lumbar pedicle screw and transpedicular transdiscal lumbar screw fixation,[63,64] C1 fracture screw fixation, multiple cervical, and high cervical screw fixation,[65−67] as well as sacral arthrodesis,[68] have all been investigated and demonstrated using patient anatomy-specific 3D printed guide templates for screw placement with favorable results.

The concept of manufacturing 3D printed patient-specific templates was also successfully applied in spine deformity by Pijpker et al.[69] The research team used an elaborate method to initially evaluate spine deformity in 3D and calculate angular reduction of kyphosis and scoliosis in a 12-year-old female patient and to digitally design custom patient-specific templates (Fig. 8.6) to mark the complex planned (and needed) closing wedge bone-disc-bone resection between T11 and T1. The designed templates as well as the patient spine model were then 3D printed in polyamide and were used intraoperatively for guidance and identification of the intended levels, while the templates were then fitted to the patient spine to identify and guide the osteotomies. This use of 3D design and prototyping of individual spine models and guiding templates facilitated the authors in safely performing a complex deformity correction operation in a young patient. Furthermore, standardizing this procedure could possibly contribute to safer and simple spinal osteotomy procedures.[69]

Novel applications

It can be considered highly probable that, in the near future, rapid prototyping would be considered for the manufacturing of patient-specific spinal implants.[70] The realization of such implants should adhere to a range of requirements, including appropriate biomechanical and biochemical properties or safety, among others. It

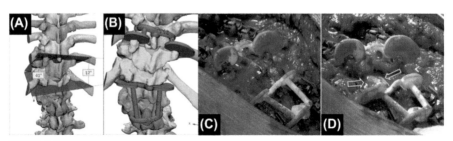

FIGURE 8.6

Design and use of three-dimensional (3D) printed osteotomy template guides for severe congenital kyphoscoliosis by Pijpker et al.[69]: (A) 3D spine model from computed tomography (CT) Digital Imaging and Communications in Medicine (DICOM) data and planned angular kyphosis and scoliosis reduction, (B) design of templates for planned osteotomy, (C) intraoperative placement of 3D printed osteotomy template guides, and (D) wedge-shaped extended pedicle subtraction osteotomy.

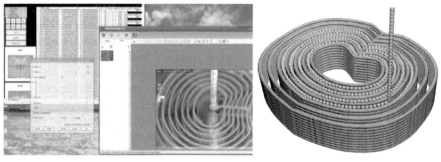

FIGURE 8.7

Digital design of layered three-dimensional (3D) printed scaffold from biodegradable polyurethane structure mimicking the natural shape and lamellar structure of intravertebral disc and schematic of spheroid deposition between the lamellae for optimization of biomechanical properties.[72]

could be expected that such implants would concern vertebral replacements or implanted templates for deformity correction. Nonetheless, researchers already work on scenarios that surpass simple spinal functional or structural replacement and envision regenerative properties to be demonstrated by possible implants.[71] In such a study, a biomimetic elastic intervertebral disc scaffold was created with 3DP technology using degradable polyurethane that demonstrated macroscopic and mechanical properties similar to natural shape, lamellar structure, and behavior of a natural intravertebral disc (Fig. 8.7) and microscopic properties able to influence cell adhesion, proliferation, and alignment.[71,72] The use of biofabrication-based techniques is a concept that recently emerged in tissue regeneration and is based on computer-designed biomaterial and cell-based scaffolds with intricate architecture and microstructure.[72] While such novel implementations cannot yet be considered mature, they nonetheless pave the way for in vivo experimentation the production of regenerative spinal implants in the future.

Anatomy, education, and prototyping in general neurosurgery

Central nervous system anatomy and education

3DP technology offers the possibility to create realistic anatomical models both of normal neuroanatomy and of pathological conditions.[73,74] Those can be prepared in order to be used not only for teaching purposes at different academic levels (by students in medical school or trainees in specialties of clinical neurosciences) but also, with the improvement in materials and model accuracy, for practical education and surgical training.[57,75] Simple 3D printed case models can provide trainees with a volume of specimens and training phantoms that cadaveric specimens simply cannot compete with due to cost and availability. The quality and accuracy of those phantoms can also currently approach that of cadaveric specimens and, in many cases, even that of living tissues, offering trainees a realistic hands-on experience and exposure to both to unique cases and to a volume of standard procedures.[76] While aforementioned quality may vary depending on the 3DP equipment used, the quality of materials, and that of the computed designed models, studies in general report very small margins of error for macroscopic structures. In General Neurosurgery, as such, not only generic models but also patient-specific phantoms can be created with a combination of techniques, using 3D MRI sequences for modeling and polylactic acid (PLA) filament for 3DP, as demonstrated in Ref[77]. The researchers in this study used PLA to print an accurate head model of a 3-year-old boy with Sturge-Weber syndrome. They also used PLA to print a mold of the pathological brain, which was then casted using styrene-ethylene-butylene-styrene in order to create a highly realistic brain with properties resembling the normal brain tissue (Fig. 8.8). The produced patient-specific phantom was qualitatively evaluated by a team of neurosurgeons who assessed, albeit subjectively, both its realism (anatomical locations, haptic response, appearance, internal consistency) and its educational utility (skills acquisition, depth sensation, orientation, learning) from good to perfect.

In a similar fashion, another research team created a skull-brain phantom of 2-year-old boy with hydrocephalus.[78] The brain in this case was casted using silicone based material, while dummy endoscope was also prototyped for training purposes, creating effectively a very low cost training model for ETV, a neurosurgical operative technique to which residents, and often specialized neurosurgeons, have limited exposure. Subjective evaluation by a team of neurosurgeons produced a strong consensus for the usefulness and the training value of the simulator phantom.[78] An even more realistic simulator for ETV training was created by another research team,[79] using patient imaging data from a 14-year-old boy with hydrocephalus. Using a combination of 3DP and casting techniques, the team innovated in the inclusion of replaceable parts (3D printed) for the simulator aiming at repeated use of the phantom, while they also produced a model realistic enough to be used with actual endoscopy equipment and able to reproduce CSF flow and pulsation. While such product design may actually lead to not so inexpensive manufacturing, this

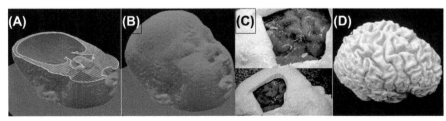

FIGURE 8.8

(A) Anatomy model for educational purposes, (B) computer-aided design (CAD)-based digital design of a pediatric head model, (C) three-dimensional (3D) printed pediatric head phantom with rubber dura and casted brain in situ as described by Grillo et al.[77] and (D) a 3D printed brain phantom from MRI data, as described by Baskaran et al.[57]

example demonstrates the feasibility of combining 3DP technology with other manufacturing techniques for the production of very accurate, "life-like" simulators for neurosurgical training, evaluated for high external and internal validity.[79] Furthermore, such hands-on training simulators can also be created for more common neurosurgical operations, such as the placement of external ventricular drainage (EVD), which are more frequently performed by trainee neurosurgeons.[80] In such a study, the research team created a very low cost, simple, and time-efficient 3D printed hollow head model for simulation training of EVD placement. A pilot objective evaluation by neurosurgical trainees revealed >100% increase in successful accurate placement of EVD after instruction and training, measured by image guidance system[80] demonstrating the high utility of 3DP simulators even for common operations. Results regarding subjective evaluation of perceived properties of a 3D printed ventriculostomy simulator are reported by Ryan et al. who also conclude that this approach can improve technique learning using low-cost realistic training phantoms and scenarios.[81]

Finally, the ability to effectively use patient-specific data for these phantoms extends their utility beyond simulation and training to the grounds of surgical planning and operation rehearsal in large possible range of operations. This can be demonstrated by the studies of Jimenez et al. and Sullivan et al. who used 3DP technology to create such operation planning phantoms for craniosynostosis and endovascular pediatric aneurysm treatment, respectively.[82,83] A large series of patient-specific 3D printed vascular models used for preoperative and intraoperative tailoring of microcatheters for endovascular coiling is reported by Ishibashi et al.[84]. The authors reported that using acrylic resin 3D printed models for 27 aneurysms, they preoperatively tailored 48 catheters and, while 81% did not require any modification to the initial shape and 71% did not require catheter replacement, the procedures were most importantly effective, safe, with no operative complications (including no aneurysm rupture), and showed high acceptance rate among operative staff.

Prototyping of materials and tools

Cranioplasty for cranial defects (due to congenital deficits, severe head injury, decompressive craniectomy, infection, or certain eclectic neurosurgical procedures) is among the few applications where the end product of 3DP techniques can be applied almost directly to the neurosurgical patient. The obvious advantages for exploring custom 3D printed cranioplasty implants in lieu of commercial implants include a combination of availability and cheaper cost (when compared to custom-printed commercial implants) with greater precision of the end product (when compared to intraoperatively molded materials). Polymethyl methacrylate (PMMA) has been commonly used as a material in cranioplasty for over half a century by neurosurgeons globally, and it is still considered a viable option and is frequently used even in modern neurosurgical practice. Recently various teams have explored the possibility of precasting PMMA into customized cranioplasty prostheses using patients' CT data according to the Digital Imaging and Communications in Medicine (DICOM) standard format. These data are used to reconstruct a stereolithography model that is then 3D printed into a physical object using PLA. This PLA model is used as a mold to cast the final PMMA cranioplasty implant. Such an approach not only reduces operative costs but also can significantly reduce operative time, especially with regard to large cranial deficits. Moreover, it retains the biocompatibility advantages of PMMA as well as the better esthetic outcome of patient-customized implants over free-hand molding of PMMA. The procedures and materials described in this approach (Fig. 8.9) seem feasible to be reproduced by commercial 3D printers (De La Peña, De La Peña-Brambila,[85] and can be used by most institutions with access to specialized computer software (DICOM viewer and CAD software) as well as typical dental lab equipment for casting. Moreover, retrospective analysis of series of patients[86] who were treated using this approach shows that not only large cranial deficits can be successfully treated but also that this method can be considered on par with current state-of-the-art cranioplasty techniques with regard to complications, esthetic results, patient satisfaction, and usability.

Prototyping of tools for common operations in general neurosurgery is also nowadays possible using 3DP technology, as was demonstrated by a study from the Barrow Innovation Center.[87] It should be noted that, in the case of prototyping material, tools and devices in general, the benefits that could factor in favor of using 3D printed ones may include the following: (a) "innovation" (a new tool or device can be prototyped and tested by 3DP tech), (b) "customization" (tools and devices that are tailored to patient anatomy *or* to surgeon's preference), (c) "troubleshooting" (existing tools' features or behavior cause inconvenience), (d) "availability" (a certain tool quickly available by demand), and finally, (e) "cost" (house developed tools with reduced material and commercial cost). While the use of 3D printed tools in the surgical fields is not yet widespread, taking into account the above factors can lead to unprecedented implications, as, for example, is the creation

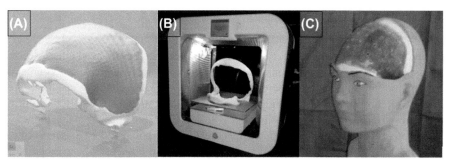

FIGURE 8.9

A wide bifrontotemporal cranial deficit due to decompressive craniectomy after traumatic brain injury, treated using three-dimensional (3D) printing technology: (A) computer-aided design (CAD)-based digital design, (B) 3D printing of polylactic acid (PLA) custom prosthesis, and (C) fitting of printed prosthesis in a mannequin as described by De La Peña et al.[85]

of operative tools out of PLA with the 1/10th of the cost of their traditional stainless steel counterparts.[88] In the case of,[87] the desired benefit fell into the category of "troubleshooting." The authors identified a common issue, during placement of ventricular catheters for hydrocephalus while using frameless image guidance systems, in the interference from ferromagnetic material-based retractors (e.g., stainless steel) that could lead to inaccurate identification of the catheter tip from the guidance system, resulting in incorrect placement and leading to multiple placement attempts at the risk of brain injury. The research team also identified that a potential simple solution would be the development of 3D printed retractors out of nonferromagnetic material, such as PLA. In the R&D process, the research team not only selected and developed a Weitlaner type retractor for prototyping but also explored the factor of "innovation" when they developed a simple addition to the tool that can function as catheter retainer. Following cadaveric tests, the team reported a patient case where the tool was successfully and safely used as intended (replacement of steel retractor that interfered with image guidance).

Patient counseling

Another recent application of 3DP models that was recently investigated is their use during patient counseling when obtaining informed consent.[89,90] To date, it is still an experimental application with a few examples reported in the literature. Concerning neurosurgery, *Alshomer et al.* used 3D printed models to improve patient comprehension during surgical counseling and education of parents of craniosynostosis patients. They reported a series of 14 parents that passed through explanation about surgery and possible complication before and after the aid of patient-specific 3D printed models. In this series, 3DP was found to be an affordable modality to provide information about craniosynostosis and to assist surgical decision-making.[91] Similar results were reported in case of posterior lumbar fixation.[92] Equally important, 3D printed models of tumors, including surrounding functional areas, have been studied in terms of doctor-to-patient communication, health literacy, decision-making, and patient satisfaction.[55] Van Belt et al. used a semistructured interview to identify facilitators and barriers in communication with the patient using such 3D models (Fig. 8.10). The authors found that the models improved patient's understanding about their situation, facilitated communication, and supported their decision about the treatment of choice. However, 3D models could be emotionally disturbing, particularly in the early phase of the disease.

Conclusions

3DP technology is gradually maturing and is currently facilitating a variety of applications in the field of Neurosurgery ranging from education and training to advanced applied techniques.[93,94] Increasing number of studies have being published during the last few years and early identified limitations, such as accuracy and speed, are

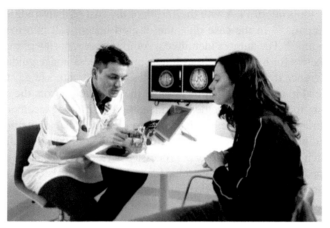

FIGURE 8.10

Enactment of patient interview—informing a patient for her pathology and obtaining consent form could be facilitated using personalized three-dimensional (3D) printed models.

From van de Belt T. H., Nijmeijer H., Grim D., Engelen L. J. L. P. G., Vreeken R., van Gelder M. M. H. J., ter Laan M. Patient-specific actual-size three-dimensional printed models for patient education in glioma treatment: first experiences. World Neurosurg. *(2018);117;e99–e105 https://doi.org/10.1016/j.wneu.2018.05.190.*

being addressed. At the current state of the art, 3DP has not only established itself as a powerful tool for stereotactical depiction of simple and complex neuroanatomical structures but has also been tested for prototyping and fabrication of materials. As such vascular and oncological neurosurgery seems to benefit the most from the advancements so far in terms of surgical planning and neurosurgical training. On the other hand, in spine surgery, functional and general neurosurgery personalized rapid prototyping can currently produce equipment and tools for intraoperative use in certain cases; while those subspecialties do trail behind in training applications, they do also focus on novel implementations.

The adoption of 3DP into the surgical fields at large can still be considered to be at an early stage, but several studies have reported promising results, especially in the fields of neurosurgery, otorhinolaryngology, and skull base. Such studies have reported benefits in terms of an accelerated learning curves.[14,95–97] Rapid prototyping with 3D printed models provides additional information to standard radiological exams and produces high-fidelity patient-specific and disease-specific models that permit visualization of complex intracranial vascular anatomy. All these features could further lead to an extensive application of 3D printed models to improve surgical planning and residents' training in the future. Consequently, an indirect improvement in treatment's effectiveness and patients' outcome can be expected, but as of yet, there is no concrete evidence in the existing literature to support this hypothesis. Despite recent developments, the technique is still expensive and time-consuming, drawbacks that currently preclude a more widespread use and its use in emergency procedures. Nonetheless, cranial deficits can already be treated using 3D printed prostheses, allowing functional, safe, and possibly aesthetically superior results at significant lower costs than traditional prostheses technology. Also, 3DP technology can serve as a tool for prototyping and production of innovative surgical devices. This envisioned application could may be more and more important in the future to create customized instruments and implants, allowing for patient-specific, personalized approaches for more effective and less invasive treatments.

All things considered, 3DP is not yet widespread in Neurological Surgery and, in spite of early adopters and certain cases, one could argue that the field is still principally dominated by traditional education and surgical training, established and repeatedly tested materials, devices and tools, and successful operative techniques backed by a lot of field experience. In this light, 3DP could potentially become a game changing technology for the future for Neurosurgery, especially in (a) significantly reducing costs and availability of materials, (b) actively involving neurosurgical research teams in prototyping and development of devices and tools, (c) greatly improving training regimens in terms of case capacity and learning curves and, finally (d) improving patient outcomes due to superior surgical planning. In achieving all these goals, 3DP could not—and should not—be fragmentally implemented—rather it should explore important synergies with other emerging technologies such as virtual/augmented reality environments for improving education, training, or operative planning,[98] as well as micro/nanofabrication technologies for creating tools, materials, and neural prostheses with desired properties[99] with regard to reducing complications and improving outcomes.

References

1. Berman B. 3-D printing: The new industrial revolution. *Bus Horiz.* 2012;55(2):155—162. https://doi.org/10.1016/j.bushor.2011.11.003.
2. Langridge B, Cantab BA, Momin S, Coumbe B, Hons BA, Woin E, et al. Systematic Review of the Use of 3-Dimensional Printing in Surgical Teaching and Assessment. *J Surg Educ.* 2017. https://doi.org/10.1016/j.jsurg.2017.06.033.
3. Randazzo M, Pisapia J, Singh N, Thawani J. 3D printing in neurosurgery: A systematic review. *Surg Neurol Int.* 2016. https://doi.org/10.4103/2152-7806.194059.
4. Yan Q, Dong H, Su J, Han J, Song B, Wei Q, Shi Y. A Review of 3D Printing Technology for Medical Applications. *Engineering.* 2018;4(5):729—742. https://doi.org/10.1016/j.eng.2018.07.021.
5. Cui T, Yan Y, Zhang R, Liu L, Xu W, Wang X. Rapid Prototyping of a Double-Layer Polyurethane—Collagen Conduit for Peripheral Nerve Regeneration. *Tissue Eng Part C: Methods.* 2009;15(1):1—9. https://doi.org/10.1089/ten.tec.2008.0354.
6. Lin J, Zhou Z, Guan J, Zhu Y, Liu Y, Yang Z, et al. Using Three-Dimensional Printing to Create Individualized Cranial Nerve Models for Skull Base Tumor Surgery. *World Neurosurg.* 2018;120:e142—e152. https://doi.org/10.1016/j.wneu.2018.07.236.
7. Zhang H, Liu G, Tong XG, Hang W. Application of three-dimensional printing technology in the surgical treatment of nasal skull base tumor. *Zhonghua Er Bi Yan Hou Tou Jing*

Wai Ke Za Zhi. 2018;53(10):780−784. https://doi.org/10.3760/cma.j.issn.1673-0860.2018.10.012.

8. Karakas AB, Govsa F, Ozer MA, Eraslan C. 3D Brain Imaging in Vascular Segmentation of Cerebral Venous Sinuses. *J Digit Imag.* 2019;32(2):314−321. https://doi.org/10.1007/s10278-018-0125-4.

9. Knoedler M, Feibus AH, Lange A, Maddox MM, Ledet E, Thomas R, Silberstein JL. Individualized physical 3-dimensional kidney tumor models constructed from 3-dimensional printers result in improved trainee anatomic understanding. *Urology.* 2015. https://doi.org/10.1016/j.urology.2015.02.053.

10. Liu YF, Xu LW, Zhu HY, Liu SSY. Technical procedures for template-guided surgery for mandibular reconstruction based on digital design and manufacturing. *Biomed Eng Online.* 2014. https://doi.org/10.1186/1475-925X-13-63.

11. Klein GT, Lu Y, Wang MY. 3D printing and neurosurgery–ready for prime time? *World Neurosurg.* 2013. https://doi.org/10.1016/j.wneu.2013.07.009.

12. Tai BL, Rooney D, Stephenson F, Liao P-S, Sagher O, Shih AJ, Savastano LE. Development of a 3D-printed external ventricular drain placement simulator: technical note. *J Neurosurg.* 2015. https://doi.org/10.3171/2014.12.JNS141867.

13. Xu WH, Liu J, Li ML, Sun ZY, Chen J, Wu JH. 3D printing of intracranial artery stenosis based on the source images of magnetic resonance angiograph. *Ann Transl Med.* 2014. https://doi.org/10.3978/j.issn.2305-5839.2014.08.02.

14. Agha RA, Fowler AJ. The role and validity of surgical simulation. *Int Surg.* 2015. https://doi.org/10.9738/INTSURG-D-14-00004.1.

15. Schaller K. Neurosurgical training under European law. *Acta Neurochir.* 2013;155(3):547. https://doi.org/10.1007/s00701-012-1579-7.

16. Stienen MN, Bartek J, Czabanka MA, Freyschlag CF, Kolias A, Krieg SM, et al. Neurosurgical procedures performed during residency in Europe—preliminary numbers and time trends. *Acta Neurochir.* 2019. https://doi.org/10.1007/s00701-019-03888-3.

17. Abla AA, Lawton MT. Three-dimensional hollow intracranial aneurysm models and their potential role for teaching, simulation, and training. *World Neurosurg.* 2015. https://doi.org/10.1016/j.wneu.2014.01.015.

18. Mashiko T, Otani K, Kawano R, Konno T, Kaneko N, Ito Y, Watanabe E. Development of three-dimensional hollow elastic model for cerebral aneurysm clipping simulation enabling rapid and low cost prototyping. *World Neurosurg.* 2015. https://doi.org/10.1016/j.wneu.2013.10.032.

19. Thawani JP, Pisapia JM, Singh N, Petrov D, Schuster JM, Hurst RW, et al. Three-dimensional printed modeling of an arteriovenous malformation including blood flow. *World Neurosurg.* 2016. https://doi.org/10.1016/j.wneu.2016.03.095.

20. Ganske IM, Schulz N, Livingston K, Goobie S, Meara JG, Proctor M, Weinstock P. Multi-modal 3D simulation makes the impossible possible. *Plast Reconstr Surg Glob Open.* 2018. https://doi.org/10.1097/GOX.0000000000001751.

21. Smith E, Prabhu SP, Flynn K, Weinstock P, Orbach DB. Optimizing cerebrovascular surgical and endovascular procedures in children via personalized 3D printing. *J Neurosurg Pediatr.* 2015. https://doi.org/10.3171/2015.3.peds14677.

22. Schultz RC, Danielson JR, Habakuk S. The use of uniform simulated models in the reconstruction of craniopagus twins. *Ann Plast Surg.* 1986. https://doi.org/10.1097/00000637-198602000-00014.

23. Christensen AM, Humphries SM, Goh KYC, Swift D. Advanced "tactile" medical imaging for separation surgeries of conjoined twins. *Childs Nerv Syst*. 2004. https://doi.org/10.1007/s00381-004-0982-7.

24. Swift DM, Weprin B, Sklar F, Sacco D, Salyer K, Genecov D, et al. Total vertex craniopagus with crossed venous drainage: Case report of successful surgical separation. *Childs Nervous System*. 2004. https://doi.org/10.1007/s00381-004-1011-6.

25. D'Urso PS, Thompson RG, Atkinson RL, Weidmann MJ, Redmond MJ, Hall BI, et al. Cerebrovascular biomodelling: A technical note. *Surg Neurol*. 1999. https://doi.org/10.1016/S0090-3019(99)00143-3.

26. Marinho P, Thines L, Verscheure L, Mordon S, Lejeune JP, Vermandel M. Recent advances in cerebrovascular simulation and neuronavigation for the optimization of intracranial aneurysm clipping. *Comput Aided Surg*. 2012. https://doi.org/10.3109/10929088.2011.653403.

27. Kimura T, Morita A, Nishimura K, Aiyama H, Itoh H, Fukaya S, et al. Simulation of and training for cerebral aneurysm clipping with 3-dimensional models. *Neurosurgery*. 2009. https://doi.org/10.1227/01.NEU.0000354350.88899.07.

28. Kondo K, Nemoto M, Masuda H, Okonogi S, Nomoto J, Harada N, et al. Anatomical reproducibility of a head model molded by a three-dimensional printer. *Neurol Med Chir*. 2015. https://doi.org/10.2176/nmc.oa.2014-0436.

29. Anderson JR, Thompson WL, Alkattan AK, Diaz O, Klucznik R, Zhang YJ, et al. Three-dimensional printing of anatomically accurate, patient specific intracranial aneurysm models. *J Neurointerventional Surg*. 2016. https://doi.org/10.1136/neurintsurg-2015-011686.

30. Khan I, Kelly P, Singer R. Prototyping of cerebral vasculature physical models. *Surg Neurol Int*. 2014. https://doi.org/10.4103/2152-7806.125858.

31. Levy EI, Snyder KV, Siddiqui AH, Bednarek DR, Varble N, Meng H, et al. Challenges and limitations of patient-specific vascular phantom fabrication using 3D Polyjet printing. *Medical Imaging 2014: Biomedical Applications in Molecular, Structural, and Functional Imaging*. 2014. https://doi.org/10.1117/12.2042266.

32. Namba K, Higaki A, Kaneko N, Mashiko T, Nemoto S, Watanabe E. Microcatheter Shaping for Intracranial Aneurysm Coiling Using the 3-Dimensional Printing Rapid Prototyping Technology: Preliminary Result in the First 10 Consecutive Cases. *World Neurosurg*. 2015. https://doi.org/10.1016/j.wneu.2015.03.006.

33. Wurm G, Tomancok B, Pogady P, Holl K, Trenkler J. Cerebrovascular stereolithographic biomodeling for aneurysm surgery. *J Neurosurg*. 2004. https://doi.org/10.3171/jns.2004.100.1.0139.

34. Ionita CN, Mokin M, Varble N, Bednarek DR, Xiang J, Snyder KV, et al. Challenges and limitations of patient-specific vascular phantom fabrication using 3D Polyjet printing. *Proc SPIE-Int Soc Opt Eng*. 2014;(716). https://doi.org/10.1117/12.2042266, 9038: 90380M.

35. Mashiko T, Kaneko N, Konno T, Otani K, Nagayama R, Watanabe E. Training in Cerebral Aneurysm Clipping Using Self-Made 3-Dimensional Models. *J Surg Educ*. 2017. https://doi.org/10.1016/j.jsurg.2016.12.010.

36. Abe M, Tabuchi K, Goto M, Uchino A. Model-based Surgical Planning and Simulation of Cranial Base Surgery. *Neurol Med -Chir*. 1998;38(11):746−751. https://doi.org/10.2176/nmc.38.746.

37. Oishi M, Fukuda M, Yajima N, Yoshida K, Takahashi M, Hiraishi T, et al. Interactive presurgical simulation applying advanced 3D imaging and modeling techniques for skull base and deep tumors. *J Neurosurg*. 2013;119(1):94−105. https://doi.org/10.3171/2013.3.JNS121109.

38. Spottiswoode BS, van den Heever DJ, Chang Y, Engelhardt S, Du Plessis S, Nicolls F, et al. Preoperative Three-Dimensional Model Creation of Magnetic Resonance Brain Images as a Tool to Assist Neurosurgical Planning. *Stereotact Funct Neurosurg*. 2013; 91(3):162–169. https://doi.org/10.1159/000345264.

39. Kondo Kosuke, Harada N, Masuda H, Sugo N, Terazono S, Okonogi S, et al. A neurosurgical simulation of skull base tumors using a 3D printed rapid prototyping model containing mesh structures. *Acta Neurochir*. 2016;158(6):1213–1219. https://doi.org/10.1007/s00701-016-2781-9.

40. Lan Q, Chen A, Zhang T, Li G, Zhu Q, Fan X, et al. Development of Three-Dimensional Printed Craniocerebral Models for Simulated Neurosurgery. *World Neurosurg*. 2016;91: 434–442. https://doi.org/10.1016/j.wneu.2016.04.069.

41. Muelleman T, Peterson J, Chowdhury N, Gorup J, Camarata P, Lin J. Individualized Surgical Approach Planning for Petroclival Tumors Using a 3D Printer. *J Neurol Surg Part B Skull Base*. 2015;77(03):243–248. https://doi.org/10.1055/s-0035-1566253.

42. Lau I, Squelch A, Wan Y, Wong A-C, Ducke W, Sun Z. Patient-specific 3D printed model in delineating brain glioma and surrounding structures in a pediatric patient. *Digital Medicine*. 2017;3(2):86. https://doi.org/10.4103/digm.digm_25_17.

43. Thawani JP, Singh N, Pisapia JM, Abdullah KG, Parker D, Pukenas BA, et al. Three-Dimensional Printed Modeling of Diffuse Low-Grade Gliomas and Associated White Matter Tract Anatomy. *Neurosurgery*. 2017;80(4):635–645. https://doi.org/10.1093/neuros/nyx009.

44. Cingoz ID, Kaya I, Kızmazoglu C, Sahin MC, Husemoglu B, Aydın HE, Yüceer N. Effects of planning with preoperative three dimensional modelling in transsphenoidal endoscopic pituitary surgery on surgical success. *Int J Sci Res*. 2018;7(10).

45. Waran Vicknes, Narayanan V, Karuppiah R, Pancharatnam D, Chandran H, Raman R, et al. Injecting Realism in Surgical Training—Initial Simulation Experience With Custom 3D Models. *Journal of Surgical Education*. 2014;71(2):193–197. https://doi.org/10.1016/J.JSURG.2013.08.010.

46. Waran V, Pancharatnam D, Thambinayagam H, Raman R, Rathinam A, Balakrishnan Y, et al. The Utilization of Cranial Models Created Using Rapid Prototyping Techniques in the Development of Models for Navigation Training. *J Neurol Surg Cent Eur Neurosurg*. 2013;75(01):012–015. https://doi.org/10.1055/s-0032-1330960.

47. Waran Vicknes, Narayanan V, Karuppiah R, Owen SLF, Aziz T. Utility of multimaterial 3D printers in creating models with pathological entities to enhance the training experience of neurosurgeons. *J Neurosurg*. 2014;120(2):489–492. https://doi.org/10.3171/2013.11.JNS131066.

48. Waran Vicknes, Narayanan V, Karuppiah R, Thambynayagam HC, Muthusamy KA, Rahman ZAA, Kirollos RW. Neurosurgical Endoscopic Training via a Realistic 3-Dimensional Model With Pathology. *Simulat Healthc*. 2015;10(1):43–48. https://doi.org/10.1097/SIH.0000000000000060.

49. Lin Q-S, Lin Y-X, Wu X-Y, Yao P-S, Chen P, Kang D-Z. Utility of 3-Dimensional–Printed Models in Enhancing the Learning Curve of Surgery of Tuberculum Sellae Meningioma. *World Neurosurgery*. 2018;113:e222–e231. https://doi.org/10.1016/j.wneu.2018.01.215.

50. Kondo Kosuke, Nemoto M, Harada N, Masuda H, Ando S, Kubota S, Sugo N. Three-Dimensional Printed Model for Surgical Simulation of Combined Transpetrosal Approach. *World Neurosurg*. 2019. https://doi.org/10.1016/J.WNEU.2019.03.219.

51. Fisher M, Applegate M, Ryalat C, Laycock M, Hulse S, Emmens M, Bell D. Evaluation of 3-D printed immobilisation shells for head and neck IMRT. *Open J Radiol*. 2014;4: 322−328. https://doi.org/10.4236/ojrad.2014.44042.

52. Laycock SD, Hulse M, Scrase CD, Tam MD, Isherwood S, Mortimore DB, et al. Towards the production of radiotherapy treatment shells on 3D printers using data derived from DICOM CT and MRI: preclinical feasibility studies. *J Radiother Pract*. 2015;14(1): 92−98. https://doi.org/10.1017/S1460396914000326.

53. Pham Q-VV, Lavallée A-P, Foias A, Roberge D, Mitrou E, Wong P. Radiotherapy Immobilization Mask Molding Through the Use of 3D-Printed Head Models. *Technol Canc Res Treat*. 2018;17. https://doi.org/10.1177/1533033818809051, 1533033818809051.

54. Brandmeir NJ, McInerney J, Zacharia BE. The use of custom 3D printed stereotactic frames for laser interstitial thermal ablation: technical note. *Neurosurg Focus*. 2016; 41(4):E3. https://doi.org/10.3171/2016.8.FOCUS16219.

55. van de Belt TH, Nijmeijer H, Grim D, Engelen LJLPG, Vreeken R, van Gelder MMHJ, ter Laan M. Patient-Specific Actual-Size Three-Dimensional Printed Models for Patient Education in Glioma Treatment: First Experiences. *World Neurosurg*. 2018;117: e99−e105. https://doi.org/10.1016/j.wneu.2018.05.190.

56. AbouHashem Y, Dayal M, Savanah S, Štrkalj G. The application of 3D printing in anatomy education. *Med Educ Online*. 2015;20(1):29847. https://doi.org/10.3402/meo.v20.29847.

57. Baskaran V, Štrkalj G, Štrkalj M, Di Ieva A. Current Applications and Future Perspectives of the Use of 3D Printing in Anatomical Training and Neurosurgery. *Front Neuroanat*. 2016;10. https://doi.org/10.3389/fnana.2016.00069.

58. Ogden K, Ordway N, Diallo D, Tillapaugh-Fay G, Aslan C. In: Yaniv ZR, Holmes DR, eds. *Dimensional accuracy of 3D printed vertebra*. 2014. https://doi.org/10.1117/12.2043489.

59. Stone JJ, Matsumoto JM, Morris JM, Spinner RJ. Preoperative Planning Using 3-Dimensional Printing for Complex Paraspinal Schwannoma Resection: 2-Dimensional Operative Video. *Oper Neurosurg (Hagerstown, Md.)*. 2019;16(3):E80. https://doi.org/10.1093/ons/opy239.

60. Sugawara T, Higashiyama N, Kaneyama S, Takabatake M, Watanabe N, Uchida F, et al. Multistep pedicle screw insertion procedure with patient-specific lamina fit-and-lock templates for the thoracic spine: clinical article. *J Neurosurg Spine*. 2013;19(2): 185−190. https://doi.org/10.3171/2013.4.SPINE121059.

61. Sugawara T, Kaneyama S, Higashiyama N, Tamura S, Endo T, Takabatake M, Sumi M. Prospective Multicenter Study of a Multistep Screw Insertion Technique Using Patient-Specific Screw Guide Templates for the Cervical and Thoracic Spine. *Spine*. 2018; 43(23):1685−1694. https://doi.org/10.1097/BRS.0000000000002810.

62. Kamishina H, Sugawara T, Nakata K, Nishida H, Yada N, Fujioka T, et al. Clinical application of 3D printing technology to the surgical treatment of atlantoaxial subluxation in small breed dogs. *PLoS One*. 2019;14(5):e0216445. https://doi.org/10.1371/journal.pone.0216445.

63. Shao Z-X, Wang J-S, Lin Z-K, Ni W-F, Wang X-Y, Wu A-M. Improving the trajectory of transpedicular transdiscal lumbar screw fixation with a computer-assisted 3D-printed custom drill guide. *PeerJ*. 2017;5:e3564. https://doi.org/10.7717/peerj.3564.

64. Kim J, Rajadurai J, Choy WJ, Cassar L, Phan K, Harris L, et al. Three-Dimensional Patient-Specific Guides for Intraoperative Navigation for Cortical Screw Trajectory

Pedicle Fixation. *World Neurosurg.* 2019;122:674−679. https://doi.org/10.1016/j.wneu.2018.11.159.

65. Burtsev AV, Pavlova OM, Ryabykh SO, Gubin AV. Computer 3D-modeling of patient-specific navigational template for cervical screw insertion. *Hirurgiâ Pozvonočnika.* 2018;15(2):33−38. https://doi.org/10.14531/ss2018.2.33-38.

66. Govsa F, Ozer MA, Biceroglu H, Karakas AB, Cagli S, Eraslan C, Alagoz AK. Creation of 3-Dimensional Life Size: Patient-Specific C1 Fracture Models for Screw Fixation. *World Neurosurg.* 2018;114:e173−e181. https://doi.org/10.1016/j.wneu.2018.02.131.

67. Nanni F de N, Vialle EN, Foggiattob JA, Silva K W S N e, Mello Neto H de O. Desenvolvimento de um guia paciente-específico para fixação de coluna cervical alta. *Revista Brasileira de Ortopedia.* 2019;54(01):020−025. https://doi.org/10.1016/j.rbo.2017.09.011.

68. Naddeo F, Naddeo A, Cappetti N, Cataldo E, Militio R. Novel Procedure for Designing and 3D Printing a Customized Surgical Template for Arthrodesis Surgery on the Sacrum. *Symmetry.* 2018;10(8):334. https://doi.org/10.3390/sym10080334.

69. Pijpker PAJ, Kuijlen JMA, Kraeima J, Faber C. Three-Dimensional Planning and Use of Individualized Osteotomy-Guiding Templates for Surgical Correction of Kyphoscoliosis: A Technical Case Report. *World Neurosurg.* 2018;119:113−117. https://doi.org/10.1016/j.wneu.2018.07.219.

70. Rankin TM, Wormer BA, Miller JD, Giovinco NA, Al Kassis S, Armstrong DG. Image once, print thrice? Three-dimensional printing of replacement parts. *Br J Radiol.* 2018. https://doi.org/10.1259/bjr.20170374, 20170374.

71. Whatley BR, Kuo J, Shuai C, Damon BJ, Wen X. Fabrication of a biomimetic elastic intervertebral disk scaffold using additive manufacturing. *Biofabrication.* 2011;3(1):015004. https://doi.org/10.1088/1758-5082/3/1/015004.

72. Whatley B. *BIOFABRICATION OF SCAFFOLDS FOR INTERVERTEBRAL DISC (IVD) TISSUE REGENERATION.* Clemson University; 2013. Available from: https://tigerprints.clemson.edu/all_dissertations/1134.

73. Ploch CC, Mansi CSSA, Jayamohan J, Kuhl E. Using 3D Printing to Create Personalized Brain Models for Neurosurgical Training and Preoperative Planning. *World Neurosurg.* 2016;90:668−674. https://doi.org/10.1016/j.wneu.2016.02.081.

74. McMenamin PG, Quayle MR, McHenry CR, Adams JW. The production of anatomical teaching resources using three-dimensional (3D) printing technology. *Anat Sci Educ.* 2014;7(6):479−486. https://doi.org/10.1002/ase.1475.

75. Vakharia VN, Vakharia NN, Hill CS. Review of 3-Dimensional Printing on Cranial Neurosurgery Simulation Training. *World Neurosurg.* 2016;88:188−198. https://doi.org/10.1016/j.wneu.2015.12.031.

76. Fredieu JR, Kerbo J, Herron M, Klatte R, Cooke M. Anatomical Models: a Digital Revolution. *Medical Science Educator.* 2015;25(2):183−194. https://doi.org/10.1007/s40670-015-0115-9.

77. Grillo FW, Souza VH, Matsuda RH, Rondinoni C, Pavan TZ, Baffa O, et al. Patient-specific neurosurgical phantom: assessment of visual quality, accuracy, and scaling effects. *3D Printing in Medicine.* 2018;4(1):3. https://doi.org/10.1186/s41205-018-0025-8.

78. Garling RJ, Jin X, Yang J, Khasawneh AH, Harris CA. Low-cost endoscopic third ventriculostomy simulator with mimetic endoscope. *J Neurosurg Pediatr.* 2018;22(2):137−146. https://doi.org/10.3171/2018.2.PEDS17671.

79. Weinstock P, Rehder R, Prabhu SP, Forbes PW, Roussin CJ, Cohen AR. Creation of a novel simulator for minimally invasive neurosurgery: fusion of 3D printing and special effects. *J Neurosurg Pediatr.* 2017;20(1):1−9. https://doi.org/10.3171/2017.1.PEDS16568.

80. Bow H, He L, Raees MA, Pruthi S, Chitale R. Development and Implementation of an Inexpensive, Easily Producible, Time Efficient External Ventricular Drain Simulator Using 3-Dimensional Printing and Image Registration. *Oper Neurosurg (Hagerstown, Md.).* 2019;16(4):496−502. https://doi.org/10.1093/ons/opy142.

81. Ryan JR, Chen T, Nakaji P, Frakes DH, Gonzalez LF. Ventriculostomy Simulation Using Patient-Specific Ventricular Anatomy, 3D Printing, and Hydrogel Casting. *World Neurosurg.* 2015;84(5):1333−1339. https://doi.org/10.1016/j.wneu.2015.06.016.

82. Jiménez Ormabera, B., Díez Valle, R., Zaratiegui Fernández, J., Llorente Ortega, M., Unamuno Iñurritegui, X., & Tejada Solís, S. (n.d.). 3D printing in neurosurgery: a specific model for patients with craniosynostosis. Neurocirugia (Asturias, Spain), 28(6), 260−265. https://doi.org/10.1016/j.neucir.2017.05.001.

83. Sullivan S, Aguilar-Salinas P, Santos R, Beier AD, Hanel RA. Three-dimensional printing and neuroendovascular simulation for the treatment of a pediatric intracranial aneurysm: case report. *J Neurosurg Pediatr.* 2018;22(6):672−677. https://doi.org/10.3171/2018.6.PEDS17696.

84. Ishibashi T, Takao H, Suzuki T, Yuki I, Kaku S, Kan I, et al. Tailor-made shaping of microcatheters using three-dimensional printed vessel models for endovascular coil embolization. *Comput Biol Med.* 2016;77:59−63. https://doi.org/10.1016/j.compbiomed.2016.07.005.

85. De La Peña A, De La Peña-Brambila J, Pérez-De La Torre J, Ochoa M, Gallardo GJ. Low-cost customized cranioplasty using a 3D digital printing model: a case report. *3D Printing in Medicine.* 2018;4(1):4. https://doi.org/10.1186/s41205-018-0026-7.

86. Morales-Gómez JA, Garcia-Estrada E, Leos-Bortoni JE, Delgado-Brito M, Flores-Huerta LE, De La Cruz-Arriaga AA, et al. Cranioplasty with a low-cost customized polymethylmethacrylate implant using a desktop 3D printer. *J Neurosurg.* 2019;130(5):1721−1727. https://doi.org/10.3171/2017.12.JNS172574.

87. Bohl MA, Xu DS, Cavallo C, Paisan GM, Smith KA, Nakaji P. The Barrow Innovation Center Case Series: A Novel 3-Dimensional−Printed Retractor for Use with Electromagnetic Neuronavigation Systems. *World Neurosurg.* 2018;116:e1075−e1078. https://doi.org/10.1016/j.wneu.2018.05.167.

88. Rankin TM, Giovinco NA, Cucher DJ, Watts G, Hurwitz B, Armstrong DG. Three-dimensional printing surgical instruments: are we there yet? *J Surg Res.* 2014;189(2):193−197. https://doi.org/10.1016/j.jss.2014.02.020.

89. Hui RW. Three-dimensional printing for patient counseling. *J Surg Oncol.* 2017;116:961. https://doi.org/10.1002/jso.24764.

90. Yoon SH, Park S, Kang CH, Park IK, Goo JM, Kim YT. Personalized 3D-Printed Model for Informed Consent for Stage I Lung Cancer: A Randomized Pilot Trial. *Semin in Thorac Cardiovasc Surg.* 2018. https://doi.org/10.1053/j.semtcvs.2018.10.017.

91. Alshomer F, AlFaqeeh F, Alariefy M, Altweijri I, Alhumsi T. Low-Cost Desktop-Based Three-Dimensional-Printed Patient-Specific Craniofacial Models in Surgical Counseling, Consent Taking, and Education of Parent of Craniosynostosis Patients: A Comparison With Conventional Visual Explanation Modalities. *J Craniofac Surg.* 2019. https://doi.org/10.1097/SCS.0000000000005401 [Published].

92. Liew Y, Beveridge E, Demetriades AK, Hughes MA. 3D printing of patient-specific anatomy: A tool to improve patient consent and enhance imaging interpretation by trainees. *Br J Neurosurg.* 2015. https://doi.org/10.3109/02688697.2015.1026799.

93. Del Castillo-Calcáneo J, Donoghue JA. A Novel Method for 3-Dimensional Printing a Brain That Feels and Looks Like One: The Next Step in the Search of the Perfect Neurosurgical Simulator. *World Neurosurg.* 2016;91:620−622. https://doi.org/10.1016/j.wneu.2016.03.086.

94. Tomasello F, Conti A, La Torre D. 3D printing in Neurosurgery. *World Neurosurg.* 2016; 91:633−634. https://doi.org/10.1016/j.wneu.2016.04.034.

95. Da Cruz MJ, Francis HW. Face and content validation of a novel three-dimensional printed temporal bone for surgical skills development. *J Laryngol Otol.* 2015. https://doi.org/10.1017/S0022215115001346.

96. Mowry SE, Jammal H, Myer C, Solares CA, Weinberger P. A novel temporal bone simulation model using 3D printing techniques. *Otol Neurotol.* 2015. https://doi.org/10.1097/MAO.0000000000000848.

97. Wen G, Cong ZX, Liu KD, Tang C, Zhong C, Li L, et al. A practical 3D printed simulator for endoscopic endonasal transsphenoidal surgery to improve basic operational skills. *Childs Nerv Sys.* 2016. https://doi.org/10.1007/s00381-016-3051-0.

98. Antoniou PE, Athanasiou A, Pickering JD, Bamidis PD. *Virtual and Augmented Reality in Neuroscience. In Neurotechnology: Methods, Advances and Applications.* The IET; 2020. in press.

99. Pampaloni NP, Giugliano M, Scaini D, Ballerini L, Rauti R. Advances in Nano Neuroscience: From Nanomaterials to Nanotools. *Front Neurosci.* 2019;12. https://doi.org/10.3389/fnins.2018.00953.

3D printing in dentistry with emphasis on prosthetic rehabilitation and regenerative approaches

Hadjichristou Christina, Bousnaki Maria, Bakopoulou Athina, Koidis Petros

Department of Prosthodontics, School of Dentistry, Faculty of Health Sciences, Aristotle University of Thessaloniki (A.U.Th), GR, Thessaloniki, Greece

Introduction

The process of three-dimensional (3D) printing any object comprises a series of procedures that begin with scanning and obtaining several two-dimensional (2D) images of the organ. The images obtained are stacked together to form a structure, followed by a processing step with the aid of processing software, and, finally, built up layer-by-layer. The first references of 3D printing are found nearly 40 years ago, in 1981, in Japan by Hideo Kodama[54]. Stereolithography (**SLA**) was introduced 2 years later by Charles Hull, describing his proposition as "successive sheets corresponding to successive cross-sectional layers dispensed and selectively exposed to synergistic stimulation and integrated with preceding layers to provide a substantially layer-by-layer build-up of the 3D object"[43].

Although dentistry is familiar to milling, the inherent deficiencies, such as material waste, slow speed, accuracy bounded by the object complexity, material properties, and the size of the cutting tools, have led to seeking alternatives to overcome these pitfalls. The so-called additive manufacturing (**AM**) or rapid prototyping has the opposite rationale to subtractive manufacturing or milling, which relies upon material removal for object formation. 3D printing offers the possibility to produce customized implants of prosthesis at a fraction of the time and cost originally entailed owing to the versatility of the printing process, introducing the advent of fully personalized treatment. In other words, 3D printing, through incremental vertical object buildup, may produce large objects passively with fine details and no material wastage[1]. Dentistry has benefited from this technology to in its every field, predominantly in oral surgery, prosthodontics, orthodontics, endodontics, and periodontics, as shown by rising numbers in publications containing the term "3D printing," although still at lower levels compared to Medicine[68]. This rising trend owes much to the expiration of the early patents, which have been related to

3D Printing: Applications in Medical Surgery. https://doi.org/10.1016/B978-0-323-66193-5.00009-5

the AM devices and processes. AM may be categorized based on the method of fabrication and this includes SLA, fused deposition modeling (FDM), binder jetting (BJ), electron beam melting (EBM), laser melting (LM), laser sintering (LS), digital light processing (DLP), and material or photopolymer jetting (PJ), which are well-known technologies of 3D printing.

Based on the nature of the **material used,** the techniques are divided into four categories: those using light-cured resin (**SLA**, DLP, and PJ), those using powder binder (**BJ**), those using sintered powder (**SLS, SLM, DMLS**, and EBM), and the one using thermoplastic materials (**FDM**). **SLA** is a 3D printing method, in which a scanning laser cures a light-sensitive polymer layer-by-layer in a vat of liquid. It is a rapid fabrication method, with low-cost material, that has the ability to create complex structures with high resolution. **DLP** uses a projector light source to cure liquid resin layer-by-layer, building the object upside down in an elevating platform. It provides high accuracy and smooth surfaces, but the materials used are expensive and the support must be removed at the end of the fabrication process. While both SLA and DLP use light as a polymerizing source, DLP provides significantly higher speed, as it has the ability to simultaneously photocure all the surface[94]. Photopolymer jetting(**PJ**)/inkjet printing/material jetting is the method that resembles the traditional household inkjet printer, but instead of the ink being absorbed on paper (2D), micrometer-sized droplets of an ink (liquid resin) are selectively jetted out of hundreds of nozzles and polymerized with ultraviolet (UV) light. Multiple print nozzles can be used with various color options and different materials. They layer thickness of such an apparatus may be as thin as 15 μm. **Selective laser melting** (**SLM**) and **selective laser sintering** (**SLS**) belong to laser powder forming methods where a laser is directed at a layer of fine powder substrate, and this laser causes full melting (for SLM) or sintering (SLS) of the powder. As soon as the layer is complete, another powder layer is deposited[85]. Among the two methods, SLM uses higher energy density; the whole procedure is carried out in closed chambers to avoid oxidation of metals and finally the fusion of the powder particles in this layer-by-layer buildup results in the 3D object[57]. During SLS, if the metal powders used are mixed, the one with lower melting points is melted and it is consequently used as a binder; this particular occasion is called **direct metal laser sintering** (**DMLS**)[88]. **FDM** is based on thermoplastic material extrusion through nozzle onto an ascending build platform. FDM results in low accuracy and can be used in limited materials, while support material must be removed at the end of the fabrication process[27]. **EBM** uses scanning electron beam that sinters powder layer-by-layer on a descending build platform. While it exhibits high processing speed, it has several disadvantages, such as extremely costly technology, production of hazardous dust, and explosive risk[27].

The large availability of devices makes it possible to expand the printable materials to a wide range, including resins, polymers, ceramics, and metals[11]. Although promising, 3D printing in Dentistry is not devoid of limitations. The so-called "staircase effect" on the finished product due to the layer-by-layer manufacturing, the aesthetically poor porous ceramic products, the low reproducibility, the need for support structures in some of the manufacturing techniques, and the need for devices tailored to dental and orofacial applications are some paradigms highlighting the need for further improvements before incorporation of these technologies as state of the art in everyday practice[11].

In this chapter, the recent advancements of 3D printing technology related to dental and orofacial applications are thoroughly reviewed and discussed, while future perspectives in oral reconstruction and regenerative dentistry are further highlighted.

Oral surgery

Based on the high number of publications in the last decade, the first and widest field of 3D printing applications in Dentistry is that of oral surgery[68]. This holds true since this is a tremendous tool in the surgeon's arsenal, helping to overcome "guesswork" of a third plane until the actual operation time, and providing insight of the surgical anatomy in a 3D environment imitating the natural case scenario. The armamentarium has been supplemented with virtual surgical planning, deriving from 3D scans (cone beam computed tomography, CBCT), where reconstruction of the missing tissues is made possible, by mirroring the contralateral nonaffected sides. Furthermore, for maxillomandibular reconstruction cases following tumor resection or trauma or orthognathic surgeries, it has been made possible to preview the final result. On top of these, the advancements in 3D imaging and planning offer options of simultaneous implant placement at the donor sites and precise transfer to the recipient site in oral cavity, minimizing the needed surgical procedures. By postoperational scanning and superimpositions, it is also possible to evaluate the final outcomes.

The procedure for maxillary or mandibular reconstruction proceeds as follows: In a computer software, data from the radiographic imaging (CBCT) of the area of interest are entered in a format called DICOM (digital imaging and communications in medicine). This allows for a complete representation of hard and soft tissue anatomy in 3D. Labor that can be implemented in this environment includes addition of the missing areas by insertion with the aid of stock mandibles manipulated for the reconstruction or even by reflection of the existing contralateral area so as to reproduce the missing anatomy, although a CBCT prior to tumor resection would be a more reliable source for the restoration. This derived model can be used as a template for prebending the titanium plates that will be used to anchor the added graft; they can also act as a template for the fabrication of osteotomy guides, with slots for the saw blade, which will be fixed to the donor site (e.g., the fibula) via monocortical screws. A second CT scan, of the donor site this time (lower extremity), is also inserted within the virtual environment to orientate the osteotomy guide production and in such a way the stents manufactured for this purpose may also serve as a drill guide for immediate implant placement at this site. The latter aid in the precise segmentation of the donor site in order to accurately fit in the area with the deficits[14].

The mostly utilized method for this model production is SLA. In addition to the above, in the case of maxillary reconstruction, navigation may also be used in assistance, due to the immobile nature of the site but not for the mandible[14].

The benefits of the above techniques are numerous. In a case control study, Hanasono et al.[39] compared the outcomes of microvascular free flap reconstruction of the mandible with the aid of CAD and rapid prototyping technique or by the conventional method, where bending the titanium plates was performed on the native mandible. The overall operative time was less for the rapid prototyping group (8.8 ± 1.0 h) than for the conventional group (10.5 ± 1.4 h). Furthermore, by measuring the mean change in postoperative length of bony landmarks of the mandible through postoperative CT scans and comparing that to the planned lengths, there was less deviation for the rapid prototyping group (4.11 ± 3.09 mm) than for the conventional group (6.92 ± 5.64 mm). Further to these, in another study, it was shown that operative time (666 ± 33.4 vs. 545 ± 12.6 min), as well as ischemia time (120 ± 19.8 vs. 73 ± 11.2 min), could be further reduced if virtual surgical planning was used in addition to the CT scans and stereolithic models for prebending the titanium plates and producing osteotomy guides. While in the cases where plates were prebent on stereolithic models (only serving as templates) but osteotomies were performed without cutting guides, the osteotomies were less accurate than virtual surgical planning cases and required the use of bone paste and grafts to replenish the gaps (27% vs. 2% of the cases, respectively).

Another field of interest where AM finds use in craniofacial operations is that of orthognathic surgery. Conventional methods of data acquisition rely on 2D radiographic imaging, as well as planning on plaster dental models mounted on semiadjustable articulators through face bow transfer. This poses obstacles in cases of facial asymmetries of the ears or eyes rendering face bow transfers inaccurate and difficult. As opposed to the above, 3D radiographic imaging, photography, dental model scanners, virtual planning, and 3D printing may assist in resolving these issues and most importantly it provides insight of the final outcome in terms of facial appearance preoperatively. A comparative study between 3D virtual model surgery with SLA versus the conventional model surgery showed that both methods had discrepancies in the predicted and the actual location of designated landmarks, but mean discrepancy was lower in the virtual model than in the conventional model (0.95 mm with SD of 0−3.2 and 1.17 mm with SD of 0−3.6 mm, respectively)[56].

Orthodontics precede and proceed the surgical procedure, initially to decompensate malocclusion, coordinate the width of the arch and rigidly stabilize the arches prior to surgery, while handling the final occlusion, and provide retention postsurgery. In between, 3D data and virtual planning aid in splint fabrication through 3D printing[89]. In this intermediate step, the surfaces of the dental casts of the maxilla and mandible are laser scanned and "mounted" on 3D CBCT scan in centric relation, the maxillomandibular readjustments are made in virtual space, and splints to guide the actual surgical practice are 3D printed using SLA[56]. In another study concerning virtual planning, it was shown that only 4% of the orthognathic virtual plans were abandoned, while 85% were completely adhered to and the rest were partially adhered to. Reasons for abandoning a virtual plan were poor communication between surgeons and engineers, misplacement of the condyle preoperatively, rapid tumor progression, and poor evaluation of the anatomy of the area preoperatively[32]. This stresses that the data acquisition needs to be obtained at a time frame close to the actual operation, so that deviations will be kept to the minimum.

Besides the oral cavity, maxillofacial surgery and dental implants seem to find purpose in cosmetic surgery, using AM to print auricular, orbital, or even nasal prostheses out of silicone. Existing contralateral segments of the respective areas are laser scanned and digitized, and their mirror images are 3D printed. They are held in place through magnetic or mechanical attachments between the dental implants and the prostheses[92]. Based on the above, 3D planning and printing are regarded as invaluable for tackling facets of craniofacial surgery and improving the quality of life of patients with serious deficiencies with improved predictability compared to conventional methods.

Prosthodontics
Fixed prosthodontics

Current progress in 3D printing technologies offers limitless possibilities in the field of prosthetic dentistry. Even though integration of 3D printing in the clinical workflow is still limited, it has already been applied in almost all aspects of prosthodontic treatment, from dental casts, metal frameworks, and removable complete and partial dentures to obturators for maxillofacial defects. The wide variety of materials used in prosthodontics necessitates the use of different AM techniques.

There are several parameters that must be taken into consideration when fabricating a dental prosthesis with the aid of 3D printing, such as dimensional accuracy, mechanical and physical properties, cost, and time. Those parameters are closely associated with factors that are defined and affected by the manufacturing technique, such as layer thickness, build orientation, and support structure[7]. More particularly, build orientation, which is defined as the orientation of printing, has been found to affect dimensional accuracy, as well as surface properties and overall fabrication time[7]. In addition, selection of build orientation affects the extent of manifestation of the "staircase effect," which further affects dimensional accuracy of the printed object[72]. As a result, it becomes apparent that slight modifications of those dominant factors can directly affect the accuracy of the restoration and by extension marginal and internal fit.

Moreover, each of the manufacturing techniques used for 3D printing bear its own characteristics that can influence processing accuracy. The accuracy of SLA is considered one of the highest among the different AM techniques[61]. The x-y planes are mainly related to the accuracy of SLA; however, z plane, which can be affected by many factors, can significantly influence printing accuracy[61]. SLA has been widely used to produce dental models. Several studies assessed trueness and precision of SLA-fabricated dental models in comparison to the original stone models[52,49,49]. Keating et al. found that despite the fact that the mean difference between the measurements made on the stone models and those made on the SLA models was not statistically significant, the mean difference of the measurements on the z plane reached a statistically significant level[52]. In a similar study, Jin et al. compared the accuracy of dental models from two different AM techniques, SLA and PJ, to the stone models[49,50]. In terms of trueness, there were no significant differences among the three different manufacturing processes, while in terms of precision, SLA- and PJ-fabricated models exhibited higher precision compared to the stone models[49].

In LM or LS techniques, such as SLS, SLM and DMLS, the characteristics of the particles, such as melting temperature, shape, and size, affect surface properties of the fabricated object[35]. Deviations in melting temperature can result in distortion and increased surface roughness, which have been associated with poor adaptation of SLM-fabricated frameworks[41,42].

LM or sintering techniques have been applied for the production of metal frameworks for fixed partial dentures (FPD) with marginal fit comparable to frameworks fabricated with the conventional workflow and within clinically acceptable values[77,98,41,42]. More specifically, in vitro studies using AM techniques for the fabrication of frameworks have had some very promising results, with improved marginal fit. Pompa et al. compared the marginal fit of 3-unit FPD, where the reported marginal gap was 43.9 µm for the SLM-fabricated cobalt-chromium (Co-Cr) frameworks and 47.5 µm for the lost-wax-fabricated nickel-chromium (Ni-Cr) frameworks[75]. However, internal adaptation was better for the Ni-Cr frameworks (54 µm) compared to the SLM-Co-Cr frameworks (58.7), though the difference was not statistically significant[75]. In a similar study, Örtorp et al. showed that DMLS-fabricated 3-unit FPD frameworks had significantly better marginal fit (84 µm) compared to conventional lost-wax-fabricated frameworks (133 µm) and milled frameworks (166 µm)[69]. Furthermore, in the study by Ucar et al., DMLS-fabricated crowns exhibited similar internal gap with cast frameworks[101]. Similarly, DMLS Co-Cr frameworks for implant-supported restoration exhibited lower values of marginal gap compared to conventionally fabricated cast Co-Cr frameworks[17]. On the other hand, Kim et al. found that the marginal and internal gap of Co-Cr FPD frameworks produced with DMLS was significantly larger compared to the conventionally fabricated cast frameworks[53]. In a clinical study, Quante et al. assessed the marginal fit of single crowns fabricated using SLM either from base metal or from precious alloy, where no statistically significant difference was found between the two alloys, with values ranging from 74 to 99 µm[77]. In addition, Huang et al. compared the marginal fit of SLM-fabricated Co-Cr crowns and cast Au-Pt crowns and found that there was no significant difference among the two types of crowns[41,42]. Furthermore, clinical assessment over a period of 47 months revealed that laser-sintered crowns exhibited a cumulative failure rate of 1.7%, with the main causes of failure being extraction of abutment teeth or need for endodontic treatment[3]. While most of the studies assessing the accuracy of 3D printed frameworks were in vitro, the superiority of SLS/SLM/DMLS-fabricated frameworks over the conventional cast or milled frameworks was revealed in terms of marginal adaptation.

Regarding post and core fabrication, only one study assessed the fracture resistance of DMLS-fabricated post and core compared to the ones produced with conventional casting and milled cast[16]. DMLS-fabricated post and core exhibited similar fracture resistance to the ones from conventional casting and lower compared to the milled cast post and core[16].

Interim prosthesis

To protect the prepared abutments against microbial attacks and the underlaying pulp from stimuli entering the oral cavity, interim prostheses need to be manufactured and worn by the patient to serve functional, esthetic, and space maintenance purposes. An alternative to the conventionally prepared provisional restorations, by means of heat pressure, may be assembled through 3D printing. Here, casts of the prepared teeth or the teeth directly need to be scanned and retrieved within the design software. The interim restorations are then designed to restore initial anatomy of the respective intact tooth/teeth and saved into an STL file, this is then exported to the printer where individual printer parameters are set[58]. Important parameters to assess are the orientation of printing, the printer itself, the technology of 3D printing, the color of the material, and the laser intensity among others.

Each millimeter of material to be printed corresponds to 15−20 layers of material to be laid and fused so that the final shape is delivered[1]. The procedure of printing of a simple restoration, such as a single crown, takes approximately 20 min, which is a significant benefit, allowing the dentist/dental technician to perform other tasks and increasing the overall productivity while the restorations are being produced[97].

The materials for this purpose seem to follow a similar classification as to those employed for conventional provisional restorations, namely those based on monomethacrylates or acrylic resins and dimethacrylate or bis-acryl/composite resins, according to their chemical composition[78]. The technique mostly utilized for this purpose is SLA and various studies have used it to study aspects of these restorations, such as their marginal fit. In a study by[64], it was found that the marginal fit produced by fused deposition using PLA (polylactic acid) was 122.89 μm (SD 26.06 μm), which is slightly above the acceptable marginal gap of 120 μm proposed by in literature[63]. Addressing the same issue of marginal discrepancy, Lee et. al. showed that 3D printed provisional crowns had lower values than those produced by milling (mean discrepancy and standard deviation for two 3D printed methods and milling, respectively, 149.1 (65.9) μm, 91.1 (36.4) μm, and 171.6 (97.4) μm[58]). It was also mentioned that milling caused exhaustion of the materials and was more time-consuming. Other published work also consider that AM enables the production of more refined geometries that may even be impossible to be produced by milling, where dimensions are limited by the bur size[78].

An aspect to keep in mind is the direction of the structure to be printed. It seems that when specimens are printed vertically, so that the testing load is directed perpendicular to the printed layers, the compressive strength of the material is higher than in the case of horizontal printing (297 ± 34 MPa and 257 ± 41 MPa, respectively)[8]. This is also beneficial because vertical printed structures require fewer supporting structures, thus there is a smaller contact area between the support structure and the printed object, subsequently less time is needed for finishing and polishing. In support of this statement, another study mentioned most accurate dimensional readings of width and length for specimens printed at 90 degrees (vertical to the build platform), and although the thickness accuracy was best for the horizontal orientation, it was thought that the ideal printing orientation was the vertical, since this would again demand less support structures[97]. In the same study, 3D printed samples were compared to commercially available materials ("Jet" and "Integrity"). Seemingly, the 3D printed samples had higher degree of conversion than conventional methods, as deduced by FTIR spectroscopy and comparable elastic modulus to "Jet" and peak stress similar to "Integrity" proving to be equally sufficient in terms of mechanical properties. A limitation was, however, that the specimens for both the abovementioned studies were cylindrical. To simulate clinical conditions more closely, Alharbi et al. fabricated crown-shaped restorations with different angulations to the support structures and with two different versions of support (thick or thin)[8]. It was deducted that the ideal configuration was when the angle between the transverse axis of the crown was at 120 degrees to the support platform with the lingual surface facing toward the support for both support occasions, as the deviation resulting from the superimposition of the printed crown compared to the scan of the reference model (designed crown) was as low as 0.031 and 0.029 mm for the thick and thin platform, respectively[8].

Another property where 3D printed interim restorations overshadow those produced conventionally or by milling is that of microhardness, as measured at 32.77 for 3D printing, 25.33 for milling, and 27.36 for conventional in Knoop hardness numbers [29]).

Ceramics

There are three ways to fabricate veneering porcelain: by layering porcelain (traditional method), by pressing (through printing or milling), and by the CAD-on technique, where the CAD file is printed simultaneously for the framework and the veneering porcelain[6]. Although milling has been widely used, especially for zirconia, it possesses the disadvantages of material waste; almost 90% of the block is thrown away, and also the possible introduction of cracks[31]. On the other hand, ceramics are the most difficult material among the ones used in dentistry for 3D printing because of their high melting point and the need for thermal treatment after shaping to achieve consolidation, thus they narrow the possible techniques of AM that can be used[74,34]. Among AM techniques, only direct inkjet printing is said to provide adequate results, whereas the rest result in porous structures[31]. This method produces the 3D structures by laying layers of the structure dropwise from a suspension, producing a green body of material that needs to be sintered subsequently.

A subset of AM especially devoted to ceramics is robocasting, which is the extrusion of a ceramic suspension from an orifice via computer-controlled layer-by-layer deposition following a CAD model to obtain a 3D structure, its green body to be exact, which then needs to follow a debunking process for the burn off of organic additives and a sintering process[74]. Since this is again a layer-by-layer deposition method, it is not devoid of the stair stepping effect and this too requires surface finishing[74].

Several parameters need to be adjusted for the suspension to avoid drawbacks such as nose clogging, printing irregularities, and compatibility with the printing unit[71]. The content of the nozzle must be able to flow under modest pressure, with the ability to remain undeformed postdeposition, then dry without shape alterations, and also sinter very densely[91]. More analytically, the requirements of the suspension for extrudability (extrusion through the nozzle) are reversible shear-thinning behavior to viscosity around $10-100$ Pa without particle agglomerates, and for printability (successive stacking of ceramic suspensions without collapsing), the suspension needs relatively high modulus (G′) with $\tau y > 200$ Pa for self-support of the printed layers[74]. The solid content of the ceramic in the slurry has to be tailored, with various values being mentioned in literature, 24.2 vol %[71], 27 vol%[31], and even as high as 47 vol% [91]. Apart from the solid content, additive content has been mentioned to be optimum at $10-12.5$ wt.% to prevent clogging and drying of the nozzles[71]. Also using dispersants and binders (organic additives < 3.0 vol %) has been advocated to reduce shrinkage[74]. If care is taken while producing the ideal slurry, the strength of the produced material may reach 763 MPa, fracture toughness of 6.7 MPa, and density as high as 96.9% of the theoretical density, which are comparable to the mechanical properties of conventionally produced 3Y-TZP resulting from cold isostatic pressing. Nevertheless, the issue of shrinkage after sintering needs to be accounted for, since this may rise up to 25%, and if not compensated for, the resulting structures will be of low trueness with dimensional alterations compared to the original design as shown by Wang et al, where the external occlusal surface and the junction of the axial and occlusal surfaces of the crown were larger and the axial surfaces were smaller than intended[104].

Although somewhat troublesome, ceramic manufacturing through 3D printing has potential, especially in the case of robocasting. This technology offers capabilities to print two discrete materials by switching the feeder of the nozzle or by utilizing multi-nozzle systems, thus allowing deposition of different compositions or even materials at different spatial geometry, such as printing metal core and veneering porcelain in the same apparatus[74]. These are improvements that need further exploration but surely deserve a spot in the near future of dental developments.

Removable prosthodontics
Complete dentures

Although progress has been made in the field of prosthodontics, the area of complete denture manufacturing with the aid of 3D printing still lags. And it is not hard to imagine the reasons for this. Complete dentures present with a need for direct interaction with the patient to transfer all the necessary information from the edentulous regions, but most importantly of the surrounding soft tissues as well. So, the simplistic transfer of data, concerning relatively immobile structures, which is the case in fixed prosthodontics or the rest of the covered fields of this chapter, does not apply here. Consideration must be taken for the support of the lips by the denture flanges, teeth positioning, and vertical dimension registration, which cannot proceed without the wax rims tryout, as well as passive and active condition of the mucosa registered by proper border molding and final impressions.

Nevertheless, some attempts have been made by research groups to examine different aspects of complete denture manufacturing process, none of which is completely devoid of traditional manufacturing steps. To start with, research groups have attempted to evaluate the precision of custom trays for final impressions by comparing 3D printed custom trays to conventional custom trays. Chen et al. used FDM and PLA filaments to print mandibular trays using scanned edentulous plaster models as a substrate[19]. Following printing, the intaglio surfaces of the trays were scanned and compared to the plaster models to evaluate the reserved space for the impression materials, which was expected to be 2 mm (thickness of a wax sheet). The mean space resulting from manual fabrication was 2.08–2.24 mm (SD: 0.26–0.56 mm), which was significantly higher than values obtained for the 3D printed trays 2.01–2.02 mm (SD: 0.09–0.10 mm), while the time spent for printing was 45 min per tray. Following this study, another team[95] used 3D printed trays (FDM) with or without tissue stops. After the impressions were made clinically, the thickness of the material was examined, showing that the digital trays had better material distribution than that of manual trays, and on top of that, the trays with tissue stops performed better. When a control group was added to simulate the classical procedure with border molding, it was evident that the flange extensions were insufficient if border molding was not performed both for digital or manual trays.

In another study, the plaster model of the maxilla was scanned and wax patterns of a complete denture were produced. The mean deviations of the tissue surfaces did not differ significantly between the 3D printed or manually produced method (average deviation of the overall area 0.29 ± 0.14 mm and 0.30 ± 0.17 mm, respectively) although the authors report that the time taken to print the 3D printed wax patten (14–16 h) and remove the support material (1–2 h) was high[18]. Inokoshi et al. tried to copy the existing dentures of patients and also make alterations within the software such as changes in the size of the artificial teeth, lip support adjustments, changes in the occlusal plane, and thereafter trial of these dentures on the patients. A deviation analysis was performed using a 3D CAD software showing that 92% of the maxillary dentures and 95% of the mandibular dentures had deviations less than 0.8 and 0.6 mm, respectively, a deviation which can be compensated by the displaceability of the mucosa (0.3 mm)[45]. Another outcome of this study, as rated by the patients and the prosthodontists, was that esthetics and stability were significantly higher when these were produced in the traditional way as opposed to the 3D printing method. The chair time was also longer with the latter[44] . An aspect stressed here was that arranging the artificial teeth in printed dentures cannot be altered at chair side, but instead several trial dentures need to be fabricated in advance to compensate for different tooth arrangements.

In an attempt for teeth set up using a 3D CAD software, Sun et al. created a database by transferring data of industrially available teeth dimensions. By scanning denture bases and wax rims obtained with the classic procedure in the clinic, they used the scanned teeth information for the set up. The components were then printed but the teeth had to be inserted one by one in their respective positions and finishing procedures (polishing and packing) had to be done in the traditional laboratory manner[96].

Furthermore, the possibility of manufacturing 3D printed denture teeth has been explored by[23]. Commercial complete denture teeth shapes were scanned and 3D printed in acrylic resin and then compared to teeth of four different companies in terms of indirect tensile fracture loads and chipping. The 3D printed teeth proved second in order concerning the first property (load-to-tensile fracture was 160.28 ± 8.83 N), whereas they did not have significant differences regarding chipping resistance (89.22 ± 14.87 N) compared to two of the four commercial teeth samples[23]. These mechanical properties were, however, deemed adequate for the use of the 3D printed teeth for complete dentures. The burden stressed in this study was again the teeth bonding to the denture base with a light-cured bonding agent. This hurdle could have been surpassed if 3D printing could perform multicolor layering to print the final draft of the complete denture. Worthy to mention, the aesthetics of the 3D printed teeth were nowhere near the artificially available denture teeth, since they were printed monochromatically in a solid resin mass without attempting layering for enamel or dentin.

This is a field where technological advancement does not seem to surpass the classical manual methodology and individual advancement that the materials and precise clinical practice have achieved through the years. This does not rule out the possibility of improvement, through new ideas and troubleshooting to achieve an ideal outcome through 3D printing in this area in the years to come.

Removable partial dentures

The first to describe CAD/CAM systems for the removable partial denture (RPD) fabrication was Williams et al., in 2006, in particular by using DMLS[106]. For this application also, an STL file with the designed RPD needs to be created and sent for printing. Prior to printing, the rest of the procedures, up to final impressions, may be carried out in the traditional manner and the data of the final cast may be scanned for the purposes of CAD. For denture designing, a software with a haptic arm may be employed for the virtual process of model survey, undercut blockout, insertion path identification, and prosthesis design[57]. Both Co-Cr alloys and titanium alloys may be used for 3D printing using different fabrication methods.

It seems that the fabrication method affects the mechanical properties of the produced frameworks. For example, when comparing SLS and DMLS for RPD fabrication out of Co-Cr alloy, although the products were more precise, accurate, harder, and with higher yield strength and fatigue resistance compared to cast alloys, the elastic modulus of SLS (202 ± 16 GPa) was significantly lower than the DMLS (225 ± 10 GPa) or cast alloys (229 ± 7 GPa), which made the authors consider the SLS method advantageous for clasp fabrication, whereas cast and DMLS would be more preferable for connectors or rests where higher stiffness is needed[5]. In a more recent study, again using Co-Cr alloy to fabricate RPDs either by 3D printing or by conventional casting, although both methods revealed clinically acceptable adaptation, the overall fit and accuracy of the conventional cast frameworks were significantly superior to the 3D printed[93]. Nevertheless, that data acquisition method did not seem to influence the accuracy and fit significantly. Among the areas which were examined, there was high accuracy (<50 μm gap) at the rests and reciprocal plates independently of the fabrication method, whereas problems occurred with major connectors and CAD printing where fit was the poorest[93].

Emphasizing on isolated clasp fabrication, SLM-fabricated clasps made of titanium show significantly higher roughness compared to milled or cast clasps, low accuracy of the outer surface, and fractures at lower test cycle numbers when tested for retentive forces, deeming them unsuitable for usage[99]. Enlightening the issue, Kajima et. al showed that the angle between the building and longitudinal directions of printing may affect these outcomes, since 90 degrees offered results comparable to the cast clasps whereas 0 and 45° provided inferior properties[51].

Although LS has many advantages, such as the absence of cutting chips production, ease of fabrication of refined shapes, independence of cutting accuracy determined by the cutting tools, simultaneous fabrication of many frameworks, automatic process, and relatively low cost[13] and[76], the surfaces produced are still too rough compared to conventional methods or milling. To combine the advantages of both milling and 3D printing, hybrid techniques have been proposed, where repeated LS and high-speed milling are combined. Two distinct studies used this hybrid method with Co-Cr alloy to produce an Akers clasp on a molar model[66,100]. Both studies deduced that the surfaces of the hybrid method were smoother than conventional cast surfaces and surfaces produced solely by repeated LS. Both studies also identified the greatest gap at the rest region rather than clasp arm or tip. The hybrid clasps also possessed higher initial and final retentive forces and lower decrease ratios after 10 000 cycles. The provided information makes it clear that further evaluation is required so that fine-tuned methods are made available for clinical use.

Maxillofacial prosthodontics

Furthermore, 3D printing has been applied in maxillofacial prosthetics facilitating treatment planning and oral rehabilitation with obturators in patients with maxillofacial defects. Generally, such cases are complicated and time-consuming and are treated by experienced prosthodontists and often provide inadequate fit and function, resulting in poor quality of life. With the development of CAD and AM technologies, presurgical digital planning, 3D visualization of the defect area, and 3D printing of customized prosthesis can enable overcome such limitations and minimize time-consuming and labor-intensive procedures[48,55]. More specifically, 3D printing has enabled the fabrication of 3D models of the defect area[47,65], surgical obturators[82,55], custom trays and molds for final impression[48], and definitive obturators[12]. In a pilot study by Jiao et al., 11 patients with maxillary defects received obturators that were fabricated with the aid of SLA technology[48]. More precisely, CT scan images from the defect area were processed with the Mimics software to create a 3D model of the patient's head, enabling the visualization of the remaining tissues around the effect area. The 3D model was further processed with the Geomagic Studio 12.0 software to design the prosthesis defect portion; SLA was used to create an acrylic resin positive mold of the defect cavity, which was further used for border molding and final impression of the residual tissues. Most of the patients were satisfied with the obturator prosthesis; none of them experienced leakage while eating, while only complained of leakage while drinking liquid and two reported that their voices were nasal[48]. In a similar study, CAD/SLA was used to fabricate custom trays for the final impressions of patients with maxillary defects. When compared with conventional trays through digital comparison, SLA custom-fabricated trays presented adequate accuracy, with acceptable discrepancies within 1 mm in most areas, except the buccal wall of the defect, where the greatest difference was observed, up to 3 mm. Additionally, the cost of fabricating a personalized obturator was assessed by Bartellas et al. In this study, low-cost desktop 3D printer and free software were used, and it was demonstrated that it is possible to create low-cost palatal obturators, making it more accessible to low-income patients in remote areas[12]. All in all, the digital workflow for the fabrication of obturator prosthesis seems to be time- and cost-efficient, with acceptable marginal fit and the ability to provide improved function and quality of life to the patients[47,55].

Orthodontics

Orthodontics is one of the fields in Dentistry that has also benefited from advances in 3D printing, enabling the transition to a fully digital workflow with the incorporation of intraoral scanners and 3D printers. With the aid of face scan, CT scan, and software programs, theoretical growth models can be applied on the tissues and predict the changes that will occur during growth and after the application of orthodontic treatment[80,46]. 3D printing can enable the presentation and visualization of these changes and, therefore, aid orthodontists foresee the biological responses following the application of orthodontic forces and patients visualize the final outcomes of orthodontics treatment[46]. Moreover, 3D printing has been used to fabricate orthodontic models, aligners, and appliances. SLA has been used to produce 3D orthodontic models from digital files, of which accuracy depends on the print layer height and the 3D printer[33]. PJ has been also used to produce orthodontic models, exhibiting very different postprocessing phases compared to SLA. The use of PJ necessitates the presence of a washing station for the removal of model's gelatinous support material after printing, while SLA requires the application of an alcohol wash, followed by exposure to ultraviolet light for complete curing[37]. The smaller (25 mm) layer height printed models, despite providing more detail and improved surface finish, exhibited the greatest deviations, compared to the larger (100 mm) layer height printed models, which exhibited the lowest deviations, all being within clinically acceptable limits[33]. Orthodontics appliances can be fabricated either directly or indirectly with the aid of 3D printing. Salmi et al. used SLA to fabricate a mold for a customized soft orthodontic aligner[84]. The accuracy of the appliance was considered adequate by the authors, with errors up to 1 mm at some points[84]. A comparison between orthodontic appliances produced either with 3D printing (PJ) or with milling showed that milled appliances had better fitting accuracy and resulted in more rapid tooth movement with more uniform stress distribution. When fabricating orthodontic aligners with 3D printing, several factors should be taken into consideration to allow a better control of tooth movement, such as a lower layer thickness (staircase effect) and a higher accuracy[62]. Multicomponent orthodontic appliances have also been produced with the aid of 3D printing, while a bending robot created the metal springs and clasps, with good clinical fit[102]. Custom brackets for lingual orthodontics have also been fabricated with 3D printing (in wax analogue followed by casting in high gold content alloy) minimizing patient discomfort and debonding incidents and problematic finishing that are usually encountered with the use of lingual brackets[105]. Even though some of these applications have been published only in limited cases as "proof of concept," they pave the future of orthodontic treatment through a digital workflow.

Endodontics

Endodontics are a less covered field in the literature concerning the utilization of 3D printing compared to the previously mentioned fields in dentistry, only receiving attention recently, mostly through case reports and a few literature reviews. Nevertheless, 3D printing may find valuable applications for nonsurgical root canal treatment with educational purposes or for the clinical retrieval of root canals through 3D printed tooth supported guides, as well as in the production of surgical guides for periapical apicectomies and lastly for tissue engineering purposes by bioprinting components for the regeneration of the dental pulp.

The traditional manner for the education of dental students in root canal treatment involves collecting natural teeth and embedding them in epoxy resin blocks. The latter is time-consuming, it involves matters of ethical approval, as well as various levels of difficulty and hazards regarding bacterial spreading. With the introduction of AM, the same teeth may be scanned using CBCT or micro-CT and printed using FDM, multijet printing/polyjet printing, DLP, or SLA[79], to produce replicates of the same teeth representing all possible scenarios for dental students before entering the clinic and also aid in a more fair skill assessment by supervisors.

Compared with the natural teeth, CBCT-scanned and SLA-printed teeth showed a 50.9 −104.3 μm variation, while there was 43.5−68.2 μm deviation between the replicas[79]. In addition to these minor deviations, when students were instructed to perform endodontic treatment on these 3D models, they reported that the sensation did not vary greatly from that on natural teeth[79]. In an attempt to simulate the natural tissues with these models more closely, Robberecht et al.[81] manufactured a hydroxy-apatite (HAp)-based root canal system with the required anatomical features that mimics the chemical composition of the mineral phase and microstructure of natural dentin. This is an example of combining 3D printing with the principles of tissue engineering toward more sophisticated models in the benefit of dental education.

Apart from student education, this type of training is also beneficial for difficult cases of trained experts who need to tackle high demanding root canal morphology, pulp canal obliteration, or dens invaginatus. A procedure involving straight line access to the root canal with the help of a guided endodontic bur is suggested for such cases. This technique of root canal access is known as "guided endodontics"[67].

Further to the nonsurgical applications of 3D printing, this technology has applications in the surgical treatment of periapical root resections, providing more accurate osteotomy perforation sites, by means of surgical guides. These guides may be produced for treatment of anatomically complex scenarios, such as roots in proximity to the sinuses, arteries, or nerves. Thermoplastic materials printed using SLS which are autoclavable due to the high melting point of the material may be safely used in surgical procedures within the oral cavity[27]. In a case series, there is a report for resecting the root apex by the use of trephine drills even without raising flaps, having simultaneously information about the depth of insertion (using stops printed within the guide), the ability to isolate the tissue for biopsies, and causing minimal loss of tissues, thus offering a faster healing period[36].

Lastly, AM has found place in bioprinting components incorporating stem cells and bioinks for regenerating the dental pulp. This makes sense since all cells in the human body are embedded in 3D tissues; hence, a 3D carrier would resemble their natural environment to a higher degree. Numerous 3D printing methods, such as microextrusion, inkjet, and laser and light lithography, have been employed for the creation and patterning of cell laden bioinks inkjet printers. A few paradigms from the literature show that 3D printing of bioscaffolds, containing mineral trioxide aggregate [22]) and biodentine[40], enhanced the differentiation of human dental pulp cells in favor of osteogenesis in in vitro models. In another study, a customized double nozzle extrusion printing system has been set up to print a mixture of sodium alginate-dentin matrix and stem cells from the apical papilla[10]. This novel bioink was advocated with high printability, cell survival, and enhanced odontogenic differentiation of the embedded cells.

All these examples are in evidence that innovative ideas have a place in Endodontics, while the dental field in general has a lot to gain by the advancements of 3D printing and tissue engineering in the future.

Periodontics

Another area in Dentistry that has been benefited from the advance of AM technologies is periodontology. Surgical implant guides, dental implants, and regenerative periodontology are the main applications of 3D printing related to periodontics. Computer-guided surgery has been an established clinically applied treatment for at least 10 years, since the 2009 consensus[38]. It is defined as the use of a surgical guide for the visualization and placement of implants, as it was planned on the CT scans. This method does not allow any deviations and offers several advantages, such as presurgical planning and optimization of implant position selection, prosthetically guided implant placement along with immediate placement of provision prosthesis, and minimal surgical trauma and discomfort[109]. However, a deviation has been observed from the planned implant position and to the implant final placement, which is an accumulation of errors from the fabrication process. Accuracy of surgical guides is affected by several different factors, such as the choice of manufacturing technique, imaging technique, type and position of surgical guide, and the fixation of the guide. Therefore, it becomes crucial to know the degree of accuracy of the method used[109,87]. In a recent systematic review and metaanalysis of clinical studies assessing the accuracy of SLA-fabricated surgical guides, it was revealed that there was 1.25 mm mean deviation at the entry point, 1.57 mm at the apex, and 4.1 degrees in angle[109]. The surgical guide system with the higher level of accuracy was a flapless one, which was totally guided and used fixation screws[109]. In a similar review, where the accuracy of mucosa-supported SLA-fabricated surgical guides was assessed, it was shown that the mean apical deviation ranged from 0.67 to 2.19 mm, the mean coronal deviation from 0.6 to 1.68 mm, and the mean angular deviation from 2.6 to 4.67 degrees[87]. The reported factors primarily affecting accuracy of implant placement were bone density, mucosal thickness, and surgical technique[87].

AM has also been used in the field of periodontics to fabricate scaffolds that mimic the properties and complex architecture of periodontium, cementum, and underlying supporting bone structure. Polycaprolactone (PCL) has been the material of choice in several studies regarding periodontal regeneration, due to its well-documented and desirable properties along with promising positive outcome from the orthopedics field[9]. Custom-fabricated 3D printed PCL scaffolds were produced by Park et al. with a fiber-guiding architecture in an attempt to mimic bone-periodontal ligament (PDL) architecture, with positive results in vivo regarding periodontal bone regeneration[73]. Furthermore, biphasic scaffolds for both bone and PDL regeneration were fabricated combining FDM technology for the construction of β-tricalcium phosphate-TCP/PCL for bone regeneration and cell sheet technology for PDL regeneration[103]. While those scaffolds showed positive results in terms of regeneration of the different tissues (bone, cementum, PDL), there was no functional orientation of the fibers, neither any specific architecture of regenerated bone[103]. To overcome those limitations, the authors modified the orientation of the fibers by modifying the fabrication of the scaffold through electrospinning for the PDL compartment and the bone architecture by adding calcium phosphate to the bone compartment of the scaffold, resulting in improved fiber orientation and increased bone formation[26]. Moreover, customized scaffolds that can precisely fit around the osseous defect area of periodontal bone have been fabricated from 3D printed PCL based on CT images of the defected area.

Guided bone regeneration has also benefited from the advances in 3D printing technologies. In the study by Shim et al., β-TCP/PCL membranes were fabricated with the aid of FDM and were assessed in vivo for their ability to guide bone regeneration[90]. The β-TCP/PCL-3D printed membranes exhibited enhanced bone regeneration and better stability when compared to collagen membranes, showing promising results for future clinical application[90]. Ciocca et al. proposed the use of a customized, DMLS-fabricated titanium mesh for prosthetically driven bone regeneration[25]. The clinical application of this customized titanium mesh in combination with bone graft of autologous and inorganic bovine bone resulted in mean bone regeneration of 3.83 mm for the mandibular arch and 3.95 mm for the maxilla, enabling implant placement[24].

AM technology has also enabled the fabrication of customized dental implants to provide patient-specific dental treatment. In vitro studies have shown the ability to produce 3D printed implants with enough accuracy and high mechanical strength, using variety of materials, such as titanium, titanium alloy, and zirconia[20,21,70,107]. More specifically, Osman et al. used DLP to fabricate zirconia dental implants with high dimensional accuracy, with deviations below 0.1 mm[70]. Comparing different build orientations, it was shown that the 0 degrees printed implant presented significantly higher strength compared to the other groups (45 and 90 degrees), indicating that the implant should be manufactured at 0-degree angle to the build platform, where the force direction will be perpendicular to the fabrication layers[70]. Moreover, microstructure assessment of the printed implant revealed the presence of cracks and porosities, indicating the need for optimization of the fabrication process to achieve better structure, which would not jeopardize the long-term prognosis[70].

Temporomandibular joint
Stabilization splint

The application of 3D printing has been also introduced in the fabrication process of occlusal stabilization splint (SS) for patients who suffer from temporomandibular disorders (TMDs)[83,15]. Salmi et al. were the first to develop SLA-fabricated SS and assess them in clinical conditions[83]. The SLA-fabricated SS presented acceptable accuracy, with dimensional errors of up to 1 mm, and the patient adapted to the SS with no reported complaints[83]. Those results were further supported by a clinical study from Berntsen et al., where conventionally manufactured SS were compared with DLP-manufactured SS[15]. Patients receiving DLP-manufactured SS were significantly more satisfied compared to those receiving conventionally manufactured SS, though the authors relate those results to the impression technique and comment that the manufacturing process did not affect patients' satisfaction[15]. The embracement of a fully digital workflow for the fabrication of SS can enable a more rapid and cost-efficient fabrication process, which will be even more useful in the future with the increasing number of patients suffering from TMD.

3D printing in TMJ replacement

Another area of Dentistry in which 3D printing is applied is the temporomandibular joint (TMJ) surgery and total replacement in cases of final-stage TMJ disease where degenerative aberrations have rendered the TMJ components unsalvageable or in cases of extensive trauma or condylar aplasia. Craniofacial anatomical models are now easily fabricated from 3D digital graphics obtained from CT data and help visualize the defected TMJ as well as presurgical planning[28]. More specifically, the CT image data are processed to produce the 3D model with the Mimics software, which differentiate among the different tissues and separates the area of interest. Once the processing has been completed, the data are transferred to the 3D printer as an STL file, and the 3D model is fabricated from acrylonitrile butadiene styrene through the FDM method[28].

Moreover, the advances in AM have offered the ability to quickly produce personalized 3D printed TMJ prosthesis for patients in need of total TMJ replacement and avoid potential intraoperative nerve damage[2,30,108]. The "Melbourne" or the OMX TMJ prosthetic total joint replacement system offers the possibility for patient-specific condylar component size, as well as fixation screw positions, providing several advantages against stock TMJ prosthesis that come in narrow span of sizes and geometries. This patient-specific TMJ prosthesis was developed to replicate patient's anatomy and to maximize fixation strength, exhibiting high sensitivity adapting to changes in prosthesis design[2]. The OMX TMJ prosthesis comprises of two components, the high-density polyethylene fossa, which is machined, and the condylar component, which is 3D printed in titanium using SLM[2]. After extensive engineering analysis, the OMX TMJ prosthesis was assessed in patients, in a prospective clinical study, exhibiting positive preliminary results, with reduction in joint pain and improvement in mandibular movement and function[4,30]. Moreover, TMJ prosthesis with customized design based on AM was also fabricated and clinically tested by Zheng et al.[108]. The CT scan files of the TMJ were processed with DICOM format and the TMJ prosthesis was designed using 3-matic research software to match the patient's specific anatomy of the glenoid fossa and articular eminence, while the condylar head component was cylinder-like shaped[108]. Furthermore, the TMJ prosthesis consisted of three parts: the fossa and the condylar head component, which were fabricated by 5-axis milling device, from ultra-high molecular weight polyethylene and cobalt-chromium-molybdenum, respectively, and the mandibular component, which was 3D printed from Ti_6Al_4V alloy[108]. Clinical application of this customized TMJ prosthesis in patients with end-stage TMJ osteoarthritis exhibited improvement in mandibular function and movements, as well as decrease in pain, with no reported complications[108].

3D printing in TMJ tissue engineering

3D printing was also used to engineer scaffolds and regenerate parts of the TMJ. In the study by Schek et al., poly-L-lactic acid/HAp composite scaffolds were manufactured from computer-designed molds that were created on a wax inkjet printer and were then seeded with BMP-7-stimulated fibroblasts and chondrocytes, showing the formation of bone and cartilage alongside a stable interface between the regenerated tissues[86]. Perfect-fitting condylar implant from nanoscale HAp /polyamide has been fabricated with rapid prototyping to replace a defective condyle[60]. Data were obtained from CT scan of the opposite, normal condyle, oriented in the correct direction and then 3D printed, while a surgical guide was also fabricated, to ensure accurate fit during surgery[60]. Legemate et al. used 3D printing to fabricate an anatomically correct TMJ disc analogue with PCL microfibers[59]. Briefly, they scanned a TMJ disc, created a CAD model, and then 3D printed the scaffold with the aid of layer-by-layer deposition technique, managing to create a TMJ disc-like construct of fibrocartilaginous tissue with regionally variant microstructure[59].

References

1. Abduo J, Lyons K, Bennamoun M. Trends in computer-aided manufacturing in prosthodontics: a review of the available streams. *Int J Dent*. 2014;2014, 783948.
2. Ackland DC, Robinson D, Redhead M, Lee PVS, Moskaljuk A, Dimitroulis G. A personalized 3D-printed prosthetic joint replacement for the human temporomandibular joint: From implant design to implantation. *J Mech Behav Biomed Mater*. 2017;69: 404−411.
3. About Tara M, Eschbach S, Bohlsen F, Kern M. Clinical outcome of metal-ceramic crowns fabricated with laser-sintering technology. *Int J Prosthodont*. 2011;24: 46−48.
4. Ackland D, Robinson D, Lee PVS, Dimitroulis G. Design and clinical outcome of a novel 3D-printed prosthetic joint replacement for the human temporomandibular joint. *Clin Biomech*. 2018;56:52−60.
5. Alageel O, Abdallah MN, Alsheghri A, Song J, Caron E, Tamimi F. Removable partial denture alloys processed by laser-sintering technique. *J Biomed Mater Res B Appl Biomater*. 2018;106:1174−1185.
6. Alghazzawi TF. Advancements in CAD/CAM technology: options for practical implementation. *J Prosthodont Res*. 2016;60:72−84.
7. Alharbi N, Wismeijer D, Osman RB. Additive manufacturing techniques in prosthodontics: where do we currently stand? a critical review. *Int J Prosthodont*. 2017;30: 474−484.
8. Alharbi N, Osman R, Wismeijer D. Effects of build direction on the mechanical properties of 3D-printed complete coverage interim dental restorations. *J Prosthet Dent*. 2016;115:760−767.

9. Asa'ad F, Pagni G, Pilipchuk SP, Giannì AB, Giannobile WV, Rasperini G. 3D-printed scaffolds and biomaterials: review of alveolar bone augmentation and periodontal regeneration applications. *Int J Dent*. 2016;2016, 1239842.

10. Athirasala A, Tahayeri A, Thrivikraman G, França CM, Monteiro N, Tran V, Ferracane J, Bertassoni LE. A dentin-derived hydrogel bioink for 3D bioprinting of cell laden scaffolds for regenerative dentistry. *Biofabrication*. 2018;10:024101.

11. Barazanchi A, Li KC, Al-Amleh B, Lyons K, Waddell JN. Additive technology: update on current materials and applications in dentistry. *J Prosthodont*. 2017;26(2):156−163.

12. Bartellas M, Tibbo J, Angel D, Rideout A, Gillis J. Three-dimensional printing: a novel approach to the creation of obturator prostheses following palatal resection for malignant palate tumors. *J Craniofac Surg*. 2018;29:e12−e15.

13. Beguma Z, Chhedat P. Rapid prototyping—when virtual meets reality. *Int J Comput Dent*. 2014;17:297−306.

14. Bell RB, Weimer KA, Dierks EJ, Buehler M, Lubek JE. Computer planning and intraoperative navigation for palatomaxillary and mandibular reconstruction with fibular free flaps. *J Oral Maxillofac Surg*. 2011;69:724−732.

15. Berntsen C, Kleven M, Heian M, Hjortsjö C. Clinical comparison of conventional and additive manufactured stabilization splints. *Acta Biomater Odontol Scand*. 2018;4: 81−89.

16. Bilgin MS, Erdem A, Dilber E, Ersoy I. Comparison of fracture resistance between cast, CAD/CAM milling, and direct metal laser sintering metal post systems. *J Pro Prosthodont Res*. 2016;60:23−28.

17. Castillo-Oyagüe R, Lynch CD, Turrión AS, López-Lozano JF, Torres-Lagares D, Suárez-García MJ. Misfit and microleakage of implant-supported crown copings obtained by laser sintering and casting techniques, luted with glass-ionomer, resin cements and acrylic/urethane-based agents. *J Dent*. 2013;41:90−96.

18. Chen H, Wang H, Lv P, Wang Y, Sun Y. Quantitative Evaluation of Tissue Surface Adaption of CAD Designed and 3D Printed Wax Pattern of Maxillary Complete Denture. *BioMed Res Int*. 2015, 453968.

19. Chen H, Yang X, Chen L, Wang Y, Sun Y. Application of FDM three-dimensional printing technology in the digital manufacture of custom edentulous mandible trays. *Sci Rep*. 2016;6:19207.

20. Chen J, Zhang Z, Chen X, Zhang C, Zhang G, Xu Z. Design and manufacture of customized dental implants by using reverse engineering and selective laser melting technology. *J Prosthet Dent*. 2014;112:1088−10895.e1.

21. Cheng YC, Lin DH, Jiang CP, Lin YM. Dental implant customization using numerical optimization design and 3-dimensional printing fabrication of zirconia ceramic. *Int J Numer Method Biomed Eng*. 2017;33.

22. Chiu YC, Fang HY, Hsu TT, Lin CY, Shie MY. The characteristics of mineral trioxide aggregate/polycaprolactone 3-dimensional scaffold with osteogenesis properties for tissue regeneration. *J Endod*. 2017;43:923−929.

23. Chung YJ, Park JM, Kim TH, Ahn JS, Cha HS, Lee JH. 3D printing of resin material for denture artificial teeth: chipping and indirect tensile fracture resistance. *Materials*. 2018;11.

24. Ciocca L, Lizio G, Baldissara P, Sambuco A, Scotti R, Corinaldesi G. Prosthetically CAD-CAM-guided bone augmentation of atrophic jaws using customized titanium mesh: preliminary results of an open prospective study. *J Oral Implantol*. 2018;44: 131−137.

25. Ciocca L, Fantini M, De Crescenzio F, Corinaldesi G, Scotti R. Direct metal laser sintering (DMLS) of a customized titanium mesh for prosthetically guided bone regeneration of atrophic maxillary arches. *Med Biol Eng Comput*. 2011;49: 1347−1352.

26. Costa PF, Vaquette C, Zhang Q, Reis RL, Ivanovski S, Hutmacher DW. Advanced tissue engineering scaffold design for regeneration of the complex hierarchical periodontal structure. *J Clin Period*. 2014;41:283−294.

27. Dawood A, Marti B, Sauret-Jackson V, Darwood A. 3D printing in dentistry. *Br Dent J*. 2015;219(11):521−529.

28. Deshmukh TR, Kuthe AM, Chaware SM, Vaibhaw B, Ingole DS. Rapid prototyping assisted fabrication of the customised temporomandibular joint implant: a case report. *Rapid Protot J*. 2011;17:362−368.

29. Digholkar S, Madhav VN, Palaskar J. Evaluation of the flexural strength and microhardness of provisional crown and bridge materials fabricated by different methods. *J Indian Prosthodont Soc*. 2016;16:328−334.

30. Dimitroulis G, Austin S, Sin Lee PV, Ackland D. A new three-dimensional, print-on-demand temporomandibular prosthetic total joint replacement system: preliminary outcomes. *J Cranio-Maxillo-Fac Surg*. 2018;46:1192−1198.

31. Ebert J, Ozkol E, Zeichner A, Uibel K, Weiss O, Koops U, Telle R, Fischer H. Direct inkjet printing of dental prostheses made of zirconia. *J Dent Res*. 2009;88:673−676.

32. Efanov JI, Roy AA, Huang KN, Borsuk DE. Virtual surgical planning: the pearls and pitfalls. *Plast Reconstr Surg Glob Open*. 2018;6:e1443.

33. Favero CS, English JD, Cozad BE, Wirthlin JO, Short MM, Kasper FK. Effect of print layer height and printer type on the accuracy of 3-dimensional printed orthodontic models. *Am J Orthod Dentofacial Orthop*. 2017;152:557−565.

34. Feilden E, Ferraro C, Zhang Q, García-Tuñón E, D'Elia E, Giuliani F, Vandeperre L, Saiz E. 3D printing bioinspired ceramic composites. *Sci Rep*. 2017;7:13759.

35. Gao B, Wu J, Zhao X, Tan H. Fabricating titanium denture base plate by laser rapid forming. *Rapid Prototyp J*. 2009;15:133−136.

36. Giacomino CM, Ray JJ, Wealleans JA. Targeted endodontic microsurgery: a novel approach to anatomically challenging scenarios using 3-dimensional-printed guides and trephine burs-a report of 3 cases. *J Endod*. 2018;44:671−677.

37. Groth C, Kravitz ND, Shirck JM. Incorporating three-dimensional printing in orthodontics. *J Clin Orthod*. 2018;52:28−33.

38. Hämmerle C, Stone P, Jung R, Kapos T, Brodala N. Consensus statements and recommended clinical procedures regarding computer-assisted implant dentistry. *Int J Oral Maxillofacial Implants*. 2009;24:126−130.

39. Hanasono MM, Skoracki RJ. Computer-assisted design and rapid prototype modeling in microvascular mandible reconstruction. *Laryngoscope*. 2013;123:597−604.

40. Ho CC, Fang HY, Wang B, Huang TH, Shie MY. The effects of Biodentine/polycaprolactone three-dimensional-scaffold with odontogenesis properties on human dental pulp cells. *Int Endod J*. 2018;51:291−300.

41. Huang Z, Wang XZ, Hou YZ. Novel method of fabricating individual trays for maxillectomy patients by computer-aided design and rapid prototyping. *J Prosthodont*. 2015a;24:115−120.

42. Huang Z, Zhang L, Zhu J, Zhang X. Clinical marginal and internal fit of metal ceramic crowns fabricated with a selective laser melting technology. *J Prosthet Dent*. 2015b; 113:623−627.

43. Hull C. *Apparatus for Production of Three- Dimensional Object by Stereolithography.* 1986. US Patent 4,575,330.

44. Inokoshi M, Kanazawa M, Minakuchi S. Evaluation of a complete denture trial method applying rapid prototyping. *Dent Mater J.* 2009;31:40−46.

45. Ishinabe S. Mucosal thickness of the denture foundation under occlusal force. *Nihon Hotetsu Shika Gakkai Zasshi.* 1991;35:111−124.

46. Jheon AH, Oberoi S, Solem RC, Kapila S. Moving towards precision orthodontics: An evolving paradigm shift in the planning and delivery of customized orthodontic therapy. *Orthod Craniofac Res.* 2017;20(1):106−113.

47. Jiang FF, Hou Y, Lu L, Ding XX, Li W, Yan AH. Functional evaluation of a CAD/CAM prosthesis for immediate defect repair after total maxillectomy: a case series of 18 patients with maxillary sinus cancer. *J Esthet Restor Dent.* 2015;27:S80−S89.

48. Jiao T, Chenyuan Z, Dong X, Gu X. Rehabilitation of maxillectomy defects with obturator prostheses fabricated using computer-aided design and rapid prototyping: a pilot study. *Int J Prosthodont.* 2014;27:480−486.

49. Jin SJ, Jeong ID, Kim JH, Kim WC. Accuracy (trueness and precision) of dental models fabricated using additive manufacturing methods. *Int J Comput Dent.* 2018;21: 107−113.

50. Jin SJ, Kim DY, Kim JH, Kim WC. Accuracy of dental replica models using photopolymer materials in additive manufacturing: in vitro three-dimensional evaluation. *J Prosthodont.* 2018. https://doi.org/10.1111/jopr.12928 (Epub ahead of print).

51. Kajima Y, Takaichi A, Nakamoto T, Kimura T, Yogo Y, Ashida M, Doi H, Nomura N, Takahashi H, Hanawa T, Wakabayashi N. Fatigue strength of Co-Cr-Mo alloy clasps prepared by selective laser melting. *J Mech Behav Biomed Mater.* 2016;59:446−458.

52. Keating AP, Knox J, Bibb R, Zhurov AI. A comparison of plaster, digital and reconstructed study model accuracy. *J Orthod.* 2008;35:191−201.

53. Kim KB, Kim WC, Kim HY, Kim JH. An evaluation of marginal fit of three-unit fixed dental prostheses fabricated by direct metal laser sintering system. *Dent Mater.* 2013; 29:e91−e96.

54. Kodama H. Automatic method for fabricating a three-dimensional plastic model with photo-hardening polymer. *Rev Sci Instr.* 1981;52:1770−1773.

55. Kortes J, Dehnad H, Kotte ANT, Fennis WMM, Rosenberg AJWP. A novel digital workflow to manufacture personalized three-dimensional-printed hollow surgical obturators after maxillectomy. *Int J Oral Maxillofac.* 2018;47:1214−1218.

56. Kwon TG, Choi JW, Kyung HM, Park HS. Accuracy of maxillary repositioning in two-jaw surgery with conventional articulator model surgery versus virtual model surgery. *Int J Oral Maxillofac Surg.* 2014;43:732−738.

57. Laverty DP, Thomas MBM, Clark P, Addy LD. The use of 3D metal printing (direct metal laser sintering) in removable prosthodontics. *Dent Update.* 2016;43(9), 826-828, 831-2, 834-5.

58. Lee WS, Lee DH, Lee KB. Evaluation of internal fit of interim crown fabricated with CAD/CAM milling and 3D printing system. *J Adv Prosthodont.* 2017;9(4):265−270.

59. Legemate K, Tarafder S, Jun Y, Lee CH. Engineering human TMJ discs with protein-releasing 3D-printed scaffolds. *J Dent Res.* 2016;95:800−807.

60. Li J, Hsu Y, Luo E, Khadka A, Hu J. Computer-aided design and manufacturing and rapid prototyped nanoscale hydroxyapatite/polyamide (n-HA/PA) construction for condylar defect caused by mandibular angle ostectomy. *Aesthetic Plast Surg.* 2011; 35:636−640.

61. Liu Q, Leu MC, Schmitt SM. Rapid prototyping in dentistry: technology and application. *Int J Adv Manuf Tech*. 2006;29:317−335.
62. Martorelli M, Gerbino S, Giudice M, Ausiello P. A comparison between customized clear and removable orthodontic appliances manufactured using RP and CNC techniques. *Dent Mater*. 2013;29:e1−10.
63. McLean JW, von Fraunhofer JA. The estimation of cement film thickness by an in vivo technique. *Br Dent J*. 1971;131:107−111.
64. Molinero-Mourelle P, Canals S, Gómez-Polo M, Solá-Ruiz MF, Del Río Highsmith J, Viñuela AC. Polylactic acid as a material for three-dimensional printing of provisional restorations. *Int J Prosthodont*. 2018;31(4):349−350.
65. Michelinakis G. The use of cone beam computed tomography and three dimensional printing technology in the restoration of a maxillectomy patient using a dental implant retained obturator. *J Indian Prosthodont Soc*. 2017;17:406−411.
66. Nakata T, Shimpo H, Ohkubo C. Clasp fabrication using one-process molding by repeated lasersintering and high-speed milling. *J Prosthodont Res*. 2017;61:276−282.
67. Nayak A, Jain PK, Kankar PK, Jain N. Computer-aided design-based guided endodontic: a novel approach for root canal access cavity preparation. *Proc Inst Mech Eng H*. 2018;232(8):787−795.
68. Oberoi G, Nitsch S, Edelmayer M, Janjić K, Müller AS, Agis H. 3D Printing—encompassing the facets of dentistry. *Front Bioeng Biotechnol*. 2018;6:172.
69. Örtorp A, Jönsson D, Mouhsen A, Vult von Steyern P. The fit of cobalt-chromium three-unit fixed dental prostheses fabricated with four different techniques: a comparative in vitro study. *Dent Mater*. 2011;27:356−363.
70. Osman RB, van der Veen AJ, Huiberts D, Wismeijer D, Alharbi N. 3D-printing zirconia implants; a dream or a reality? an in-vitro study evaluating the dimensional accuracy, surface topography and mechanical properties of printed zirconia implant and discs. *J Mech Behav Biomed Mater*. 2017;75:521−528.
71. Ozkol E, Ebert J, Uibel K, Watjen AM, Telle R. Development of high solid content aqueous 3Y-TZP suspensions for direct inkjet printing using a thermal inkjet printer. *J Eur Ceram Soc*. 2009;29:403−409.
72. Pandy PM, Reddy NV, Dhande SG. Slicing procedures in layerd manufacturing: a review. *Rapid Prototyp J*. 2003;9:274−288.
73. Park CH, Rios HF, Jin Q, Sugai JV, Padial-Molina M, Taut AD, Flanagan CL, Hollister SJ, Giannobile WV. Tissue engineering bone ligament complexes using fiber-guiding scaffolds. *Biomaterials*. 2012;33:137−145.
74. Peng E, Zhang D, Ding J. Ceramic robocasting: recent achievements, potential, and future developments. *Adv Mater*. 2018;30:e1802404.
75. Pompa G, Di Carlo S, De Angelis F, Cristalli MP, Annibali S. Comparison of conventional methods and laser-assisted rapid prototyping for manufacturing fixed dental prostheses: an in vitro study. *BioMed Res Int*. 2015;2015, 318097.
76. Prabhu R, Prabhu G, Baskaran E, Arumugam EM. Clinical acceptability of metal-ceramic fixed partial dental prosthesis fabricated with direct metal laser sintering technique-5year follow-up. *J Indian Prosthodont Soc*. 2016;16:193−197.
77. Quante K, Ludwig K, Kern M. Marginal and internal fit of metal-ceramic crowns fabricated with a new laser melting technology. *Dent Mater*. 2008;24:1211−1315.
78. Revilla-León M, Meyers MJ, Zandinejad A, Özcan M. A review on chemical composition, mechanical properties, and manufacturing work flow of additively manufactured current polymers for interim dental restorations. *J Esthet Restor Dent*. 2019;31:51−57.

79. Reymus M, Fotiadou C, Kessler A, Heck K, Hickel R, Diegritz C. 3D printed replicas for endodontic education. *Int Endod J*. 2019;52(1):123−130.
80. Reynolds M, Reynolds M, Adeeb S, El-Bialy T. 3-d volumetric evaluation of human mandibular growth. *Open Biomed Eng J*. 2011;5:83−89.
81. Robberecht L, Chai F, Dehurtevent M, Marchandise P, Bécavin T, Hornez JC, Deveaux E. A novel anatomical ceramic root canal simulator for endodontic training. *Eur J Dent Educ*. 2017;21:e1−e6.
82. Rodney J, Chicchon I. Digital Design and Fabrication of Surgical Obturators Based Only on Preoperative Computed Tomography Data. *Int J Prosthodont (IJP)*. 2017;30: 111−112.
83. Salmi M, Paloheimo KS, Tuomi J, Ingman T, Mäkitie A. A digital process for additive manufacturing of occlusal splints: a clinical pilot study. *J R Soc Interface*. 2013;10, 20130203.
84. Salmi M, Tuomi J, Sirkkanen R, Ingman T, Mäkitie A. Rapid tooling method for soft customized removable oral appliances. *Open Dent J*. 2012;6:85−89.
85. Santos EC, Shiomi M, Osakada K, Laoui T. Rapid manufacturing of metal components by laser forming. *Proc ASME Int Conf Manuf Sci Eng*. 2006;46:1459−1468.
86. Schek RM, Taboas JM, Hollister SJ, Krebsbach PH. Tissue engineering osteochondral implants for temporomandibular joint repair. *Orthod Craniofac Res*. 2005;8: 313−319.
87. Seo C, Juodzbalys G. Accuracy of guided surgery via stereolithographic mucosa-supported surgical guide in implant surgery for edentulous poatient: a systematic review. *J Oral Maxillofac Res*. 2018;9 e1.
88. Shellabear M, Nyrhil. O. DMLS − development history and state of the art. In: *Proceedings of the Fourth Laser Assisted Net Shape Engineering (LANE) 2004, September 21−24 2004*. Erlangen, Germany: Bamberg-Meisenbach; 2004:393−404. ISBN 3-87525-202-0.
89. Shetye PR. Chapter 9.2: Computerized surgical planning in orthographic surgery. In: *Plastic surgery: volume 3: Craniofacial, head and Neck Surgery and pediatric plastic surgery*. 4 ed. Elsevier; 2017:230−240.
90. Shim JH, Won JY, Park JH, Bae JH, Ahn G, Kim CH, Lim DH, Cho DW, Yun WS, Bae EB, Jeong CM, Huh JB. Effects of 3D-printed polycaprolactone/β-tricalcium phosphate membranes on guided bone regeneration. *Int J Mol Sci*. 2017;18:E899.
91. Silva NR, Witek L, Coelho PG, Thompson VP, Rekow ED, Smay J. Additive CAD/CAM process for dental prostheses. *J Prosthodont*. 2011;20:93−96.
92. Sim F, Over LM, Dierks EJ, Cheng A, Patel AA, Bell B. Chapter 12: maxillofacial reconstruction and prosthetic rehabilitation. In: *Oral, Head and Neck Oncology and Reconstructive Surgery*. 1 ed. Elsevier; 2018:221−267.
93. Soltanzadeh P, Suprono MS, Kattadiyil MT, Goodacre C, Gregorius W. An in vitro investigation of accuracy and fit of conventional and CAD/CAM removable partial denture frameworks. *J Prosthodont*. 2018. https://doi.org/10.1111/jopr.12997 (Epub ahead of print).
94. Stansbury JW, Idacavage MJ. 3D printing with polymers: challenges among expanding options and opportunities. *Dent Mater*. 2016;32(1):54−64.
95. Sun Y, Chen H, Li H, Deng K, Zhao T, Wang Y, Zhou Y. Clinical evaluation of final impressions from three-dimensional printed custom trays. *Sci Rep*. 2017;7:14958.
96. Sun Y, Lü P, Wang Y. Study on CAD&RP for removable complete denture. *Comput Methods Programs Biomed*. 2009;93:266−272.

97. Tahayeri A, Morgan M, Fugolin AP, Bompolaki D, Athirasala A, Pfeifer CS, Ferracane JL, Bertassoni LE. 3D printed versus conventionally cured provisional crown and bridge dental materials. *Dent Mater*. 2018;34:192−200.

98. Tamac E, Toksavul S, Toman M. Clinical marginal and internal adaptation of CAD/CAM milling, laser sintering, and cast metal ceramic crowns. *J Prosthet Dent*. 2014; 112:909−913.

99. Tan FB, Song JL, Wang C, Fan YB, Dai HW. Titanium clasp fabricated by selective laser melting, CNC milling, and conventional casting: a comparative in vitro study. *J Prosthodont Res*. 2018;63:58−65.

100. Torii M, Nakata T, Takahashi K, Kawamura N, Shimpo H, Ohkubo C. Fitness and retentive force of cobalt-chromium alloy clasps fabricated with repeated laser sintering and milling. *J Prosthodont Res*. 2018;62(3):342−346.

101. Ucar Y, Akova T, Akyl MS, Brantley WA. Internal fit evaluation of crown prepared using a new dental crown fabrication technique: laser-sintered Co-Cr crowns. *J Prosthet Dent*. 2009;102:253−259.

102. van der Meer WJ, Vissink A, Ren Y. Full 3-dimensional digital workflow for multicomponent dental appliances: a proof of concept. *J Am Dent Assoc*. 2016;147:288−291.

103. Vaquette C, Fan W, Xiao Y, Hamlet S, Hutmacher DW, Ivanovski S. A biphasic scaffold design combined with cell sheet technology for simultaneous regeneration of alveolar bone/periodontal ligament complex. *Biomaterials*. 2012;33:5560−5573.

104. Wang W, Yu H, Liu Y, Jiang X, Gao B. Trueness analysis of zirconia crowns fabricated with 3-dimensional printing. *J Prosthet Dent*. 2019;121:285−291.

105. Wiechmann D, Rummel V, Thalheim A, Simon JS, Wiechmann L. Customized brackets and archwires for lingual orthodontic treatment. *Am J Orthod Dentofacial Orthop*. 2003;124:593−599.

106. Williams RJ, Bibb R, Eggbeer D, Collis J. Use of CAD/CAM technology to fabricate a removable partial denture framework. *J Prosthet Dent*. 2006;96:96−99.

107. Yang F, Chen C, Zhou Q, Gong Y, Li R, Li C, Klämpfl F, Freund S, Wu X, Sun Y, Li X, Schmidt M, Ma D, Yu Y. Laser beam melting 3D printing of Ti6Al4V based porous structured dental implants: fabrication, biocompatibility analysis and photoelastic study. *Sci Rep*. 2017;7:45360.

108. Zheng J, Chen X, Jiang W, Zhang S, Chen M, Yang C. An innovative total temporomandibular joint prosthesis with customized design and 3D printing additive fabrication: a prospective clinical study. *J Transl Med*. 2019;17:4.

109. Zhou W, Liu Z, Song L, Kuo CL, Shafer DM. Clinical factors affecting the accuracy of guided implant surgery-a systematic review and meta-analysis. *J Evid Based Dent Pract*. 2018;18:28−40.

Three-dimensional printing in plastic and reconstructive surgery

Efterpi Demiri[1], Georgia-Alexandra Spyropoulou, MD, PhD[2], Antonios Tsimponis[3], Dimitrios Dionyssiou, MD, PhD[4]

[1]*Professor in Plastic Surgery of Aristotle University of Thessaloniki, Chief of the Department of Plastic Surgery, Papageorgiou Hospital, Thessaloniki, Greece;* [2]*Associate Professor in Plastic Surgery, Aristotle University of Thessaloniki, Thessaloniki, Greece;* [3]*Plastic Surgeon, Department of Plastic Surgery of the Aristotle University of Thessaloniki, Thessaloniki, Greece;* [4]*Associate Professor in Plastic Surgery, Aristotle University of Thessaloniki, Thessaloniki, Greece*

Introduction

During the last three decades, advancements in bioprosthetics, biomaterials and tissue engineering have been accompanied by an outbreak in three-dimensional (3D) technology applications in several medical disciplines including plastic, reconstructive and aesthetic surgery. The philosophy behind plastic surgery lies on how basic surgical techniques attempt to close a wound defect and treat congenital anomalies by harvesting, molding ("$\pi\lambda\acute{\alpha}\sigma\sigma\epsilon\iota\nu$") and moving tissues with similar characteristics into the defect area, while maintaining its functionality and aesthetics. The same philosophy embraces the 3D technology principles, which ultimately aim to reproduce with extreme precision anatomical structures and tissues that are absent from the human body, borrowing only a few cells from the body and thus avoiding the creation or limiting the need for donor regions.

Taking one step back, 3D imaging technology is a primary and integral stage in the 3D printing process and has been used for several decades in the preoperative design of many plastic surgery interventions. Burn surgery first introduced the use of 3D tissue printing in plastic surgery; the need for immediate availability of skin substitutes gave birth to the idea of culturing large keratinocyte lines from a smaller number of cells, which were used to cover extensive burn defects in patients lacking available donor areas.[1] Thereafter, improvement in design and extrusion methods made the 3D printing technologies much more affordable, with numerous applications in surgery.

Three-dimensional printing technologies

3D printing is the process by which computer software obtained from 3D imaging is used to guide a machine into manufacturing a detailed 3D model. The process

3D Printing: Applications in Medical Surgery. https://doi.org/10.1016/B978-0-323-66193-5.00010-1

includes fabricating prototypes by laying down sequential layers of material. The different types of 3D printing technologies include selective laser melting, fused deposition modeling (FDM), binder jetting and bioprinting.[2]

In selective laser melting, a laser beam strikes on a fine metal powder bed causing the particles to fuse and join together; then, a roller or blade spreads extra powder onto the build tray and the process is repeated until the form is completed. In FDM, the object is created from a plastic filament or metal wire that is unwound from a coil, melted and deposited in layers. Binder jetting refers to a process where the molding material is applied layer by layer on the build area and the printer head spreads the binder in between to create a solid form.[3] Finally, in bioprinting, successive layers of cells, matrix and nutrients are sprayed from the printer head to create tissue-like 3D structures. Rapid prototyping refers to the technology where objects or models are designed and derived through 3D printing from a computed tomography (CT) scan, magnetic resonance imaging (MRI), or optical scan after a computer-aided 3D modeling stage.[4] As these technologies rapidly evolve, 3D printing can provide an individual product in a short period of time, which suits the goal of individualized medicine where each patient is given a specific, tailored, therapeutic approach.

The highly expanding use of 3D printing technologies in various fields of plastic and reconstructive surgery allows the surgeons to create customized patient-tailored products and replace tissues using individualized artificial and biologic implants.[5] Moreover, 3D printing is being increasingly employed in order to improve patients' care and advance surgical training. Recent published data demonstrate promising alternative to current reconstructive surgical treatments, while a huge volume of ongoing research studies on 3D printing applications are being elaborated worldwide.

Areas of biological and surgical applications of 3D printing in plastic surgery include surgical planning and teaching,[6] mandible and maxilla reconstruction after oncological resection,[7] trauma reconstruction,[5] reconstruction of craniofacial congenital anomalies,[8] orthognathic surgery,[9] oculoplastic surgery,[10] breast reconstruction,[11] hand surgery,[12] facial aesthetics and microtia correction,[13] and burns reconstruction.[14]

Three-dimensional printing technologies for preoperative planning in plastic surgery

In plastic and reconstructive surgery, 3D printed models may be widely used in preoperative planning and intraoperative guidance; extended oncological resections, major traumas or congenital anomalies often result in tissue defects that necessitate complex tissue transfer and/or combination of various reconstructive techniques. CT, MRI and other two-dimensional (2D) modalities have been used for several decades in the past and are still being used as tools to help the plastic surgeon to analyze the tissue loss and identify the ideal tissue donor sites.

A typical example of using the 3D imaging technology is its application in reconstructive breast surgery, where the introduction of computed tomographic angiography (CTA) has enabled the surgeon to improve clinical practice and reduce intraoperative time, through the accurate and reliable preoperative imaging and identification of the ideal perforators of a deep inferior epigastric perforator flap[15,16] (Fig. 10.1). The novel introduction of the fourth dimensions in the CTA has led to the development of the four-dimensional (4D) CTA, which allows even more information to be obtained beforehand on the dynamic flow of perforators in certain perforasomes.[17]

Moreover, 3D imaging of facial vascular malformations is being used in preoperative planning and navigating surgical excision (Fig. 10.2). Combining conventional imaging techniques with 3D printed models may lead to improved diagnosis of vascular lesions and should be considered a useful adjunct to surgical management.[18]

Generally, 3D printed models representing the exact amount of any tissue defect that must be replaced may provide the surgeon with more information considering the size, shape and depth of the defect, its relationship with the surrounding anatomical structures and the different types of tissues that are missing after severe traumas or oncological resections.[19] In this way, 3D printing can be an extremely valuable tool in assessing the tissue loss, literally quantifying the volume difference and, thus, accurately planning the whole reconstructive procedure[20] (Fig. 10.3).

Furthermore, patient-unique pathologies depicted in 3D printed models help both young and experienced surgeons to preoperatively predict potential intraoperative challenges and postoperative outcomes. Accomplishing all these, they are capable of developing a thorough surgical plan required to perform complex reconstructive surgeries, especially microsurgical procedures and to gain more expertise, while decreasing the intraoperative time and enhancing final results.

Three-dimensional printing technologies for education and training

3D printed constructions are increasingly used for medical teaching, doctors training, and patients' education, as they realistically simulate tissue structures and allow for exact understanding, handling, and operating.

Plastic surgery requires excellent knowledge of applied surgical anatomy. Spending numerous hours over human cadavers in anatomy labs was the standard medical training during the past years for medical students and residents. The scarcity of human cadavers, however, led to more technology-dependent educational programs. Medical students' and young doctors' training can be boosted using 3D printed objects, such as models for in-depth understanding the human anatomy, while residents' surgical skills are enhanced by practicing on tissues or organs' replicas, which simulate human ones, before operating on real patients.[5]

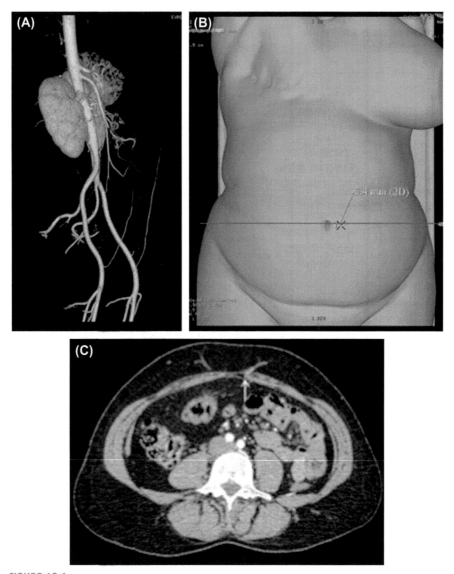

FIGURE 10.1

Use of three-dimensional (3D) imaging of the abdominal wall (A, B) and computed tomographic angiography data (C) in preoperative identification of the ideal deep inferior epigastric perforator for a delayed deep inferior epigastric perforator (DIEP) flap-based breast reconstruction.

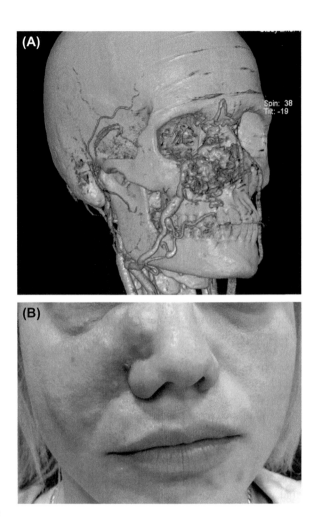

FIGURE 10.2

Three-dimensional imaging of a facial vascular malformation of the right cheek (A, B).

Initially, realistic educational models of the facial bony and soft tissue structures have been produced for facial surgery training. Cleft lip and palate simulators have been created to enable young surgeons to perform cleft lip and palate surgical reconstructions, as well as secondary nasal deformity repairs; the surgeons gave a positive feedback on the simulators realism and anatomic accuracy.[6,21] Elastic two-layer models, made from polyurethane on the outer side and silicone on the inner side, have been constructed for teaching residents to perform facial local skin flaps and cheiloplasty; again, young doctors reported their experiences to be really enjoyable and realistic.[22]

Pediatric patient-specific costal cartilage models have also been produced by utilizing computer-aided design (CAD) and 3D printing technology for microtia skills

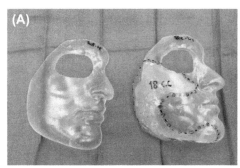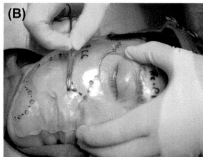

FIGURE 10.3

Three-dimensional printed model of the right hemifacial area, presenting a soft tissue defect of the right cheek, comparing to the healthy contralateral one that is used for preparing a 3D printed "reverse" model (A); models are used to accurately assess the volume difference and plan the surgical correction (B).

Courtesy to Professor Mimis Cohen, University of Illinois at Chicago.

training and neoauricle reconstruction; thus, the trainees can learn to successfully carve the silicone composite ribs that have similar geometry, pliability, texture, and suturing characteristics compared to human cartilaginous tissue, while this was confirmed by experienced ear plastic surgeons.[23]

Training in aesthetic surgery, an area that residents usually lack hands-on experience, can also be assisted with the use of 3D printed scaffolds. Nasal models, based on prominent dorsum humped noses, have been created and used as hands-on rhinoplasty training modules; acrylonitrile butadiene styrene was used for simulating the bony skeleton and different types of medical silicone for the cartilage, skin and mucosa.[24]

During the recent years, 3D printing emerging technologies were used to develop impressive virtual reality surgical systems, which provide opportunities for better visualization of the patients' anatomy and structural anomalies (Fig. 10.4). Virtual surgery planning assists surgeons to develop their accurate surgical plans before entering the operating room, practice on surgical techniques, anticipate difficulties, minimize surgical errors, reduce the length of surgeries, predict postoperative results and—finally—improve the overall quality of their clinical praxis.[25,26] Furthermore, 3D printing of perforator vascular anatomy may be extremely helpful for training and teaching dissection of perforator flaps; Gillis and Morris manufactured a model of internal mammary artery perforators and the neighboring ribs using a binder jet 3D printer.[27] The ability of physically interacting with the model and visualizing it in multiple planes significantly helped surgeons through dissection and identification of the dominant perforator.

Very recently, 3D microsurgical endoscopes using 3D monitors and special 3D glasses have been built to enhance microsurgical training and facilitate microsurgical vascular anastomoses and peripheral nerve sutures (Fig. 10.5).

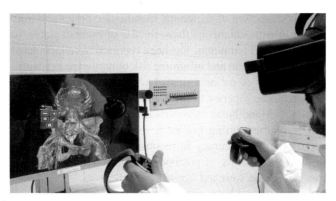

FIGURE 10.4

An example of a virtual reality surgical system using three-dimensional (3D) printing technology.

Courtesy to Professor Mimis Cohen, University of Illinois at Chicago.

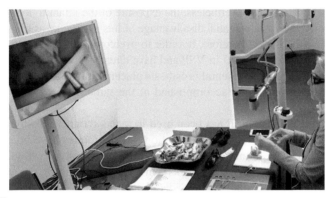

FIGURE 10.5

Three-dimensional (3D) microsurgical system using 3D monitors and special 3D glasses built to enhance microsurgical training and facilitate microvascular anastomoses.

On the other hand, 3D printed models may be extremely helpful for patients themselves, to understand better their problems and get a more detailed knowledge of the intended procedures, surgical treatment modalities and outcomes; patients can use their senses, namely vision and touch, to see, hold and compare the pre- and postoperative 3D models and, therefore, they may have more realistic expectations from the planned surgery.[20]

Three-dimensional printing in head and neck reconstruction

Applications of 3D printing technologies in head and neck reconstruction are multiple and include craniofacial anomalies of variable severities, i.e., from simple localized soft tissue defects to large and composite 3D tissue losses.[28]

Regarding reconstruction of segmental mandibulectomies and maxillary defects with free osseous or osteocutaneous flaps, the use of prebent plates, based on accurate mandible 3D printed templates, has been reported to reduce general anesthesia time, achieve better occlusion and minimize risk of hardware exposure.[25,29,30] Moreover, the facial contour of patients treated with prebent reconstruction plates has been demonstrated to be superior to the contour of patients treated with intraoperatively bent plates.[31] Mandibular reconstruction with vascularized free fibula flaps assisted by 3D printable cutting guides is reported not only to reduce operating time but also to optimize accuracy in reconstruction, enhance bone consolidation and increase the predictability of postoperative results; additional costs, however, should be considered and weighed against those benefits.[32,33]

3D printed models have been manufactured and used for mandibular distraction osteogenesis in infants suffering from Pierre Robin sequence. 3D printing guided mandible distraction has demonstrated significantly shorter operating time and hospital stay compared to the traditional surgical procedure, with no increase in postoperative complications.[34] Printable cutting guides provided with virtual surgical planning (VSP) also help the surgeon to avoid damage to the inferior alveolar nerve and/or developing dental structures.[35] Nevertheless, the exposure of the infant to ionizing radiation should be considered as a potential disadvantage of this technique, as CT scan is necessary for the VSP process; therefore, in order to overcome this disadvantage, some authors suggested the use of MRI in VSP and have already reported promising results.[36]

Dental implantation and dental prosthesis placement may also be assisted by 3D printing technologies and is accomplished at the same surgical time as mandible resection and reconstruction.[37]

The use of CAD and VSP has been used in facial symmetry restoration procedures; reduced surgical time and optimization of osteotomies have been reported as some of the most important advantages of this methodology, while higher cost, longer production time (days to weeks) and lack of flexibility to intraoperative changing of the surgical plan are considered as drawbacks.[38-40]

Another recent application of 3D printing in head and neck reconstruction is the creation of orbital implant templates for secondary orbital reconstructions in posttraumatic cases or following oncological excisions; 3D technology was used to fashion patient-specific stenciled and molded orbital implants with successful outcome.[10] Custom-made CAD-based orbital implants are reported to provide the most precise orbital reconstruction, as well as shorter operation time compared to the standard preformed orbital implants.[41]

3D printed patient-specific neck splints have been manufactured and successfully used for the treatment of postburn neck contractures; although their production costs are higher compared to standard neck splints, 3D printed splints can be fabricated precisely to have a perfect contact to the patient and can be adjusted after anatomical changes during wound healing.[41,42]

Finally, forehead and temporal augmentation using 3D printing-assisted methyl methacrylate implants has been used for aesthetic purposes to enhance facial features of Asian patients.[43]

Three-dimensional printing in breast surgery

Breast operations including augmentation, reduction, correction of asymmetry and gynecomastia, and breast reconstruction after mastectomy constitute nowadays the most frequent plastic surgery procedures performed worldwide. Breast augmentation is the most common aesthetic breast operation, while breast reconstruction is characterized as an integral phase of the total breast cancer management.[44] Breast symmetry, size and shape are key components of aesthetic outcomes of any breast surgical procedure and can be optimized by accurate preoperative measurements and intraoperative planning.[45]

The usual practice for estimating and selecting the ideal volume and shape of breast implants in breast augmentation, asymmetry or reconstruction is based on surgeons' ability and experience, and is limited to clinical measurements and analysis of 2D photographs; various objective quantitative means of calculating breast volume have been reported, such as the use of prefilled bags of water or rice, a selection of multiple size implants, or the use of the contralateral breast as a template for unilateral delay breast reconstruction.[46] The same principles are also applied in autologous flap-based breast reconstruction, while the analysis of the contralateral breast is intended for both immediate and delayed reconstruction procedures; the aesthetic outcome and symmetrical shape of the reconstructed breast is dictated by the footprint, conus and skin envelope of the contralateral breast.[47]

3D imaging technology is currently a valuable tool in breast surgery, while the use of 3D printed models provides quantitative breast measurements and volumetric calculations, as well as visual assessment of the size, shape, contour and symmetry of the breasts.[48-50] However, the high cost and lack of access are the main reasons that prevent 3D scanning from wide application in breast surgery.

Comparing techniques measuring the breast, the 3D surface imaging (SI) photography has distinguished advantages over the CT/MRI modalities: the 3D SI photography is noninvasive and free of adverse health effects, while it eliminates X-ray exposure for patients and—more importantly—for medical personnel; moreover, recording time of the measurement is significantly shorter comparing to the CT/MRI-based techniques.[51] On the other hand, the use of CTA/MRA is still valuable for preplanning free tissue flap's perforators).[47]

Although 3D scanning techniques that measure directly the breast volumes are reported to be superior to anthropometric measuring in accuracy, precision and reproducibility, according to Yang et al., 3D scanning methods are not accurate in looking through the breast substances, reaching the interspace between the chest and posterior border of the breast, and/or correctly imaging the inframammary fold, especially in large and ptotic breasts.[51]

An interesting approach for volumetric analysis of the breast mound has been described by Chae et al.; based on scanned data of CT or MRI, they created software-generated 3D reconstructions and produce biomodels of the breasts using a 3D printer for tactile appreciation of the breast characteristics. The authors reported promising results in terms of better preoperative planning and surgical guidance, reduction of operative times and improvement of the final aesthetic outcomes.[44]

Hummelink et al. used the 3D stereophotogrammetry technology to create 3D printed breast molds for intraoperative use in autologous breast reconstruction; the flap is placed inside the patient-specific printed template in order to aid the surgeon to determine the shape and volume of the autologous tissue, which will create the desired breast mound. According to the authors' preliminary experience, this easy and inexpensive method may provide very satisfying results; however, patients' characteristics and donor sites' availability should be preoperatively considered in order to be able to use the template to its full potential.[11]

Another application of the 3D printing technology in breast surgery has been reported by Patete et al. regarding autologous fat grafting in the breast. The geometry of fat tissue deposition within the receiving area is believed to represent a crucial element in maximizing the surgical outcome and minimizing complications, such as cysts, implanted tissue necrosis and fat resorption. The authors describe a computer-assisted surgical planning tool to quantify and analyze the grafting geometry by means of a genetic algorithm that allows optimization of fat tissue transfer. Based on MRI scans, a 3D model of the patient's thorax is created, while the developed software generates a uniform fat graft distribution; optimizing the position and direction of the insertion pathways of the fat may limit complications and enhance quality of the surgical outcome.[52]

Three-dimensional printing in reconstructive surgery of the extremities

3D printing of the bony and soft tissue pathology of the hand and foot is an interesting example of 3D technology in reconstructive surgery of the extremities. Manufacturing a 3D model can offer multiple information to the surgeon regarding the volume of the osseous structures, the angle, the type and the fragments of a fracture, the surrounding soft tissue damage, and the biomechanics of the optimal method of surgical treatment. Chae et al. reported on the use of 3D printed haptic "reverse" models for preoperative planning in soft tissue reconstruction of the ankle. A 3D "reverse image" model was created based on the CT findings of the contralateral healthy ankle; a radial forearm free flap was then planned according to the printed model and executed effectively to precisely reconstruct the wound defect.[53]

3D technologies have been used to create new customized instruments for hand surgery, like bone reduction clamps for managing finger fractures,[54] as well as patient-specific splints for hand rehabilitation, prostheses and robotic hands.[55,56]

Recently, the concept of 4D printing was introduced, with time as the fourth dimension; Chae et al. used 3D printed models of the thumb and first metacarpal during various movements and demonstrated 4D printing. This new evolution in CT-guided stereolithographic modeling may deliver complex spatiotemporal anatomical details and, therefore, improve even more preoperative planning.[57]

Bioprinting—tissue engineering

Application of advanced 3D printing technologies to biocompatible materials, cells and supporting matrix has recently allowed the development of bioprinting, an exciting 3D printing field. Although, at the moment it is in an embryonic stage, bioprinting holds great promise for tissue regeneration, tissue engineering and artificial organ creation. The obvious advantage of biomanufacturing autologous tissue in plastic and reconstructive surgery is the dramatic reduction for need of donor sites and/or immunosuppression.[58] Many studies have reported the use of stem cells for the production of 3D bioprinted controlled tissue scaffolds, which may be used to replace complex tissue defects.[59]

Cartilage and osteochondral tissue engineering is a rapidly expanding field of 3D bioprinting applications that—if successful—may allow the regeneration, rather than the replacement, of damaged or absent cartilage, bone and joints with numerous clinical applications.[60] Theodoridis et al. used adipose-derived mesenchymal stem cells on different 3D printed scaffold patterns to develop in vitro hyaline cartilage; newly constructed cartilaginous implants were found to exhibit mechanical properties that approximated those from physiological cartilaginous tissue.[61]

Zorpf et al. implanted in a porcine model nasal and auricular porous anatomic 3D printed scaffolds, using SLS technology with polycaprolactone (PCL) and a resorbable biopolymer; after being seeded in vitro with chondrocytes, the scaffolds developed cartilage growth, and when implanted subcutaneously in pigs, they maintained foundation support and appearance.[62]

Using a rabbit model, Kim et al. implanted subperiosteally, on the nasal dorsum, 3D printed nasal scaffolds; these scaffolds were printed in PCL using FDM technology and based on CT scans of the rabbit nasal dorsum. Histologic evaluation at 4 and 12 weeks showed neovascularization into the implanted scaffolds, maintenance of implanted chondrocytes, and maturation of the cartilage with minimal inflammation; no implant extrusion was recorded.[63]

Tissue engineering has great potential for hand surgery and reconstruction after trauma, oncological resections, and congenital anomalies. As the hand represents an extremely complex structure to regenerate, hand tissue engineering focuses toward bioprinted scaffolds, which provide 3D frameworks that mimic the natural extracellular environment and enhance specific cell attachment and growth into highly functioning units.[64]

Laser-assisted bioprinting technology has been used to create fully cellularized skin substitutes, providing the possibility to position different cell types in an exact 3D spatial pattern. Using a rat model, Michael et al. positioned fibroblasts and keratinocytes on a stabilizing matrix to produce new skin; after being tested in vivo to cover skin defects, bioprinted skin showed formation of multilayer epidermis and proliferation of printed keratinocytes and collagen production by the printed fibroblasts with new blood vessels found to grow from the wound in direction of the printed cells.[14]

3D bioprinted skin, produced either in situ or in vitro, maybe an extremely promising and helpful tool in reconstructing skin defects, especially in burn patients. Its advantages, comparing to the conventional skin substitutes, are mainly due to the presence of differentiated printed cell types in precise layer-by-layer deposition, which facilitates recapitulation of native skin physiology and improves functional outcome.[65] Although skin tissue engineering is an evolving field with numerous reconstructive and cosmetic applications, several issues, i.e., vascularity, cell and scaffold combinations, and cost, need to be overcome before the wide clinical applicability of ready-to-use bioprinted skin can be realized.[66]

Overall, 3D bioprinting is a rapidly developing and very transformative technology, and its use in reconstructive surgery will lead to a paradigm shift in patient outcomes.

References

1. Freeman AE, Igel HJ, Herrman BJ, Kleinfeld KL. *In Vitro.* 1976;12(5):352−362.
2. Kamali P, Dean D, Skoracki R, Koolen PGL, Paul MA, Ibrahim AMS, Lin SJ. The current role of three-dimensional printing in plastic surgery. *Plast Reconstr Surg.* 2016; 137(3):1045−1056.
3. Hanasono MM, Jacob RF, Bidaut L, Robb GL, Skoracki RJ. Midfacial reconstruction using virtual planning, rapid prototype modeling, and stereotactic navigation. *Plast Reconstr Surg.* 2010;126(6):2002−2006.
4. Ganry L, Quilichini J, Bandini CM, Leyder P, Hersant B, Meningaud JP. Three-dimensional surgical modeling with an open source software protocol: study of precision and reproducibility in mandibular reconstruction with the fibula free flap. *Int J Oral Maxillofac Surg.* 2017;46(8):946−957.
5. Baumeister AJ, Zuriarrain A, Newman MI. Three-dimensional printing in Plastic and reconstructive surgery: a systematic review. *Ann Plast Surg.* 2016;77(5):569−576.
6. Lioufas PA, Quayle MR, Leong JC, McMenamin PG. 3D printed models of cleft palate pathology for surgical education. *Plast Reconstr Surg Glob Open.* 2016;4(9):e1029.
7. Shenaq DS, Matros E. Virtual planning and navigational technology in reconstructive surgery. *J Surg Oncol.* 2018;118(5):845−852.
8. Jacobs CA, Lin AY. A new classification of three-dimensional printing technologies: systematic review of three-dimensional printing for patient-specific craniomaxillofacial surgery. *Plast Reconstr Surg.* 2017;139(5):1211−1220.
9. Zhang C, Ma MW, Xu JJ, Lu JJ, Xie F, Yang LY, Li SY, Wu HH, Sun H, Yang B, Teng L. Application of the 3D digital ostectomy template (DOT) in mandibular angle ostectomy (MAO). *J Craniomaxillofac Surg.* 2018;46(10):1821−1827.
10. Callahan AB, Campbell AA, Petris C, Kazim M. Low-cost 3D printing orbital implant templates in secondary orbital reconstructions. *Ophthalmic Plast Reconstr Surg.* 2017; 33(5):376−380.
11. Hummelink S, Verhulst AC, Maal TJJ, Ulrich DJO. Applications and limitations of using patient- specific 3D printed molds in autologous breast reconstruction. *Eur J Plast Surg.* 2018;41(5):571−576.

12. Osagie L, Shaunak S, Murtaza A, Cerovac S, Umarji S. Advances in 3D modeling: pre-operative templating for revision wrist surgery. *Hand.* 2017;12(5):NP68−NP72.
13. Flores RL, Liss H, Raffaelli S, Humayun A, Khouri KS, Coelho PG, Witek L. The technique for 3D printing patient-specific models for auricular reconstruction. *J Craniomaxillofac Surg.* 2017;45(6):937−943.
14. Michael S, Sorg H, Peck CT, Koch L, Deiwick A, Chichkov B, Vogt PM, Reimers K. Tissue engineered skin substitutes created by laser-assisted bioprinting form skin-like structures in the dorsal skin fold chamber in mice. *PLoS One.* 2013;8(3):e57741.
15. Rozen WM, Anavekar NS, Ashton MW, Stella DL, Grinsell D, Bloom RJ, Taylor GI. Does the preoperative imaging of perforators with CT angiography improve operative outcomes in breast reconstruction? *Microsurgery.* 2008a;28(7):516−523.
16. Rozen WM, Ashton MW, Grinsell D, Stella DL, Phillips TJ, Taylor GI. Establishing the case for CT angiography in the preoperative imaging of abdominal wall perforators. *Microsurgery.* 2008b;28(5):306−313.
17. Nie JY, Lu LJ, Gong X, Li Q, Nie JJ. Delineating the vascular territory (perforasome) of a perforator in the lower extremity of the rabbit with four-dimensional computed tomographic angiography. *Plast Reconstr Surg.* 2013;131(3):565−571.
18. Paul MA, Opyrchal J, Witowski J, Ibrahim AMS, Knakiewicz M, Jaremkow P. The use of a three-dimensional printed model surgical excision of a vascular lesion in the head and neck. *J Craniofac Surg.* 2019. https://doi.org/10.1097/SCS.0000000000005541.
19. Brouwers L, Teutelink A, van Tilborg FAJB, de Jongh MAC, Lansink KWWW, Bemelman M. Validation study of 3D-printed anatomical models using 2 PLA printers for preoperative planning in trauma surgery, a human cadaver study. *Eur J Trauma Emerg Surg.* 2018. https://doi.org/10.1007/s00068-018-0970-3 [Epub ahead of print].
20. Gerstle TL, Ibrahim AS, Kim PS, Lee BT, Lin SJ. A plastic surgery application in evolution: three-dimensional printing. *Plast Reconstr Surg.* 2014;133(2):446−451.
21. Podolsky DJ, Wong Riff KW, Drake JM, Forrest CR, Fisher DM. A high fidelity cleft lip simulator. *Plast Reconstr Surg Glob Open.* 2018;6(9):e1871.
22. Ueda K, Shigemura Y, Otsuki Y, Fuse A, Mitsuno D. Three-dimensional computer assisted two-layer elastic models of the face. *Plast Reconstr Surg.* 2017;140(5):983−986.
23. Berens AM, Newman S, Bhrany AD, Murakami C, Sie KC, Zopf DA. Computer-aided design and 3D printing to produce a costal cartilage model for simulation of auricular reconstruction. *Otolaryngol Head Neck Surg.* 2016;155(2):356−359.
24. Zabaneh G, Ledeer R, Grosvenor A, Wilkes G. Rhinoplasty: a hands-on training module. *Plast Reconstr Surg.* 2009;124(3):952−954.
25. Patel A, Levine J, Brecht L, Saadeh P, Hirsch DL. Digital technologies in mandibular pathology and reconstruction. *Atlas Oral Maxillofac Surg Clin North Am.* 2012;20(1):95−106.
26. Arias E, Huang YH, Zhao L, Seelaus R, Patel P, Cohen M. Virtual surgical planning and three-dimensional guide for soft tissue correction in facial asymmetry. *J Craniofac Surg.* 2019;30(3):846−850.
27. Gillis JA, Morris SF. Three-dimensional printing of perforator vascular anatomy. *Plast Reconstr Surg.* 2014;133(1):80−82e.
28. Crafts TD, Ellsperman SE, Wannemuehler TJ, Bellicchi TD, Shipchandler TZ, Mantravadi AV. Three-dimensional printing and its applications in otorhinolaryngology-head and neck surgery. *Otolaryngol Head Neck Surg.* 2017;156(6):999−1010.
29. Sieira Gil R, Roig AM, Obispo CA, Morla A, Pages CM, Perez JL. Surgical planning and microvascular reconstruction of the mandible with a fibular flap using computer-aided

design, rapid prototype modelling, and precontoured titanium reconstruction plates: a prospective study. *Br J Oral Maxillofac Surg*. 2015;53(1):49—53.

30. Largo RD, Garvey PB. Updates in head and neck reconstruction. *Plast Reconstr Surg*. 2018;141(2):271—285e.

31. Azuma M, Yanagawa T, Ishibashi-kanno N, Uchida F, Ito T, Yamagata K, Hasegawa S, Sasaki K, Adachi K, Tabushi K, Sekido M, Bukawa H. Mandibular reconstruction using plates prebent to fit rapid prototyping 3-dimensional printing models ameliorates contour deformity. *Head Face Med*. 2014;10:45.

32. Weitz J, Bauer FJ, Hapfelmeier A, Rohleder NH, Wolff KD, Kesting MR. Accuracy of mandibular reconstruction by three-dimensional guided vascularized free fibula flap after segmental mandibulectomy. *Br J Oral Maxilofac Surg*. 2016;54(5):506—510.

33. Weitz J, Wolff KD, Kesting MR, Nobis CP. Development of a novel resection and cutting guide for mandibular reconstruction using free fibula flap. *J Craniomaxillofac Surg*. 2018;46(11):1975—1978.

34. Mao Z, Zhang N, Cui Y. Three-dimensional printing of surgical guides for mandibular distraction osteogenesis in infancy. *Medicine*. 2019;98(10):e14754.

35. Resnick CM. Precise osteotomies for mandibular distraction in infants with Robin sequence using virtual surgical planning. *Int J Oral Maxillofac Surg*. 2018;47(1):35—43.

36. Shui W, Zhou M, Chen S, Pan Z, Deng Q, Yao Y, Pan H, He T, Wang X. The production of digital and printed resources from multi-ple modalities using visualization and three-dimensional printing techniques. *Int J Comput Assist Radiol Surg*. 2017;12(1):13—23.

37. Levine JP, Bae JS, Soares M, Brecht LE, Saadeh PB, Ceradini DJ, Hirsch DL. Jaw in a day: total maxillofacial reconstruction using digital technology. *Plast Reconstr Surg*. 2013;131(6):1386—1391.

38. Hirsch DL, Garfein ES, Christensen AM, Weimer KA, Saddeh PB, Levine JP. Use of computer-aided design and computer-aided manufacturing to produce orthognathically ideal surgical outcomes: a paradigm shift in head and neck reconstruction. *J Oral Maxillofac Surg*. 2009;67(10):2115—2122.

39. Zweifel DF, Simon C, Hoarau R, Pasche P, Broome M. Are virtual planning and guided surgery for head and neck reconstruction economically viable? *J Oral Maxillofac Surg*. 2015;73(1):170—175.

40. Ritschl LM, Mucke T, Fichter A, Gull FD, Schmid C, Duc JMP, et al. Functional outcome of CAD/CAM-assisted versus conventional microvascular, fibular free flap reconstruction of the mandible: a retrospective study of 30 cases. *J Reconstr Microsurg*. 2017;33(4):281—291.

41. Zimmerer RM, Ellis E, Aniceto GS, Schramm A, Wagner ME, Grant MP, Cornelius CP, Strong EB, Rana M, Chye LT, Calle AR, Wilde F, Perez D, Tavassol F, Bittermann G, Mahoney NR, Alamillos MR, Basic J, Dittmann J, Rasse M, Gellrich NC. A prospective multicenter study to compare the precision of posttraumatic internal orbital reconstruction with standard preformed and individualized orbital implants. *J Craniomaxillofac Surg*. 2016;44(9):1485—1497.

42. Visscher DO, te Slaa S, Jaspers ME, van de Hulsbeek M, Borst J, Wolff J, Forouzanfar T, van Zuijlen PP. 3D printing of patient-specific neck splints for the treatment of post-burn neck contractures. *Burns Trauma*. 2018;6:15. https://doi.org/10.1186/s41038-018-0116-1. eCollection 2018.

43. Hirohi T, Nagai K, Ng D, Harii K. Integrated forehead and temporal augmentation using 3d printing-assisted methyl methacrylate implants. *Aesthet Surg J*. 2018;38(11):1157—1168.

44. Chae MP, Hunter-Smith DJ, Spychal RT, Rozen WM. 3D volumetric analysis for planning breast reconstructive surgery. *Breast Cancer Res Treat*. 2014;146(2):457−460.

45. Blondeel PN, Hijjawi J, Depypere H, Roche N, Van Landuyt K. Shaping the breast in aesthetic and reconstructive surgery: an easy three-step principle. *Plast Reconstr Surg*. 2009;123(2):455−462.

46. Dionyssiou D, Demiri E, Davison J. A simple method for determining the breast implant size in augmentation mammoplasty. *A esth Plast Surg*. 2005;29(6):571−573.

47. Dionyssiou D, Demiri E, Tsimponis A, Boorman J. Predesigned breast shaping assisted by multidetector row CT angiography in autologous breast reconstruction. *Plast Reconstr Surg*. 2014;133(2):100−108e.

48. Tepper OM, Small K, Rudolph L, Choi M, Karp N. Virtual 3-dimensional modeling as a valuable adjunct to aesthetic and reconstructive breast surgery. *Am J Surg*. 2006;192(4):548−551.

49. Tepper OM, Small KH, Unger JG, Feldman DL, Kumar N, Choi M, Karp NS. 3D analysis of breast augmentation defines operative changes and their relationship to implant dimensions. *Ann Plast Surg*. 2009;62(5):570−575.

50. Eder M, Waldenfels FV, Sichtermann M, Schuster T, Papadopulos NA, Machens HG, Biemer E, Kovacs L. Three-dimensional evaluation of breast contour and volume changes following subpectoral augmentation mammaplasty over 6 months. *J Plast Reconstr Aesthet Surg*. 2011;64(9):1152−1160.

51. Yang J, Zhang R, Shen J, Hu Y, Lv Q. The three-dimensional techniques in the objective measurement of breast aesthetics. *Aesthetic Plast Surg*. 2015;39(6):910−915.

52. Patete P, Rigotti G, Marchi A, Baroni G. Computer assisted planning of autologous fat grafting in breast. *Comput Aided Surg*. 2013;18(1−2):10−18.

53. Chae MP, Lin F, Spychal RT, Hunter-Smith DJ, Rozen WM. 3D-printed haptic "reverse" models for preoperative planning in soft-tissue reconstruction: a case report. *Microsurgery*. 2015b;35(2):148−153.

54. Fuller SM, Butz DR, Vevang CB, Makhlouf MV. Application of 3-dimensional printing in hand surgery for production of a novel reduction clamp. *J Hand Surg Am*. 2014;39(9):1840−1845.

55. Cui Lei, Phan A, Allison G. Design and fabrication of a three dimensional printable non-assembly articulated hand exoskeleton for rehabilitation. *Conf Proc IEEE Eng Med Biol Soc*. 2015;2015:4627−4630.

56. Vujaklija I, Farina D. 3D printed upper limb prosthetics. *Expert Rev Med Devices*. 2018;15(7):505−512.

57. Chae MP, Hunter-Smith DJ, De-Silva I, Tham S, Spychal RT, Rozen WM. Four-dimensional (4D) printing: a new evolution in computed tomography-guided stereolithographic modeling. Principles and application. *J Reconstr Microsurg*. 2015a;31(6):458−463.

58. Jessop ZM, Al-Sabah A, Gardiner MD, Combellack E, Hawkins K, Whitaker IS. 3D bioprinting for reconstructive surgery: principles, applications and challenges. *J Plast Reconstr Aesthet Surg*. 2017;70(9):1155−1170.

59. Ong CS, Yesantharao P, Huang CY, Mattson G, Boktor J, Fukunishi T, Zhang H, Hibino N. 3D bioprinting using stem cells. *Pediatr Res*. 2018;83(1−2):223−231.

60. Daly AC, Freeman FE, Gonzalez-Fernandez T, Critchley SE, Nulty J, Kelly DJ. 3D bioprinting for cartilage and osteochondral engineering. *Adv Healthc Mater*. 2017;6(22). https://doi.org/10.1002/adhm.201700298 [Epub 2017 Aug 14].

61. Theodoridis K, Aggelidou E, Vavilis T, Manthou ME, Tsimponis A, Demiri EC, Boukla A, Salpistis C, Bakopoulou A, Mihailidis A, Kritis A. Hyaline cartilage next

generation implants from adipose-derived mesenchymal stem cells: Comparative study on 3D-printed polycaprolactone patterns. *J Tissue Eng Regen Med.* 2019;13(2): 342−355.

62. Zopf DA, Mitsak AG, Flanagan CL, Wheeler M, Green GE, Hollister GJ. Computer aided-designed, 3-dimensionally printed porous tissue bioscaffolds for craniofacial soft tissue reconstruction. *Otolaryngol Head Neck Surg.* 2015;152(1):57−62.

63. Kim YS, Shin YS, Park DY, Choi JW, Park JK, Kim DH, Kim CH, Park SA. The application of three-dimensional printing in animal model of augmentation rhinoplasty. *Ann Biomed Eng.* 2015;43(9):2153−2162.

64. Kloczko E, Nikkhah D, Yildirimer L. Scaffolds for hand tissue engineering: the importance of surface topography. *J Hand Surg Eur.* 2015;40(9):973−985.

65. Varkey M, Visscher DO, van Zuijlen PPM, Atala A, Yoo JJ. Skin bioprinting: the future of burn wound reconstruction? *Burns Trauma.* 2019;7:4. https://doi.org/10.1186/s41038-019-0142-7. eCollection 2019.

66. Tarassoli SP, Jessop ZM, Al-Sabah A, Gao N, Whitaker S, Doak S, Whitaker IS. Skin tissue engineering using 3D bioprinting: An evolving research field. *J Plast Reconstr Aesthet Surg.* 2018;71(5):615−623.

Three-dimensional printing in colorectal surgery

Constantine P. Spanos, MD, FACS, FASCRS, MBA [1], **Marianna P. Spanos, BA** [2]

[1]*Doctor, Surgery, Aristotelian University, Thessaloniki, Greece;* [2]*Center for Human Genetics, Cambridge, Massachusetts, United States*

Introduction

Three-dimensional (3D) printing is an engineering process during which a 3D object is created by applying various materials using a computer-generated model.[1] Materials are usually applied layer by layer.[1,2] The process can be broken down into the following components:

- Image acquisition/creation
- Modeling: In which computer-aided design (CAD) software, a scanner, or a digital camera creates a digital 3D rendering of an object
- Printing: Several modalities are currently available for 3D printing. Stereolithography uses a liquid photoactive resin that is solidified by ultraviolet light. Fuel deposition modeling uses heat to create object from molten plastics. Multijet modeling uses multiple materials to create color-coded objects at high resolution. These modalities vary in their resolution quality, time to print, and cost.[1−3]

3D printing has application in a multitude of industries. Product design and engineering as well as the automotive industry were initial adopters of the discipline.[4] In medicine, 3D printing has the potential to be useful in several aspects. Anatomic models, especially those based on individual patient anatomy, can be used for educational purposes, preoperative planning, and training.[3] Surgical instruments and implants and prostheses can be manufactured using 3D printing.[3] In many instances, these "prints" can be customized to a patient's anatomic characteristics.

This segment will focus on the current application of 3D printing in the specialty of colorectal surgery.

Colorectal surgery

The specialty of colorectal surgery is unique in several aspects. It covers a large part of the visceral anatomy. Many disorders in colorectal surgery are associated with or

3D Printing: Applications in Medical Surgery. https://doi.org/10.1016/B978-0-323-66193-5.00011-3

located in the pelvis, a part of the human body with intricate anatomical detail, involving the digestive tract, complex vascular anatomy, and the nervous system. The anorectal region is also intricate in its anatomy. Surgery on any part of the anatomical structures associated with colorectal surgery may affect the anatomical integrity, as well as function of one or more structures aforementioned. In theory, this specialty may lend itself to several applications of 3D printing. Several reports have been published demonstrating the feasibility of 3D printing in colorectal surgery.

Preoperative planning in rectal cancer

Hanabe and Ito[5] used a 3D printed model of the pelvis to facilitate the understanding of anatomy in rectal cancer. The end goal was to aid the surgeon in laparoscopic rectal cancer resection. A multidetector CT scan was used to acquire arterial and venous images with axial thin-slice reconstruction. With the aid of CAD software and a 3D printer, pelvic models with all vital structures (bones, muscles, iliac vessels and branches, nerves, and urogenital organs) were created. Even though the model was of high quality, the long printing time of 40 h and the inelastic nature of the printing material were limiting factors. The model demonstrated the complex special relationships between the pelvic structures but could not replicate the texture of live tissue, as well as the mechanics of an actual surgical procedure realistically.

Preoperative planning in total mesocolic excision for right colon cancer

Total mesocolic excision is employed as a surgical method of extended mesocolic lymphadenectomy for potential optimal oncologic outcomes in right colon cancer resections. One of the key aspects of the operation is careful dissection of the middle colic artery and vein, the venous gastrocolic trunk. This anatomic structure has great variability from patient to patient. Garcia-Granero et al[6] used a 3D model printed after CT scanning of a patient with right colon cancer. Initially, a multidetector CT scan of the patient was obtained. Arterial and venous images were acquired. Thin-sliced axial images were then reconstructed using CAD software. Major vascular structures were identified (aorta, vena cava, inferior mesenteric artery and vein, superior mesenteric artery and vein). The gastrocolic venous trunk structures were depicted, as were the viscera. A 3D model was printed, and the patient underwent laparoscopic right hemicolectomy with complete mesocolic excision based on the model. In a similar fashion, Luzon et al[7] used 3D printing to evaluate the linear dimensional differences in the anatomical landmarks of the superior mesenteric artery and vein among 3D virtual models, 3D printed models, and preoperative measurements. This study concluded that there were acceptable correlations between 3D printed models, 3D virtual models, and live tissue, thus providing for a potentially useful visual aid preoperatively or intraoperatively.

3D printing in colorectal metastatic disease

3D printing can be employed in the preoperative planning of colorectal hepatic metastases. Tumor location, relationship to vascular structures, and tumor volume can be depicted to facilitate development of the surgical strategy to be followed. Witowski et al[8] printed a 3D model of the liver in a patient with a single metastatic lesion 2 years postlaparoscopic colectomy. The printing process took 72 h. The model was carefully examined by the operating team preoperatively, and it was used during surgery for guidance. Igami et al[9] used a 3D printed liver model in two patients with colorectal metastases who received preoperative chemotherapy. The resections of the lesions were performed using the 3D printed model for guidance.

Finally, 3D printing has been used to evaluate the response of colorectal liver metastases to chemotherapy. Choi et al[10] used a personalized 3D printed tumor model to assess the accuracy of 3D ultrasound in the evaluation of hepatic metastases from colorectal cancer. In this study, there was a correlation between tumor volume on CT and a 3D ultrasound study of the printed liver "tumors" before and after chemotherapy. The investigators concluded the model was accurate and reliable in the evaluation of tumor response to therapy.

Sacral neuromulation: 3D printed guidance for electrode implantation

Sacral neuromodulation is an established modality for the treatment of fecal incontinence and constipation. It involves the implantation of a special tined electrode through the sacral foramina. The tined electrode is connected to a temporary neuromodulator/generator for a test trail. If the test trial proves successful (i.e., 50% improvement in symptoms of incontinence or constipation), a permanent neuromodulator/generator is connected to the tined electrode and implanted usually in the subcutaneous tissue of the patient's lower lumbar region. The critical portion of the entire procedure is the correct placement of the tined electrode through the sacral foramen. This is greatly dependent on the patient's individual sacral anatomy. Cui et al[11] used 3D printing to help guide the placement of the electrodes for neuromodulation utilizing a 3D image of sacrum in two patients with intractable constipation. The 3D sacral image was used as a template to help print guiding test needles for the insertion of the tined electrodes. This was in essence a guiding device that facilitated determination of the appropriate sacral foramen (from S2 to S4) through which optimal placement of the electrode could be achieved.

Anal fistula surgery

Anal fistulae can be the bane of many a colorectal surgeon. Fistula anatomy is highly individualized and frequently complex. Recurrence is common when secondary extensions of fistula tracts are not dealt with. There is always a potential for surgical iatrogenic sphincter complex injury with resulting fecal incontinence and poor quality of life. Furthermore, there is no standard of care in fistula surgery, with a multitude of procedures available and variable outcomes. Preoperative imaging of the precise individual fistula anatomy and the relationship of fistula to the sphincter complex may be of great value in the planning of anal fistula surgery. Sahnan et al[12] used MRI sequences of anal fistulae in three patients to allow for segmentation of the fistula tracts and subsequent 3D printing of the fistula anal sphincters and levator ani plate. This study proved the feasibility of 3D reconstruction of anal fistula tracts and the potential benefits it may have in surgical planning, patient education, and surgical training. Bageas et al[13] also used a 3D printed fistula model of a patient to facilitate training of resident surgeons in randomized, prospective study.

Lateral pelvic lymph node dissection using a 3D printed pelvic model for education

Lateral pelvic lymph node dissection is the standard surgical technique in the treatment of locally advanced rectal cancer in Japan. This procedure is technically demanding and has a steep learning curve. This is secondary to the complexity of the pelvic anatomy and the close relationship between lymphatic tissue and major vascular structures and nerves. Cadaveric dissection has been considered helpful in the mastery of pelvic anatomy and surgery. Limited supply of cadavers has led to alternative methods to facilitate learning pelvic anatomy. Hojo et al[14] created a 3D pelvic model to educate medical students, surgical residents, and young surgeons in pelvic anatomy in rectal cancer patients. The investigators performed a single-center, open-label randomized controlled trial comparing a 3D printed model to a textbook in pelvic anatomy education. They found the utilization of the 3D model superior to the textbook in this aspect.

Conclusion

The application of 3D printing in colorectal surgery is at an embryonic stage of development. There have been few reports demonstrating the feasibility of using this technology in various aspects of the specialty. The most notable examples are utilization in preoperative planning and surgical education. There have been no prospective, randomized trials that demonstrate improved patient outcomes as a result of using 3D printing in colorectal surgery. Two randomized controlled studies reported an improvement in aspects of education in pelvic anatomy and fistula surgery.[13,14] In theory, 3D printed models can augment the study of images and textbook when reviewing a specific patient for surgical treatment. A significant limitation of 3D printing is the time to produce a model for use, as well as the cost. The widespread adoption of 3D printing in colorectal surgery remains to be seen.

References

1. Emile SH, Wexner SD. Systematic review of the applications of three-dimensional printing in colorectal surgery. *Colorectal Dis*. 2018;21:261−269.
2. Papazarkadas X, Spartalis E, Patsouras D, et al. The role of 3D printing in colorectal surgery: current evidence and perspectives. *In Vivo*. 2019;33:297−302.
3. Malik HH, Darwood AR, Shaunak S, et al. Three-dimensional printing in surgery: a review of current surgical applications. *J Surg Res*. 2015;199:512−522.
4. Kroll E, Artzi D. Enhancing aerospace engineering students' learning with 3D printing and wind-tunnel models. *Rapid Prototyp J*. 2011;17:393−402.
5. Hanabe A, Ito M. A three-dimensional pelvic model made with a three-dimensional printer: applications for laparoscopic surgery to treat rectal cancer. *Tech Coloproctol*. 2017;21:383−387.
6. Garcia-Granero A, Sanchez-Guillen L, Fletcher-Sanfeliu D, et al. Application of three-dimensional printing in laparoscopic dissection to facilitate D3-lympadenectomy for right colon cancer. *Tech Coloproctol*. 2018;22:129−133.
7. Luzon JA, Andersen BT, Stimec BV, et al. Implementation of 3D printed superior mesenteric vascular models for surgeical planning and/or navigation in right colectomy with extended D3 mesenterectomy: comparison of virtual and physical models to the anatomy found at surgery. *Surg Endosc*. 2018. https://doi.org/10.1007/s00464-018-6332-8.
8. Witowski JS, Pedziwiatr M, Major P, et al. A cost-effective, personalized, 3D-printed liver model for preoperative planning before laparoscopic liver hemihepatectomy for colorectal cancer metastases. *Int J Comput Assist Radiol Surg*. 2017;12:2047−2054.
9. Igami T, Nakamura Y, Hirose T, et al. Application of a three-dimensional print of liver in hepatectomy for small tumors invisible by intraoperative ultrasonography: preliminary experience. *World J Surg*. 2014;38:3163−3166.
10. Choi YR, Kim JH, Park SJ, et al. Threapeutic response assessment using 3D ultrasound for hepatic metastasis from colorectal cancer: application of a personalized, 3D-printed tumor model using CT images. *PLoS One*. 2017;12:c0182596.
11. Cui Z, Wang Z, Ye G, et al. A novel three-dimensional printed guiding device for electrode implantation of sacral neuromodulation. *Colorectal Dis*. 2018;20:O26−O29.
12. Sahnan K, Adegbola SO, Tozer PJ, et al. Innovation in the imaging of perianal fistula: a step towards personalized medicine. *Therap Adv Gastroenterol*. 2018;11, 17562848187.
13. Bangeas P, Drevelegas K, Agorastou C, et al. Thre-dimensional printing as an educational tool in colorectal surgery. *Front Biosci*. 2018. https://doi.org/10.2741/13487.
14. Hojo D, Murono K, Nozawa H, et al. Utility of a three-dimensional printed pelvic model for a lateral pelvic lymph node dissection education: a randomized controlled trial. *J Am Coll Surg*. 2019;229:522−559.

3D printing in adult and pediatric neurosurgery: the present and the future

12

Stavros Polyzoidis, MD, PhD [1]**, Laura Stone McGuire, MD** [2]**, Dimitrios Nikas, MD** [2]**,**
Keyoumars Ashkan, FRCS, MD [3]

[1]*Department of Neurosurgery, AHEPA Hospital, Aristotle University of Thessaloniki, Thessaloniki, Greece;* [2]*Department of Neurosurgery University of Illinois at Chicago, Chicago, IL, United States;* [3]*Department of Neurosurgery, King's College Hospital London, King's College London, London, United Kingdom*

Abbreviations

2D	Two-dimensional
3D	Three-dimensional
AR	Augmented reality
AVM	Arteriovenous malformation
CT	Computed tomography
CTA	Computed tomography angiography
FDA	Food and Drug Administration
LITT	Laser interstitial thermal therapy
MCA	Middle cerebral artery
MRI	Magnetic resonance imaging
TOF MRA	Time-of-flight magnetic resonance angiography
VR	Virtual reality

Introduction

The technology of three-dimensional (3D) printing has emerged since a few decades now and it has been described as a transformative technology with the potential to reform medicine. In neurosurgery, with the wide variety of pathologies and the broad use of innovative technologies, 3D printing has gradually been introduced as an adjunct tool to daily practice. Still, it has not been integrated as yet in the clinical routine or as part of standard of care in the vast majority of neurosurgical activities worldwide. Although 3D printed custom-made xenografts for cranioplasty are a fine example of its applications, presently the use of 3D printing technology is relatively not widespread and is mainly being used for educational, patient consultation, and preoperative planning purposes.

However, technological advances have streamlined the manufacturing processes and decreased purchase and production costs, while the range of materials used has expanded. Undoubtedly, the above have rendered 3D printing technology very promising and more accessible, with a great potential to play a core role in the concept of personalized medicine in the ever-evolving field of neurosurgery. In this respect, numerous potential applications of 3D printing have been proposed both in adult and pediatric neurosurgery, crystallizing the transition from the "one-size-fits-all" to the "tailor-made" concept of neurosurgical clinical practice.

As mentioned above, the introduction and expansion of 3D printing within the field of neurosurgery has prompted multiple new uses of this technology, from preoperative planning to surgical teaching and assessment. However, while earlier uses of 3D printing in neurosurgery primarily focused on the development of accurate patient-specific models, more recent studies integrate 3D printed models into neurosurgical training, in the manufacturing of implants, and in combining 3D printed features with virtual reality (VR) or augmented reality (AR) for enhanced simulated cases.

This chapter will review the current clinical applications described in the literature, the modalities of 3D printing implemented, and the advantages and limitations of its use and will further discuss potential future directions of the technology within both adult and pediatric neurosurgery. While specific 3D printing modalities utilized in neurosurgery may be briefly described, a detailed discussion of these printing methodologies and the 3D printing software available will be beyond the scope of this chapter.

Applications

In a recent systematic review, Randazzo et al.[1] described the applications of 3D printing as falling within the following categories: surgical planning and modeling, training and simulation, and neurosurgical devices and implants. These uses of 3D printing have been examined within the full spectrum of neurosurgical subspecialties, from spine and neuro-oncology to cerebrovascular and functional. Another recent review by Langridge et al.[2] further details the uses of 3D printing within surgical teaching and assessment, identifying neurosurgery as one of the most common specialties in which this technology has been employed for this purpose. The following sections highlight some of the applications of 3D printing within the subspecialties of adult and pediatric neurosurgery.

Adult neurosurgery

Spinal surgery

As we are further entering the era of patient-specific spinal surgery, the ultimate target is further improving outcomes. 3D printed custom-made spinal implants, biometric magnetic resonance imaging (MRI) along with simulated training, and robotic surgery can offer better accuracy and precision and thus improve outcomes, while at the same time reduce surgery time, implant failures, intraoperative radiation exposure, and hospitalization lengths. In spinal surgery, 3D printing has been implemented for the development of surgical implants, training simulators, models for preoperative planning, and intraoperative screw and osteotomy guides.

Biomechanically optimal spinal implants should address the need (1) for correcting angles for sagittal, coronal, and axial balance; (2) for ideal distribution of forces and loads; (3) for proportional intervertebral height, width, and shape; (4) for as much as possible motion preservation; and (5) for protection of nervous tissue and neurological function. The task of manufacturing such implants is both complex and demanding. Current, uniform implants abound in beneficial properties, but also have their limitations and cannot always address the specific needs of each individual patient.

Multiple implants have been designed for use in spinal surgery, and some have been commercially adapted within the past few years. Cheng et al.[3,4] developed 3D printed scaffolds with polylactic acid plastic coated with bone morphogenic protein to promote osteogenesis in spine surgery. An example of a commercially available and the Food and Drug Administration (FDA)-approved product, Osseus Fusion Systems designed and 3D printed the titanium implant, called Aries-L interbody fusion device, to mimic the natural architecture of bone matrix. As another FDA-approved example, a multilevel cervical cage has been produced by Emerging Implant Technologies GmbH using its trademark Cellular Titanium technology. Additionally, tissue-engineered solutions using 3D printing have also been explored in the spine subspecialty of neurosurgery, including the treatment of intervertebral disc degeneration with an elastic scaffold.[5]

Additionally, training models for a variety of spinal procedures have been developed. Apart from the traditional saw bone model for pedicle screw placement, which can be readily produced via 3D printing, more advanced systems have been created. A cervical laminectomy simulation has been produced with a multilayered surgical phantom, fabricated by filling molds with hydrogels, plaster, and fiberglass, with a pressure transducer to measure spinal cord manipulation.[6] Additional simulators modeled the technique for sacral screw placement using custom-made surgical instruments[7] and developed a model for procedural training in cervical myelography.[8]

Furthermore, 3D printed models guide preoperative planning. A novel synthetic spine model for use in corrective scoliosis surgery accurately mimicked anatomy and biomechanical properties in two adult patients and found comparable surgical correction performed on the 3D printed model to the later operative findings.[9] Revision surgeries pose a complex challenge to spine surgeons, and a 3D printed patient-specific template aided surgeons in safe pedicle screw placement in revision pediatric kyphoscoliosis surgery.[10] In a series of seven patients, Lador et al.[11] demonstrated multiple uses of 3D printing technology in spine oncology— from producing custom-made titanium implants to generating replicas of spinal pathology for surgical planning.

Similar to the use of 3D printed models in other subspecialties, it has been found to strengthen patient–physician communication. A study of 45 patients found that 3D printed models of lumbar spine advanced patient education;[12] personalized 3D printed models not only enhanced understanding of lumbar anatomy, physiology, and patients' disease and surgical plan but they also improved patients' subjective satisfaction.

Neuro-oncology

The field of surgical neuro-oncology has similarly implemented 3D printing in surgical planning and training simulators. While improvements in visualization of neuroanatomy, including the advancement of MRI, have granted better understanding of tissue planes between normal brain and abnormal tumor, this two-dimensional (2D) representation of the pathology remains limited in demonstrating physical relationships between structures; even 3D reconstructions are depicted on a flat monitor or, at best, with VR or AR devices. Thus, patient-specific modeling with 3D printing technology helps to provide surgeons with a better understanding of anatomical landmarks. Further, 3D printers may use a variety of materials to produce the model to mimic the texture and consistency of different tissue and tumor types, which strengthens the realism of the reproduction.[13] Additionally, some studies have combined 3D prototyping with other visualization techniques. Spottiswoode et al.[14] added functional MRI to 3D printed brain models in preoperative planning to highlight eloquent cortex. Oishi et al.[15] combined an interactive VR simulation with a 3D printed replication of patient anatomy for presurgical preparation in skull base tumors and found utility in determining the optimal surgical strategy.

In addition to the production of models for preoperative planning and training simulators, neurosurgical devices have also been produced. Recently, Mirani et al.[16] fabricated a 3D printed drug-eluting hydrogel mesh laden with all-trans retinoic acid for the treatment of glioblastoma, warranting further research into this modality of adjuvant therapy delivery. Another application of 3D printing created a proton range compensator, providing a conformal dose distribution during proton therapy and protecting tissue surrounding the tumor; this 3D printed technology minimized the space and cost requirements of a proton facility and its manufacturing processes, with concomitant improvements in accuracy.[17]

Tailor-made radiotherapy and radiosurgery (Cyberknife, Novalis, Gamma Knife, etc.) treatments can be further improved by use of 3D printing. 3D prototypes depicting the precise anatomy and proximity of tumors to crucial and eloquent structures help simulate and stratify the physics, treatment strategy, radiation dose, and number of sessions of radiotherapy and radiosurgery. The use of frame-based masks in radiotherapy is a current application of 3D printing in neuro-oncology, while treatments such as tumor treating fields and laser interstitial thermal therapy (LITT) are already benefiting from 3D prototyping and can be further evolved by use of it.

Vascular neurosurgery

As endovascular and radiosurgical therapies for intracranial tumors, aneurysms, and vascular malformations increase, opportunities for training in microsurgical approaches decrease; however, the advancement of 3D printing technologies facilitates such education through simulation. The advent of 3D printing enabled the production of patient-specific vascular networks within patients, representing 2D medical imaging in a tangible, physical form that could be integrated into surgical planning and training.[18] The literature describes 3D printing in producing models for cerebrovascular anatomy, intracranial aneurysms, vascular malformations, and intracranial stenosis.

Throughout the literature, studies have shown that 3D printing can accurately and reliably reproduce complex vascular networks from patient source imaging. Mashiko et al.[19,20] used preoperative imaging studies to create both solid and hollow 3D configurations in less than 24 h and demonstrated excellent correlations between the models and the intraoperative anatomy. Thawani et al.[21] produced a 3D model of an arteriovenous malformation (AVM) with a 0.1 mm accuracy when compared to source imaging, with fast throughput, and colored according to blood flow (arterial vs. venous).

While some models include only vascular networks, others include the skin, skull, dura, and brain tissue to enhance realism. For instance, Nagassa et al.[22] constructed a patient-derived middle cerebral artery (MCA) aneurysm training model combining 3D printing with casting techniques—including components of the skin, skull, brain, and vasculature—to generate an aneurysm surgery simulator, which could be further implemented in training. Earlier 3D prototypes of vascular structures typically used CT or rotational angiography as source images; however, newer studies have sought to validate magnetic resonance—based imaging modalities also, most recently with 3D time-of-flight magnetic resonance angiography.[23] Multiple methods to validate the vasculature printed to actual anatomy have been implemented, including qualitative visual comparison and quantitative measurements.[1]

The use of these models in preoperative planning and rehearsal confers benefit in improved patient outcomes. In aneurysm surgery, for example, when the time required to choose a clip corresponds to the time required to temporarily occlude a parent vessel, effective preoperative planning matters. In another study, with the incorporation of aneurysm models into preoperative practice, simulation resulted in few number of clips applied or removed in the operating room.[19,20] In a study using computed tomography angiography—based 3D printed models of seven MCA aneurysm patients, the simulator proved useful for choosing the clips before surgery.[24] In two cases of pediatric AVM extirpations when compared to matched control cases, Weinstock et al.[25] reduced intraoperative time by 12%.

Additionally, in stereotactic radiosurgical treatment of vascular lesions, 3D printing decreased the time required for contouring target AVMs.[26] Endovascular applications in treatment planning have also emerged, whereby rehearsing the intervention can decrease procedural time, radiation dose, and possible complications. Namba et al.[27] used 3D printing of both solid and hollow aneurysm models to plan and shape the microcatheter required for coiling and further successfully implemented its use in 10 consecutive cases.

With 3D printing, cerebrovascular bioimplants have also been developed. Using biocompatible silver nanoparticles and polyamide, Herbert et al.[28] developed a low-profile, 3D printed, wireless electronic, implantable biodevice to measure and monitor cerebral aneurysm hemodynamics.

Along similar lines, in the future, vascular lesions could be treated with custom-made clips and endovascular devices/implants. As aneurysms either complex or not are crucial cerebral pathologies, their treatment, either surgical or endovascular, requires special instruments and special clips, grafts, coils, stents, or diverters. The special anatomy of parent vessels and the presence of arterial branches arising from the aneurysm dome warrant the use of devices with special architecture adapting to the actual architecture, caliber, and angles of the pathology. This perspective along with preoperative case-based simulation points toward the direction of less vascular injuries, less operative time, less clip removals and revisions, less radiation exposures, and subsequently improved outcomes.

Functional neurosurgery

Functional neurosurgery also represents a field with numerous potential applications of 3D printing. It relies on precision, which is a threefold process based on detailed anatomical illustration, recognition of surgical target, and accurate intervention. The more meticulous the insertion of electrodes and grids, the more targeted is the stimulation and recording of brain activity. That is achieved with individualized planning for each patient, as it is well known that the brain (cortex and deeper structures) is characterized by morphological and functional variability,[29] while gyral and sulcal patterns are unique for each individual as fingerprints. Ono et al in 1990 provided in their atlas standardized morphological criteria to define and identify each sulcus of the human brain. Still, there are significant variations in the shape, size, and spatial pattern of gyri and sulci between normal individuals, which is even more pronounced in pathological conditions.[30–33] With the use of 3D printing, preoperative planning and simulation can be furthermore detailed, while custom-made electrodes and grids based on patient-specific anatomical and functional imaging (MRI, functional MRI, and transcranial magnetic stimulation) can definitely enhance precision and contribute toward the elimination of technique and treatment side effects and failures, and therefore improve patient outcomes.

Stereotactic frame placement has also been examined with 3D printing technology. Several companies have emerged in this sphere; for instance, both the NeuroBlate and also STarFix systems utilize 3D printing to rapidly produce patient-specific frames. A study of 263 patients using the STarFix microTargeting platform for deep brain stimulation found comparable clinical accuracy and patient outcome when compared to traditional stereotactic frame systems.[34] In two studies, each with five patients requiring LITT, 3D printed stereotactic frames were effectively rendered to guide LITT catheter placement.[35,36]

With epilepsy surgery, 3D printing strengthens precision to best target regions of the brain for electrode placement and subsequently identify the epileptogenic focus or foci. To plan depth electrode placement in epilepsy surgery, Javan et al.[37] developed a novel 3D printed brain model with a mesh-like surface to visualize the deep structures. Naftulin et al.[38] created a cost-effective model for simulation of the placement of surface electrodes, whereby surgeons placed electrodes directly onto the model to optimize surgical coverage. Furthermore, researchers have printed personalized silicone sheets to embed electrodes, for instance, for brain—machine interfaces (Hirata et al.[39]; Morris et al.[40]).

Neurotrauma

The most commonly studied use of 3D printing in neurotrauma involves repair of skull defects following craniectomies. In this domain, recent studies focus on the development of low-cost cranioplasties.[41,42] Others have trialed different materials in the development of implants, such as calcium phosphate.[43] In order to address temporalis muscle hollowing, a modified 3D printed cranial implant was designed, where the anteroinferior border of the implant was extended and elevated between the frontozygomatic suture and root of zygomatic process, which led to superior aesthetic outcomes.[44] Advances in the printing of cranial flaps include biological implants. 3D printing hydrogels and skull scaffolds may improve patient outcomes by promoting cell growth around an implant and decreasing risk of infection or inflammation that may occur with other implant materials.[43] Chen et al.[45] developed a multilevel customized 3D printing strategy to apply an autogenous bone matrix for the repair of skull defects; in this, in vivo implants integrated tightly to the defects' margin, facilitated mineralization, and generated vascularized mature bone.

In addition to the studies regarding cranioplasties, other studies in neurotrauma have examined 3D printing in training residents. Ryan et al.[46] developed a low-cost simulator for the placement of external ventricular drains using patient-specific, 3D printed ventricular anatomy, in combination with a gravity-driven pump for the fluid to provide normal and abnormal ventricular pressures. Another system for ventriculostomy training employs a mixed reality setting, linking an electromagnetic tracking system to a virtual depiction of the positioning of the catheter.[47] Beyond training of neurosurgical residents, Bishop et al.[48] focused on the training of rural practitioners who are based at hospitals remote from tertiary neurosurgical centers. They generated a 3D printed simulator for burr holes and craniotomies for the treatment of head trauma requiring immediate surgery, aiming for potentially getting these operations performed by rural practitioners in case when transfer delays can be detrimental.

Custom-made skin, skull, and dura grafts for scalp, skull, and dura gaps

Tissue engineering combined with 3D printing technologies could render possible the less costly and more massive production of autologous and homologous skin, bone, and dura grafts. Skin grafting, mainly in the form of acellular scaffolds combined with autologous skin cells, has been shown to provide a very valid option for wound closure in burns.[49] 3D printing can contribute to the development of more stable vascular and lymphatic networks enabling the production of full-thickness skin grafts to cover skin gaps of traumatic or infectious etiology. Bone graft technologies have been significantly advancing since more than 4 decades now and have been mentioned in previous sections. Additionally, Liu et al.[50] reported the use of artificial 3D printed dura for the treatment of sacral canal (Tarlov) cysts. These dura matter patches were used for dural wrapping after cyst wall was open and removed, while no CSF leak, infection, or meningitis was reported. Such dura grafts can have numerous applications and can be used at any site along the neuroaxis.

Pediatric neurosurgery

If there is one field of neurosurgery that highlights the impact of 3D printing on better training and improved outcomes, that is pediatric neurosurgery. The almost absolute lack of cadaveric teaching options and the absence of a realistic alternative for hands-on training render rapid prototyping a unique option for the development of surgical skills and planning off theater. This need is even more pronounced in the case of skull deformities and trauma, which present in high rates in the pediatric population.[51]

In general, the literature on 3D printing in pediatric neurosurgery overlaps with uses in neuro-oncology, cerebrovascular,[25,52] spine,[10,53] trauma,[41] and functional surgery. However, 3D printing most often described in pediatric neurosurgery falls within craniofacial surgery, including the treatment of craniosynostosis and the generation of custom implants. Garcia-Mato et al.[54] recently proposed a workflow in the management of craniosynostosis that combines multiple techniques, utilizing virtual surgical planning, computer-aided design of osteotomy guides, 3D printed templates, and intraoperative navigation.

Other studies have similarly described the use of 3D printed osteotomy templates in the treatment of synostosis to improve cosmetic results,[41,55,56] as well as the production of patient-specific implants through a variety of 3D printing modalities.[41,57,58] In resident training, the use of 3D printed skulls of children with craniosynostosis, as well as mandibular and Le Fort I distraction cases, improved the time and accuracy to complete written and marked surgical plans of surgical trainees.[59] Simulations have been generated for training in pediatric neurosurgery via 3D printing. An inexpensive, synthetic simulator for endoscope-assisted repair of metopic and sagittal synostosis has also been developed with realistic anatomic features and also with representative procedural steps required in real surgery.[60] Moreover, others have developed realistic 3D prototypes based on actual craniosynostosis cases for extraoperative resident training and courses.[3,4]

Beyond craniosynostosis, however, a neonatal phantom skull was generated to mimic its morphological and acoustic properties, allowing for measurement of temperature variations during ultrasound examination and use as an ultrasound training tool.[61] Additionally, a full-scale, lifelike model for endoscopic third ventriculostomy, modeled after a 14-year-old adolescent, has also been described; using a combination of 3D printing with special effects techniques provided both anatomical and haptic accuracy to neurosurgery residents and fellows.[62]

As an educational tool, not only does 3D printing improve surgical trainee understanding of anatomy and surgical strategy but it also enhances patient−physician or parent−physician communication. Alshomer et al.[63] found that personalized 3D printed models aided in the description of the surgical procedure with parents, improving their knowledge and understanding of the child's disease and surgical plan and aiding in decision-making.

Advantages and limitations

3D printing techniques offer practical and accurate methods of producing patient-specific models for surgical planning, simulation and training, and tissue-engineered implants or devices. The rapidity of prototyping, its accessibility, and generally low costs associated with the production also place 3D printing at an advantage. The accuracy of these models in comparison to actual anatomy has been verified across multiple studies. Further, 3D printing provides an additional benefit in better understanding anatomy spatially. Medical images have traditionally been viewed in 2D format, while even 3D reconstructions of images still must be interpreted on a 2D computer monitor. VR and AR have provided an opportunity to view medical images in 3D format. Newer VR and AR platforms and programs do offer the ability to view and virtually manipulate patient-specific images; however, these technologies currently lack the kinesthetic appreciation of patient-specific surgical anatomy and relationships between critical structures.

The application of 3D printing to neurosurgical education allows for surgical training in a no-risk environment. Compared to other educational tools, including cadaver laboratories, 3D printing offers an affordable and easily reproducible option. As demonstrated above, studies have shown that the incorporation of 3D printing into preoperative training improved the trainee understanding of surgical anatomy and reduced operative time. Additionally, patient-specific, 3D printed models aid in patient−physician communication; the use of 3D models has been shown to result in higher understanding and satisfaction of preoperative patient education during the informed consent process.[12,63,64]

In neurosurgery, submillimeter accuracy to depict disease processes remains critical for effective modeling and simulation, and while published studies validate the replication of pathologies, certain 3D printers may grant better resolution of the finished product than others. The fused deposition modeling method, for instance, utilized by the Makerbot Replicator, has less resolution along the z axis and may have a rough surface; yet, this method remains the most affordable and uses durable materials.[65] Other systems, such as stereolithography, employed by the 3D Systems ProJet, generate models with finer resolution than fused deposition modeling;[65] although inaccuracies in vessel wall thickness and elasticity were previously described as limitations,[20] later studies employed stereolithography with <0.1 mm discrepancy from imaging in the production of AVMs.[21] A third common 3D printing technique used in neurosurgery, polyjet matrix modeling, or multijet modeling offers the highest precision, requires less time, and prints simultaneously with multiple materials of differing qualities, like firmness or texture;[65] the Stratasys Objet Connex series of printers uses this method and has been studied in the creation of models of the brain, skull, cranial nerves, vascular network, aneurysm, and brain tumors [8,13,66-68].

3D printed models of aneurysms and AVMs have been shown to accurately depict anatomical morphology of the lesions; however, at this point, current models can neither perfectly depict the consistency of different aneurysm or tumor types nor the dissection of surrounding tissue. Vasculature poses a challenge when reproducing lifelike pliability, texture, and thickness, but hollow elastic arteries and aneurysms attempt to reconcile this discrepancy. Additionally, simulators do not depict complications well, such as intraoperative aneurysmal rupture, with 3D printed models, although the integration of VR and AR technologies may allow for such enactments.

Over the past few years, advancements in simulators have allowed for more lifelike experiences and examples of surgical cases, and these simulators often combine 3D printed elements with other materials to depict body fluids and computer-based programs that can provide haptic or tactile feedback, measure force applied by the surgeon, or mirror image guidance or fluoroscopy. A model of endoscopic third ventriculostomy used a 3D printed skin, skull, and brain model; fabricated a replaceable third ventricular floor; and filled the ventricular system with fluid to reproduce a realistic setting for the procedure.[62] Bohl et al.[9,69,70] developed "The Living Spine Model," which incorporates 3D printed bone to mirror biomechanical performance of pedicle screw placement as well as radiopacity for realistic fluoroscopic views of the spine. In addition, to simulate real operative views and challenges, the authors equipped this model with bleeding bone capable of achieving hemostasis with a mimic hemostatic agent, electrically conductive nerve roots, a synthetic thecal sac, and surrounding radiolucent soft supportive tissue.

While 3D printed implants, such as synthetic bone flaps for cranioplasties, offer a customized, well-fitted device for seamless integration, this customization may conversely pose a limitation in spine surgery. For example, after tissue dissection, manipulation, and preparation, a single custom-made implant for interbody fusions may not be adequate as surgical anatomy may have changed throughout the procedure; thus, a range of interbody products would need to be manufactured for a single patient, which may not prove practical.[71]

The length of time required to print limits its utility in emergency situations, such as aneurysmal rupture or intracerebral hemorrhage. Several printers boast printing capabilities within a few hours; however, the speed of printing may sacrifice the precision of the 3D model. Likewise, more affordable printers, for individual consumer use and available for purchase online, also come with the trade-off of the resolution of the printed object. 3D printers now may be sold online for several hundred dollars, although these may only be compatible with a single plastic material; however, more advanced 3D printers range from several thousand to hundreds of thousands of dollars. In addition, a range of different materials may be used to generate the object; however, more complex materials or their combinations require more advanced 3D printers. Thus, while some 3D printers have become available for relatively low cost, those that integrate medical-grade materials for implantations, including biomaterials or metals, may remain expensive.

Notably, as 3D printers become more accessible and as hospitals purchase equipment for local, on-site use to produce custom surgical equipment and implants, hospitals must implement a quality management system to evaluate materials for safety, biocompatibility, and more. Further, the size of objects produced is also limited by the size of the 3D printer, which can prevent large structures such as the entire neuroaxis from being produced easily.

Future directions

A number of future directions of 3D printing in neurosurgery have already been mentioned above in each subspecialty section. Broadly, the development of 3D printing in neurosurgery involves the advancement of simulators. 3D printing will likely be combined with other forms of visualization, such as VR and AR for both planning and practice.[15,47] Mixed reality experiences will provide low-cost, no-risk training to neurosurgical residents and may be incorporated into the assessment of surgical technique and precision. Using such simulators may even be integrated into a formal evaluation process, such as board examinations. Newer techniques of 3D printing and the materials used will continuously improve the realism, kinesthetics, and haptic feedback.

Another future direction of 3D printing within the neurosciences derives from the use of advanced polymers, whereby natural and synthetic polymers or their combination may provide constructs for replacement of human organ tissue.[72] Examples of such 3D bioprinting includes use of the printing of autogenous bone matrix for cranioplasty implants.[45] Shahriari et al.[73] developed a porous, multichannel scaffold for axon growth, providing a synthetic conduit for nerve regeneration. The future may see the production of better artificial blood vessels for vascular bypass procedures.[74,75] Furthermore, in situ 3D printing may improve wound healing in the setting of complex wound revisions.[76]

Low-cost, 3D printed personalized implants will become more commonplace in the future, as hospitals invest in on-site 3D printers and as companies develop more options for implants in both cranial and spine surgeries. In addition to the development of patient-specific models and implants, custom printing surgical tools will also likely evolve.[77] Patient-specific templates for osteotomies and screw placement will continue to evolve, especially as the field of robotics within neurosurgery expands.

Conclusion

The future of 3D printing in neurosurgery is very promising and challenging. The applications are extensive and diverse, with the potential to transform daily practice both inside and outside surgery, training, and patient–doctor interactions. The rapidity of production of realistic, unique, patient-specific, anatomically correct, 3D models allows for the practical application of this technique in daily neurosurgical education and practice, which could effectively improve surgical outcomes and decrease surgical complications. Additionally, 3D printing technology improves not only the surgeon's understanding of 3D anatomy and spatial relationships between the lesion and surrounding tissue but it also fosters better patient–physician relationships, as models allow patients and their families to better understand their pathology.

Furthermore, 3D printing provides neurosurgical trainees with a low-cost alternative with fewer ethical issues in comparison to cadaver-based models. In addition, it increases the experience of surgical trainees in a low-risk scenario, practicing on lifelike models of real patient anatomy eliminating the expense of the potential complications from intraoperative learning. The future applications of 3D printing within neurosurgery span from integrated models with VR and AR for preoperative planning and surgical training to the development of new bio-implants and instruments, while lower costs and more massive productions remain a prerequisite.

References

1. Randazzo M, Pisapia JM, Singh N, Thawani JP. 3D printing in neurosurgery: A systematic review. *Surg Neurol Int*. November 14 2016;7(Suppl 33):S801–S809.
2. Langridge B, Momin S, Coumbe B, Woin E, Griffin M, Butler P. Systematic review of the use of 3-dimensional printing in surgical teaching and assessment. *J Surg Educ*. January–February 2018;75(1):209–221.
3. Cheng CH, Chen YW, Kai-Xing Lee A, Yao CH, Shie MY. Development of mussel-inspired 3D-printed poly (lactic acid) scaffold grafted with bone morphogenetic protein-2 for stimulating osteogenesis. *J Mater Sci Mater Med*. June 20 2019;30(7):78.

4. Cheng D, Yuan M, Perera I, O'Connor A, Evins AI, Imahiyerobo T, Souweidane M, Hoffman C. Developing a 3D composite training model for cranial remodeling. *J Neurosurg Pediatr.* September 20 2019:1−10.

5. Whatley BR, Kuo J, Shuai C, Damon BJ, Wen X. Fabrication of a biomimetic elastic intervertebral disk scaffold using additive manufacturing. *Biofabrication.* March 2011; 3(1):015004.

6. Weiss MY, Melnyk R, Mix D, Ghazi A, Vates GE, Stone JJ. Design and validation of a cervical laminectomy simulator using 3D printing and hydrogel phantoms. *Oper Neurosurg (Hagerstown).* February 1 2020;18(2):202−208.

7. Bow H, Zuckerman SL, Griffith B, Lewis S, McGruder C, Pruthi S, Parker SL. A 3D-printed simulator and teaching module for placing S2-alar-iliac screws. *Oper Neurosurg (Hagerstown).* March 1 2020;18(3):339−346.

8. Clifton W, Nottmeier E, Damon A, Dove C, Pichelmann M. The future of biomechanical spine research: conception and design of a dynamic 3D printed cervical myelography phantom. *Cureus.* May 3 2019;11(5):e4591.

9. Bohl MA, McBryan S, Nakaji P, Chang SW, Turner JD, Kakarla UK. Development and first clinical use of a novel anatomical and biomechanical testing platform for scoliosis. *J Spine Surg.* September 2019;5(3):329−336.

10. Gadiya A, Shah K, Nagad P, Nene A. A technical note on making patient-specific pedicle screw templates for revision pediatric kyphoscoliosis surgery with sublaminar wires In Situ. *J Orthop Case Rep.* January-February 2019;9(1):82−84.

11. Lador R, Regev G, Salame K, Khashan M, Lidar Z. Use of 3-dimensional printing technology in complex spine surgeries. *World Neurosurg.* 2020;133:e327−e341.

12. Zhuang YD, Zhou MC, Liu SC, Wu JF, Wang R, Chen C2. Effectiveness of personalized 3D printed models for patient education in degenerative lumbar disease. *Patient Educ Counsel.* October 2019;102(10):1875−1881.

13. Waran V, Narayanan V, Karuppiah R, Owen SL, Aziz T. Utility of multimaterial 3D printers in creating models with pathological entities to enhance the training experience of neurosurgeons. *J Neurosurg.* February 2014;120(2):489−492.

14. Spottiswoode BS, van den Heever DJ, Chang Y, Engelhardt S, Du Plessis S, Nicolls F, Hartzenberg HB, Gretschel A. Preoperative three-dimensional model creation of magnetic resonance brain images as a tool to assist neurosurgical planning. *Stereotact Funct Neurosurg.* 2013;91(3):162−169.

15. Oishi M, Fukuda M, Yajima N, Yoshida K, Takahashi M, Hiraishi T, Takao T, Saito A, Fujii Y. Interactive presurgical simulation applying advanced 3D imaging and modeling techniques for skull base and deep tumors. *J Neurosurg.* July 2013;119(1):94−105.

16. Mirani B, Pagan E, Shojaei S, Duchscherer J, Toyota BD, Ghavami S, Akbari M. A 3D bioprinted hydrogel mesh loaded with all-trans retinoic acid for treatment of glioblastoma. *Eur J Pharmacol.* July 5 2019;854:201−212.

17. Ju SG, Kim MK, Hong CS, Kim JS, Han Y, Choi DH, Shin D, Lee SB. New technique for developing a proton range compensator with use of a 3-dimensional printer. *Int J Radiat Oncol Biol Phys.* February 1 2014;88(2):453−458.

18. Abla AA, Lawton MT. Three-dimensional hollow intracranial aneurysm models and their potential role for teaching, simulation, and training. *World Neurosurg.* January 2015;83(1):35−36.

19. Mashiko T, Otani K, Kawano R, Konno T, Kaneko N, Ito Y, Watanabe E. Development of three-dimensional hollow elastic model for cerebral aneurysm clipping simulation enabling rapid and low cost prototyping. *World Neurosurg.* March 2015;83(3):351−361.

20. Mashiko T, Konno T, Kaneko N, Watanabe E. Training in Brain Retraction Using a Self-Made Three-Dimensional Model. *World Neurosurg.* August 2015;84(2):585−590.
21. Thawani JP, Pisapia JM, Singh N, Petrov D, Schuster JM, Hurst RW, Zager EL, Pukenas BA. Three-dimensional printed modeling of an arteriovenous malformation including blood flow. *World Neurosurg.* June 2016;90:675−683.e2.
22. Nagassa RG, McMenamin PG, Adams JW, Quayle MR, Rosenfeld JV. Advanced 3D printed model of middle cerebral artery aneurysms for neurosurgery simulation. *3D Print Med.* August 1 2019;5(1):11.
23. Acar T, Karakas AB, Ozer MA, Koc AM, Govsa F. Building three-dimensional intracranial aneurysm models from 3D-TOF MRA: a validation study. *J Digit Imag.* December 2019;32(6):963−970.
24. Wang L, Ye X, Hao Q, Ma L, Chen X, Wang H, Zhao Y. Three-dimensional intracranial middle cerebral artery aneurysm models for aneurysm surgery and training. *J Clin Neurosci.* April 2018;50:77−82.
25. Weinstock P, Prabhu SP, Flynn K, Orbach DB, Smith E. Optimizing cerebrovascular surgical and endovascular procedures in children via personalized 3D printing. *J Neurosurg Pediatr.* November 2015;16(5):584−589.
26. Conti A, Pontoriero A, Iatì G, Marino D, La Torre D, Vinci S, Germanò A, Pergolizzi S, Tomasello F. 3D-printing of arteriovenous malformations for radiosurgical treatment: pushing anatomy understanding to real boundaries. *Cureus.* 2016 April 29;8(4):e594.
27. Namba K, Higaki A, Kaneko N, Mashiko T, Nemoto S, Watanabe E. Microcatheter shaping for intracranial aneurysm coiling using the 3-dimensional printing rapid prototyping technology: Preliminary result in the first 10 consecutive cases. *World Neurosurg.* July 2015;84(1):178−186.
28. Herbert R, Mishra S, Lim HR, Yoo H, Yeo WH. Fully printed, wireless, stretchable implantable biosystem toward batteryless, real-time monitoring of cerebral aneurysm hemodynamics. *Adv Sci.* August 7 2019;6(18):1901034.
29. Mellerio C, Lapointe M-N, Roca P, Charron S, Legrand L, Meder J-F, Oppenheim C, Cachia A. Identification of reliable sulcal patterns of the human rolandic region. *Front Hum Neurosci.* 2016;10:410.
30. Blanton RE, Levitt JG, Thompson PM, Narr KL, Capetillo-Cunliffe L, Nobel A, Singerman JD, McCracken JT, Toga AW. Mapping cortical asymmetry and complexity patterns in normal children. *Psychiatr Res.* 2001;107:29−43.
31. Ono M, Kubik S, Abernathey CD. *Atlas of the Cerebral Sulci.* Stuttgart: Thieme; 1990.
32. Rademacher J, Caviness Jr VS, Steinmetz H, Galaburda AM. Topographical variation of the human primary cortices: implications for neuroimaging, brain mapping and neurobiology. *Cerebr Cortex.* 1993;3:313−329.
33. Rajkowska G, Goldman-Rakic PS. Cytoarchitectonic definition of prefrontal areas in the normal human cortex: II. Variability in locations of areas 9 and 46 and relationship to the talairach coordinate system. *Cerebr Cortex.* 1995;5:323−337.
34. Konrad PE, Neimat JS, Yu H, Kao CC, Remple MS, D'Haese PF, Dawant BM. Customized, miniature rapid-prototype stereotactic frames for use in deep brain stimulator surgery: initial clinical methodology and experience from 263 patients from 2002 to 2008. *Stereotact Funct Neurosurg.* 2011;89(1):34−41.
35. Brandmeir NJ, McInerney J, Zacharia BE. The use of custom 3D printed stereotactic frames for laser interstitial thermal ablation: technical note. *Neurosurg Focus.* October 2016;41(4):E3.

36. Dadey DY, Kamath AA, Smyth MD, Chicoine MR, Leuthardt EC, Kim AH. Utilizing personalized stereotactic frames for laser interstitial thermal ablation of posterior fossa and mesiotemporal brain lesions: a single-institution series. *Neurosurg Focus*. October 2016;41(4):E4.

37. Javan R, Schickel M, Zhao Y, Agbo T, Fleming C, Heidari P, Gholipour T, Shields DC, Koubeissi M. Using 3D-printed mesh-like brain cortex with deep structures for planning intracranial EEG electrode placement. *J Digit Imag*. April 2020;33(2):324−333.

38. Naftulin JS, Kimchi EY, Cash SS. Streamlined, Inexpensive 3D Printing of the Brain and Skull. *PloS One*. August 21 2015;10(8):e0136198.

39. Hirata M, Morris S, Sugata H, Matsushita K, Yanagisawa T, Kishima H, Yoshimine T. Patient-specific contour-fitting sheet electrodes for electrocorticographic brain machine interfaces. *Conf Proc IEEE Eng Med Biol Soc*. 2014;2014:5204−5207.

40. Morris S, Hirata M, Sugata H, Goto T, Matsushita K, Yanagisawa T, Saitoh Y, Kishima H, Yoshimine T. Patient-specific cortical electrodes for sulcal and gyral implantation. *IEEE Trans Biomed Eng*. 2015 April;62(4):1034−1041.

41. De La Peña A, De La Peña-Brambila J, Pérez-De La Torre J, Ochoa M4, Gallardo GJ. Low-cost customized cranioplasty using a 3D digital printing model: a case report. *3D Print Med*. 2018;4(1):4.

42. Tan ET, Ling JM, Dinesh SK. The feasibility of producing patient-specific acrylic cranioplasty implants with a low-cost 3D printer. *J Neurosurg*. May 2016;124(5):1531−1537.

43. Klammert U, Gbureck U, Vorndran E, Rödiger J, Meyer-Marcotty P, Kübler AC. 3D powder printed calcium phosphate implants for reconstruction of cranial and maxillofacial defects. *J Cranio-Maxillo-Fac Surg*. December 2010;38(8):565−570.

44. Park SE, Park EK1, Shim KW2, Kim DS1. Modified cranioplasty technique using 3-dimensional printed implants in preventing temporalis muscle hollowing. *World Neurosurg*. June 2019;126:e1160−e1168.

45. Chen H, Zhang J, Li X, Liu L, Zhang X, Ren D, Ma C, Zhang L, Fei Z, Xu T. Multi-level customized 3D printing for autogenous implants in skull tissue engineering. *Biofabrication*. July 10 2019;11(4):045007.

46. Ryan JR, Chen T, Nakaji P, Frakes DH, Gonzalez LF. Ventriculostomy simulation using patient-specific ventricular anatomy, 3D printing, and hydrogel casting. *World Neurosurg*. November 2015;84(5):1333−1339.

47. Bova FJ, Rajon DA, Friedman WA, Murad GJ, Hoh DJ, Jacob RP, Lampotang S, Lizdas DE, Lombard G, Lister JR. Mixed-reality simulation for neurosurgical procedures. *Neurosurgery*. October 2013;73(Suppl 1):138−145.

48. Bishop N, Boone D, Williams KL, Avery R, Dubrowski A. Development of a three-dimensional printed emergent burr hole and craniotomy simulator. *Cureus*. April 3 2019;11(4):e4373.

49. Boyce ST, Lalley AL. Tissue engineering of skin and regenerative medicine for wound care. *Burns Trauma*. 2018;6:4. Published 2018 Jan 24.

50. Liu B, Wang Z, Lin G, Zhang J. Radiculoplasty with reconstruction using 3D-printed artificial dura mater for the treatment of symptomatic sacral canal cysts: two case reports. *Medicine (Baltim)*. 2018;97:e13289.

51. Hutchison BL, Hutchison LA, Thompson JM, Mitchell EA. Plagiocephaly and brachycephaly in the first two years of life: a prospective cohort study. *Pediatrics*. 2004 October;114(4):970−980.

52. Sullivan S, Aguilar-Salinas P, Santos R, Beier AD, Hanel RA. Three-dimensional printing and neuroendovascular simulation for the treatment of a pediatric intracranial aneurysm: case report. *J Neurosurg Pediatr*. December 1 2018;22(6):672−677.

53. Pacione D, Tanweer O, Berman P, Harter DH. The utility of a multimaterial 3D printed model for surgical planning of complex deformity of the skull base and craniovertebral junction. *J Neurosurg*. November 2016;125(5):1194−1197.

54. García-Mato D, Ochandiano S, García-Sevilla M, Navarro-Cuéllar C, Darriba-Allés JV, García-Leal R, Calvo-Haro JA, Pérez-Mañanes R, Salmerón JI, Pascau J. Craniosynostosis surgery: workflow based on virtual surgical planning, intraoperative navigation and 3D printed patient-specific guides and templates. *Sci Rep*. November 27 2019;9(1): 17691.

55. Kobets AJ, Ammar A, Nakhla J, Scoco A, Nasser R, Goodrich JT, Abbott R. Virtual modeling, stereolithography, and intraoperative CT guidance for the optimization of sagittal synostosis reconstruction: a technical note. *Childs Nerv Syst*. May 2018;34(5): 965−970.

56. Soleman J, Thieringer F, Beinemann J, Kunz C, Guzman R. Computer-assisted virtual planning and surgical template fabrication for frontoorbital advancement. *Neurosurg Focus*. May 2015;38(5):E5.

57. Borghi A, Rodgers W, Schievano S, Ponniah A, Jeelani O, Dunaway D. Proof of concept study for the design, manufacturing, and testing of a patient-specific shape memory device for treatment of unicoronal craniosynostosis. *J Craniofac Surg*. January 2018;29(1): 45−48.

58. Day KM, Gabrick KS, Sargent LA. Applications of computer technology in complex craniofacial reconstruction. *Plast Reconstr Surg Glob Open*. March 6 2018;6(3):e1655.

59. Lobb DC, Cottler P, Dart D, Black JS. The use of patient-specific three-dimensional printed surgical models enhances plastic surgery resident education in craniofacial surgery. *J Craniofac Surg*. March/April 2019;30(2):339−341.

60. Eastwood KW, Bodani VP, Haji FA, Looi T, Naguib HE, Drake JM. Development of synthetic simulators for endoscope-assisted repair of metopic and sagittal craniosynostosis. *J Neurosurg Pediatr*. August 2018;22(2):128−136.

61. Gatto M, Memoli G, Shaw A, Sadhoo N, Gelat P, Harris RA. Three-dimensional printing (3DP) of neonatal head phantom for ultrasound: thermocouple embedding and simulation of bone. *Med Eng Phys*. September 2012;34(7):929−937.

62. Weinstock P, Rehder R, Prabhu SP, Forbes PW, Roussin CJ, Cohen AR. Creation of a novel simulator for minimally invasive neurosurgery: fusion of 3D printing and special effects. *J Neurosurg Pediatr*. July 2017;20(1):1−9.

63. Alshomer F, AlFaqeeh F, Alariefy M, Altweijri I, Alhumsi T. Low-cost desktop-based three-dimensional-printed patient-specific craniofacial models in surgical counseling, consent taking, and education of parent of craniosynostosis patients: a comparison with conventional visual explanation modalities. *J Craniofac Surg*. September 2019; 30(6):1652−1656.

64. Kim PS, Choi CH, Han IH, Lee JH, Choi HJ, Lee JI. Obtaining informed consent using patient specific 3D printing cerebral aneurysm model. *J Korean Neurosurg Soc*. July 2019;62(4):398−404.

65. Pucci JU, Christophe BR, Sisti JA, Connolly Jr ES. Three-dimensional printing: technologies, applications, and limitations in neurosurgery. *Biotechnol Adv*. September 2017; 35(5):521−529.

66. Waran V, Pancharatnam D, Thambinayagam HC, Raman R, Rathinam AK, Balakrishnan YK, Tung TS, Rahman ZA. The utilization of cranial models created using rapid prototyping techniques in the development of models for navigation training. *J Neurol Surg Cent Eur Neurosurg*. January 2014;75(1):12−15.

67. Waran V, Narayanan V, Karuppiah R, Pancharatnam D, Chandran H, Raman R, Rahman ZA, Owen SL, Aziz TZ. Injecting realism in surgical training-initial simulation experience with custom 3D models. *J Surg Educ*. March−April 2014;71(2):193−197.

68. Waran V, Narayanan V, Karuppiah R, Thambynayagam HC, Muthusamy KA, Rahman ZA, Kirollos RW. Neurosurgical endoscopic training via a realistic 3-dimensional model with pathology. *Simulat Healthc J Soc Med Simulat*. February 2015; 10(1):43−48.

69. Bohl MA, Zhou JJ, Mooney MA, Repp GJ, Cavallo C, Nakaji P, Chang SW, Turner JD, Kakarla UK. The Barrow Biomimetic Spine: effect of a 3-dimensional-printed spinal osteotomy model on performance of spinal osteotomies by medical students and interns. *J Spine Surg*. March 2019;5(1):58−65.

70. Bohl MA, Morgan CD, Mooney MA, Repp GJ, Lehrman JN, Kelly BP, Chang SW, Turner JD, Kakarla UK. Biomechanical testing of a 3D-printed L5 vertebral body model. *Cureus*. January 15 2019;11(1):e3893.

71. Sheha ED, Gandhi SD, Colman MW. 3D printing in spine surgery. *Ann Transl Med*. September 2019;7(Suppl 5):S164.

72. Wang X. Advanced polymers for three-dimensional (3D) organ bioprinting. *Micromachines*. November 25 2019;10(12).

73. Shahriari D, Loke G, Tafel I, Park S, Chiang PH, Fink Y, Anikeeva P. Scalable fabrication of porous microchannel nerve guidance scaffolds with complex geometries. *Adv Mater*. July 2019;31(30):e1902021. Epub 2019 Jun 6.

74. Abdollahi S, Boktor J, Hibino N. Bioprinting of freestanding vascular grafts and the regulatory considerations for additively manufactured vascular prostheses. *Transl Res*. September 2019;211:123−138.

75. Papaioannou TG, Manolesou D, Dimakakos E, Tsoucalas G, Vavuranakis M, Tousoulis D. 3D bioprinting methods and techniques: applications on artificial blood vessel fabrication. *Acta Cardiol Sin*. May 2019;35(3):284−289.

76. Chouhan D, Dey N, Bhardwaj N, Mandal BB. Emerging and innovative approaches for wound healing and skin regeneration: Current status and advances. *Biomaterials*. September 2019;216:119267.

77. Rankin TM, Giovinco NA, Cucher DJ, Watts G, Hurwitz B, Armstrong DG. Three-dimensional printing surgical instruments: are we there yet? *J Surg Res*. June 15 2014; 189(2):193−197.

Index